THE PRIVILEGE OF CARING

A DOCTOR'S URGENT CALL TO HEAL THE U.S. HEALTHCARE SYSTEM

ERIC DANIEL FETHKE, M.D.

Publishing Services provided by Paper Raven Books LLC
Printed in the United States of America
First Printing, 2023

Paperback ISBN: 979-8-9891704-0-1
Hardback ISBN: 979-8-9891704-1-8

DEDICATION

I owe the world to my family, without whom I would be unworthy of this lofty project.

To my wife and best friend, I love that you remain my most brutally honest and supportive critic—you keep me grounded.

To my boys, who give my life meaning and orientation—you grant me life-sustaining focus.

To my mother, whose strength through life's challenges taught me the meaning of true love.

To my mother-in-law, whose respect for American medicine reminds me constantly that my profession is at its core deeply honorable.

To my late father-in-law, who lived and breathed a life in the service of his family and others less fortunate—you define honest dedication.

To my sister whose talents and moral strength serve as a guiding beacon in my life.

To my late father, who remains my purest model of true kindness and taught me to seek the beauty rather than the darkness in others—you remain the brightest light in my life.

TABLE OF CONTENTS

INTRODUCTION

CARE ENOUGH TO BE CURIOUS

When Gilbert Tremain was born in 1942, he came out blue. It's common for babies, who get oxygen from their mothers via the umbilical cord before birth, to be a little purple here and there. A healthy baby's skin will pink up once the baby takes some breaths, but little Gilbert's skin remained blue—a condition known as cyanosis. Because the sonogram of the heart, known as an echocardiogram, would not be invented until 1953,[1] it took a few days and several tests for the doctors to determine Gilbert's problem. They discovered that his cyanosis was caused by a relatively rare heart defect, called Tetralogy of Fallot, affecting one in 2000 newborns.

There was no universally accepted treatment for infants and children with Tetralogy of Fallot, nor any significant heart problem, at the time. The New York doctors did not tell Gilbert's family that, two years prior in 1940, some researchers at Johns Hopkins University in Baltimore, Maryland had just completed the first successful operation for Tetralogy[2] on 15-month-old Eileen Saxon. These pioneers had thus

1 Singh, Siddharth; Goyal, Abha (2007), "The Origin of Echocardiography: A Tribute to Inge Edler," *Tex Heart Inst J.* 34 (4): 431–438, PMC 2170493. PMID 18172524, https://www.ncbi.nlm.nih.gov/pmc/articles/PMC2170493/.

2 Neil, Clark (1994), "Tetralogy of Fallot. The First 300 years," Tex Heart Inst J. 21 (4): 272–279, https://www.ncbi.nlm.nih.gov/pmc/articles/PMC325189/.

ushered in the era of heart surgery that would spread across the nation and the world for the next four decades.

They told his parents that he wouldn't live very long—10 years, maybe 15 if they were lucky. That's not something any parent wants to hear, so it's no wonder that when Gilbert was small, his mother was very protective. She was fearful. She didn't want him to hurt himself, often scolding him to be more careful. His mom reminded him a lot not to do things because he had a "bad heart."

Gilbert's father took the opposite approach. He told his wife to let their child play like everybody else and encouraged his son to be normal during the limited time he had. Gilbert soon distinguished himself as a plucky kid and a natural-born troublemaker. He followed his father's advice, always outside playing in the street or at the park with the rest of the kids. Increasingly, after playing particularly hard, Gilbert suddenly became very short of breath, dizzy, and fatigued. Those around him were struck by how blue his face became as the blood in his heart temporarily rushed away from his lungs directly into his body without receiving oxygen first.

These episodes had been described by physicians as "Tet spells" and were the hallmark of a worsening condition. Gilbert stopped his activities for a few moments and instinctively bent over into a squat, resting his elbows on his knees. His symptoms gradually resolved, and his face pinked up, allowing him to return to his playtime activities and return to being a "normal" kid.

The first time Gilbert and his parents visited the clinic at Columbia-Presbyterian Hospital was in 1947. He was five years old. When the doctor, Kenneth Lum, a large Chinese man, walked in, Gilbert's father abruptly stood and put a hand on his son's shoulder, ready to pick him up and walk out of the clinic. He didn't want some foreigner in a big city hospital experimenting on his kid.

"Does he get down and hug his knees when he gets tired?" Dr. Lum asked quietly. Gilbert's parents nodded. Then the doctor turned to

Gilbert's mom and said, "When you were about three months pregnant, you thought you'd lost him, didn't you?"

His father's eyes widened with astonishment. That's exactly what had happened. How did this man know exactly what his son did when he got tired? How did he know that his wife had indeed thought that she'd lost the baby during their pregnancy? Gilbert's father sat down just as abruptly as he'd stood, somewhat embarrassed that he was so quick to judge. Dr. Lum clearly knew more than he did about his son's condition. Maybe he could help.

I have the good fortune to be a pediatric cardiologist who has been caring for children with potentially life-threatening heart conditions for over two decades. My best teachers and role models instilled in me the fundamental belief that giving my patients the best chance of success means teaching them everything they need to know about their healthcare. In 1998, after completing my studies in pediatric cardiology at the very same department in Columbia University where Gilbert had first been taken by his parents, I took my mentors' philosophy with me back to the suburban community outside of New York City where I was raised. This was just five years before Gilbert Tremain would enter my life as a grown man with grandchildren. Our paths would remain aligned for the next 15 years, learning valuable medical and life lessons from each other along the way.

No one in my family had been a doctor. My father, Walter, was an American Navy officer. Faded pictures I found from the 1960s show a dashing, green-eyed, short-cut, dark-haired lieutenant looking much the part of *An Officer and a Gentleman*. Three years after graduating the top of his class at Princeton with a degree in chemical engineering, while on shore leave in the south of France, he met my mom, Monique Weisz.

She had come along from their home in the outskirts of Paris with her family for their annual summer vacation. Her uncle lived in the small town of Saint-Aubin-sur-Mer, a shoreside village where, just 20 years earlier, the great D-Day invasions changed the course of world history. Sun-scorched and slightly balding, in his skimpy bathing suit that was then the European fashion, Uncle Lulu walked up to the young lieutenant's ship just as he disembarked.

"Is this your ship?" he asked in French laden with a thick Normandy drawl. Walter learned proper French in high school in Rockland County, New York, but this man's accent made it hard to decipher his words. Lulu gently indicated for my father to wait right there. He was going to get someone who spoke a little English to help translate. This someone was my then-21-year-old mom who, coincidentally, was born the same year as Gilbert Tremain.

I am told that when my parents met, they instantly fell in love and, over the next five days, went out on a series of highly chaperoned dates filled with endless conversations. Within a week, Walter asked Monique's father, Adalbert Weisz, a Hungarian Jew who survived the Holocaust of Europe, for his permission to marry Monique and take her back to the States. After a series of international spy operations, during which Adalbert's distant family friends in America knocked on the house door of Walter's parents to inquire about his family, a good report came back to my grandfather, and he blessed their union.

Walter returned to his ship to complete his last few days of Navy service and rushed back to Monique, whereupon the marriage was made official at the local Justice of the Peace in the Parisian suburb of Bagnolet. After two weeks of celebration, the couple voyaged across the Atlantic back to New York. Four days after leaving France, Monique stepped onto the western shore of Manhattan, pale and green from sea sickness. She vowed never to board a ship again.

My parents eventually settled down in Cincinnati, Ohio, where my father took a position at the headquarters of a century-old consumer goods company—the industry giant Procter & Gamble. I was born two years later at one of our nation's best medical institutions, Cincinnati Children's Hospital. We moved from our apartment complex to a beautiful home in the suburbs just two years later after my sister arrived. As I started to run and bicycle, my parents noted that my legs rotated outward at the hip. This did not deter my inclination for activity, including climbing and jumping out of the huge crabapple tree in the backyard, even while wearing robotic-looking, 10-pound metal leg braces. My hips never did fully rotate to a normal position, but they never stopped me. I often experienced typical childhood orthopedic injuries and my share of stitches.

During my preschool years, my mother returned to France by airplane with my sister and me in tow to stay with her parents. I vividly and fondly remember spending hours with my grandfather Adalbert in the small, immaculate fruit garden behind his house in the suburbs of Paris. Here he taught me the discipline of considering a job finished only when your tools and body were completely clean. You never knew, looking at his immaculately clean hands at the dinner table, that he and his son, my mother's older brother Alecs, ran a precision machine parts shop they referred to as the "atelier."

In the early 1940s, Adalbert was forced by the Nazis during their occupation of France to fabricate small machine parts in his atelier, which the Germans used to repair their tanks and other weapons of war. This sacrifice against his own sense of ethics tore through his soul. Years later, during a home break from my second year of college at Princeton, sitting alone together at our kitchen table, he told me about his experiences through tears. Our family also returned regularly to France for the ritual of long summer days on the Normandy coast beaches. I used to play in the now-abandoned Nazi cement bunkers, stopping to eat long strands of saltwater taffy we called Gui-Gui, and harvest buckets of mussels for the evening's dinner at low tide amongst the abandoned D-Day docks.

My father took a position at a large chemical engineering firm, Union Carbide, in 1969, and we moved back to his parents' home in Rockland County, New York while our house was built in the Greater Hudson Valley suburbs. I attended kindergarten across the street from this house—all of the neighborhood elementary school children assumed the fond title of "walkers." Years later, I would fondly recall my favorite crossing guard when, in all types of weather, I saw my newly retired patient, Gilbert Tremain, working as a crossing guard outside another local school. My father advanced through the ranks of Union Carbide, and my mother went from being a full-time housewife to a teacher's assistant for 15 years in my elementary school.

I was an outgoing child intellectually and physically, playing multiple sports and becoming an early songwriter on my family's upright piano during the early days of MTV. I graduated second in my high school class, only 0.1 percentage points behind my friend in first position. I earned a coveted position at several universities, but I eventually chose to attend my father's *alma mater*, Princeton University, where I pursued premedical studies and majored in music. My sister followed her heart and completed a degree in fashion design at New York's prestigious Fashion Institute of Technology. After a brief one-year pause to consider an arduous career in music, and a life-changing trip to the Philippines during the rise of the People's President Corazon Aquino,[3] I began my medical education at Columbia University's College of Physicians and Surgeons in 1987.

For many years, I didn't quite understand why I was so drawn to medicine. All my high school friends were convinced that I would become a doctor, but I was not so certain that I had what it took. Deep down, I always knew that I wanted to be a doctor, but there

3 I was invited on this trip by my Princeton University classmate, Maria Ressa, who would go onto have an amazing career in journalism, including being awarded the 2021 Nobel Peace Prize for her work to "safeguard freedom of expression."

remained a significant lack of confidence that a suburban kid from a public school system could rise to the challenge.

During college, I volunteered in the local hospital that decades later would become the backdrop for the TV series *House*. I completed a course outside of my college studies to become a local emergency medical technician. I worked several overnight shifts per week with a local ambulance corps. I loved the combination of intellectual and physical skills required to care for patients. Most of all, I liked helping people.

While in medical school, I was also drawn to learning from and working with a handful of what I felt were particularly special physicians. This included my classmate, Viyada, the most intelligent and powerful woman I have ever met, who soon became my best friend and life partner. Unlike many doctors who carried out their daily responsibilities in an almost detached and mechanical way, these noteworthy physicians just had this *je ne sais quoi* way of caring for patients that resonated with me. I later recognized the value in their simple but magical approach. Like Dorothy says so poignantly in *The Wizard of Oz*, I sensed that "there's no place like home." In the shadow cast by these compassionate physicians, I knew I made the right choice to be a doctor. I was home.

I trained with many bright, caring, and exceptional physicians for 12 years after college. The work ethic I learned from my parents and my grandfather carried me through the long study and hospital shift hours. I was often delirious from lack of sleep. I learned to maximize my time, including taking energy-boosting catnaps or an hour to sweat it out on a run or my bike. I found my confidence boosted as those mentors I admired most gave me positive feedback. This support played no small part in my decision to join Dr . Welton Gersony's Pediatric Cardiology Program at Columbia University, where I remained for over a decade. Most importantly, my patients appeared to respond well to my interactions with them, sensing that I yearned to get to know them as people in my endeavors to treat and heal them. I now knew that I had indeed found my calling. I could be a doctor after all and make a difference.

Those mentors I admired most did not hold themselves above others because of their knowledge. On the contrary, they saw themselves as servants to their patients. They discovered that healthcare is not a game of cards where giving away your hand means you lose. They knew and exemplified that the best outcomes were ensured when they laid their cards on the table, fully engaging their patients and their families along the way. They felt obligated to impart their knowledge and wisdom not only to cure but to heal.

Many of my colleagues are very adept at the technical aspects of pediatric cardiology, including complex testing and difficult surgeries. Yet I have known only a handful of cardiologists who rise above the role of simple technician to that of healing physician. These doctors understand that the education process that enables us to become physicians does not innately make us elite. Their lessons continue to guide me with the conviction that the profession of medicine is only noble because we have the privilege of caring for others.

In the end, after all is said and done, who am I? Basically, I am the product of a public education in a small suburb of New York City and the first physician in my immediate and extended family. I am an Ivy League-trained medical doctor who cares deeply about healing people, and I love what I do. Though I have over 20 years of experience treating people with heart problems beginning in childhood, I remain curious about many of life's influences on my patients and how I can best serve them. My curiosity leads me to explore, listen, and challenge myself and others to always constructively question the *status quo* in pursuit of how we can help to make the world of medicine meet its full potential to improve our lives.

I am also a teacher. I give regular talks and lectures, and one or two students shadow me in the office or at the hospitals every day. These medical and nursing students, technicians, interns, and residents challenge me and keep me mentally sharp. As a teacher of the next generation of healthcare workers, I am passionate about helping them find joy in their profession. My students are worried about their futures. They often feel lost, overwhelmed, and uncertain about the career they chose. It is my hope that this book helps them reignite the passion that initially led them to enter the health profession.

Most importantly, I am a concerned citizen who, like others, is often frustrated by the dialogue about the future of US healthcare. As fraught with problems as it is for us doctors, our system can be even worse for consumers. My patients and non-physician friends understandably need help in navigating the confusing US healthcare landscape. They are uneasy about where it is heading. They have become cynical.

A common theme among everyone involved—physicians, medical school students, and the general public—is a feeling of powerlessness. We can all feel that the human element is carelessly left behind in the struggle to determine the future of the American health system. Complex factors out of our control, instead of the welfare of individuals and the population, increasingly dictate our healthcare policy. This book contains support for these concerns while also suggesting several solutions.

Over the past almost 30 years, I trained and worked in some of the most prestigious institutions of learning in our country. I have also had the privilege of providing basic healthcare, as well as more complex subspecialty care, in developing countries, including Guatemala and South Africa. I worked with colleagues from around the globe of many different cultural and spiritual backgrounds. Some of these colleagues are leading experts in the world and in their fields. Others are less in the limelight and more focused on the delivery of care at the ground level. Yet every medical professional I worked with has shared the same desire—to help heal the person we treat so that they may return to their loved ones better than we found them.

The views expressed in this book are the sum of my interactions with professional colleagues and my patients. It has always been my goal to absorb and embody the best aspects of my colleagues' skills because I believe medicine should be a continual apprenticeship that evolves and is reshaped by every such exchange. I make no claim that this book and its contents are based upon intensive research in the field of healthcare policy or other administrative areas of medicine. On the contrary, I intentionally endeavored to present the experience of those on the forefront of healthcare delivery. As with any battle—in this case, against disease—there are always soldiers fighting on the front lines. These warriors, including myself, often wonder whether those at the higher echelons truly understand what it's like on the ground. At the center of our endeavors to improve America's healthcare should always be a nonpartisan commitment to the best interests of those for whom we care. In the end, those of us involved in the delivery of healthcare should strive to ensure that we do so with compassion, humility, and honesty.

Our nation is in the midst of a decades-long struggle to determine the future of American healthcare policy and delivery. Even before the COVID-19 pandemic, healthcare became a mainstream topic in the American consciousness. We are engaged in a tug-of-war across political, economic, and ethical lines with the future of our nation's healthcare riding on the line. The issues in this book couldn't be more timely. As the Mayor of Jackson, Mississippi, Chokwe Antar Lumumba, recently remarked, "The right to vote was the particularly strong push of the 20th century. Then, I think access to healthcare has to be the right that we must pledge to fight for in the 21st century."[4]

To address this challenge, it is imperative that physicians responsibly reflect upon the choices we make—personally, professionally, and nationally. Our collective professional influence is being reawakened at a time of dire need in our nation that current historians compare[5] to the Civil War of the 1860s and the Great Depression of the 1930s. This book is in part dedicated to urging American physicians to heed this call to wage their collective clout on behalf of our people. Like others before me, I support a separation of health and state in America that will allow our ethical healthcare standards to remain based upon scientifically sound evidence and evolve free of political or economic bias. The pandemic has made it all too evident that the status of our healthcare can no longer afford to be tossed in the waves of political campaigns, racist and religious fervors, or medicolegal liability concerns.

Over the past two decades, I have experienced many examples of these effects on my professional life.

I couldn't believe what I was hearing. In that moment I felt like I was seriously living in an alternate reality. The tall, well-suited, new nurse administrator in my main local hospital repeated for the third time, "We have never done this before. We are not equipped to handle a newborn baby with such a tachycardia. We cannot give you permission to treat this patient in our hospital."

As was par for the course, at 4 p.m. on a Friday evening after a long week of work, I received an urgent call from my colleague at the now-three-year old local community hospital just two miles from my

4 Candace Smith, et al., "In Mississippi, Families of COVID-19 Victims Say Poverty and Race Determine Survival," ABC News, May 21, 2020 (online), https://abcnews.go.com/US/mississippi-families-covid-19-victims-poverty-race-determine/story?id=70817722.

5 Griffin, Jeff, "The History of Medicine and Organized Healthcare in America," *HUB International Limited* (online), Mar 27, 2020, https://www.griffinbenefits.com/blog/history-of-healthcare.

office. With an air of concern, he methodically presented the situation to me. "We have a full-term newborn who was noted by the well baby nursery to be breathing fast. When vital signs were taken, the heart rate was over 250 BPM. The baby is stable, otherwise healthy, and I have faxed you a copy of the ECG done about 15 minutes ago. What should I do? Can you come see the baby?"

Upon reviewing the ECG, I noted that this baby's heart was indeed beating very fast from an abnormal location in the top atrial chambers of the heart. On close inspection, I noted that the atria of the heart were beating at almost 400 beats per minute, while the bottom ventricular chambers were beating and creating the pulse the nurses counted of about 250 beats per minute. I immediately recognized this relatively rare condition as electrical pattern know as idiopathic atrial flutter of the newborn. I had successfully treated it before in my training in New York City and twice over the past five years. The most recent case had been just about a year ago in the very same new hospital that was now calling me. In the newborn, a quick jolt of electricity from a device known as a defibrillator—a procedure known as electrical cardioversion—immediately terminates this abnormal electrical impulse of the heart and literally resets the pattern back to the normal sinus rhythm. One and done, never to return again, and avoiding toxic medications. If left untreated for days, the young heart muscles will become tired and result in a condition known as congestive heart failure.

I patiently, but with some intentional degree of authority, replied, "Once again, this is not true. I have successfully and safely performed this cardioversion on other newborn babies in this hospital's neonatal nursery. This condition is easy to treat and must be done as soon as possible to prevent this baby's heart from getting tired."

Despite my pleas at now 6 p.m. in the evening, she stood firm and would not let me care for the baby. She added further salt to the wound by adding, "I know, Doctor, that you think you can do this procedure, but we must think about what's best for the patient. Don't you agree?"

This comment took my last breath away. I did not know if I was now more angry or just bewildered. Why on earth would anyone think I would not be considering what was in the patient's best interest? Was her attitude purely condescending or just ignorant? In the end, the baby was transferred out to a city hospital several hours later. By the time they arrived, his little heart was tired but did respond well to the same treatment I had offered. Because the atrial flutter had persisted so long, he ended up being sent home on a several-month course of potentially toxic medications that would not have been required if I could have treated him sooner at the local hospital.

When I shared this story with a physician colleague and friend one late evening at a neighborhood gathering, he confided, "I too am exhausted and completely frustrated trying to do what's best for my patients. " He went on to explain, "The local hospitals do not have the resources to care for some of my sickest residents. To make things worse, the city hospitals often have no longterm beds for my patients. If they come back to the Center too early, they will just turn around and have to be readmitted to the hospital, often within 24 hours. It's a never-ending revolving door. I just want what's best for my patients."

Dr. Wilson is the medical director of The Center for Discovery, a pioneering and unique chronic care residential facility for young people with complex medical problems, including severe autism and developmental delays. Over the past 30 years, this upstate New York-based facility, known fondly as "The Center," has helped lead and revolutionize the advancement of care for such individuals and their families. Dr. Wilson is a middle-aged, experienced, and highly trained doctor with the wonderful combination of compassion, gentility, and boundless energy that makes him the ideal physician to head the medical efforts of a place as special as the Center. This institution has been so successful in improving the quality and duration of life for their residents that they are just now beginning the expansion of their facilities to include a new hospital on their 1,500-acre campus.

While the Center has proven to be the ideal model of a medically successful and economically efficient medical home for their extremely medically complex residents, as we begin 2022, those who run it now find themselves stranded and isolated from the other elements of their region's healthcare.

At the time of this book, we find ourselves at a critical juncture where we must decide if our healthcare reform is legitimately patient-centered. The exasperating and discouraging problems my colleague and his administrative leadership now face in managing patients, like Alex, under their care are sadly becoming more widespread. Alex's medical needs require a skillset and resources beyond that available in the local hospitals. The resources that these hospitals lack are not simply technical or intellectual in nature. By restricting the number of hospital days for which the health insurance will pay, the current healthcare system itself fundamentally prohibits the most valuable of resources that patients like Alex need—time.

In this book, I will strive to explain how the organization and funding of our current healthcare system leaves patients like Alex and exceptional institutions like The Center with little option but to go it alone. I openly call out the hypocrisy of the current policymakers who claim to seek improvements in access and quality of the public's health while simultaneously leaving places like The Center to battle against money-driven policies and standards that fly in the face of true healthcare advancement and reform. As the medical profession successfully forges ahead to tackle complex medical conditions, time becomes an ever more critical resource that any healthcare reform policies must address if we are to be successful.

Decisions made today will determine the direction that US healthcare will take for generations to come, and the stakes are high for all parties. The answers to such important questions as healthcare reform are best found when we enter into a public discourse empowered by such knowledge as I hope you attain from this book. I invite all who care about our nation's health to join me in identifying that which makes our American healthcare system valued and special to us as a people. I hope that you will come to believe, as I do, that this system is ultimately worth nurturing rather than discarding.

I remind my students and patients daily that to find the solutions to any important problem, we must first care enough to be curious. Only then can we step up and ask the important questions clearly and thoughtfully. Once the answers are discovered, we must act boldly and decisively, which often calls for radical change. It has always been my experience that, after taking the initial big leap, success and happiness are then best ensured through the combination of our collective smaller steps that consistently and reliably lead us forward. A kernel of hope is far more valuable than a tear of despair. I thus share my optimism and the insights contained in this work on behalf of all with a stake in the future of healthcare—every one of us. In so doing, I hope to empower as many Americans as possible to take the necessary steps to reclaim, reimagine, and improve our unique health system.

Gilbert Tremain far outlived his original doctors' expectations. His entire seven decades of life were a testament to both the intellectual and emotional effectiveness of the American medical system's sound approach to the treatment of his severe congenital heart defect. Gilbert did not hesitate to repeatedly remind me that he chose to keep his doctors, including me, only if they agreed to work side by side with him and his family as allies. This was his key to survival, and he refused to give an inch to anyone who fought him on this philosophy.

Over the years, he convinced me that doctors who adopt this approach are the best equipped to benefit tens of thousands of individuals like himself worldwide who would otherwise die prematurely. In a strong partnership with physicians, Gilbert's generation and their parents blazed new territory, literally inventing the field of complex heart surgery. Gilbert was not just "fixed" by his doctors. He was empowered to live a full and active life. Time and time again, he was healed.

Throughout the book, I include the stories of the most influential individuals I encountered in my career—my patients, especially my oldest patient, Gilbert Tremain. His particular story embodies all that I cherish in my field of pediatric cardiology, and I owe much of my philosophy about the art of medicine to my relationship with him. Together, we shared the unsettling recognition that much has been lost in the relationships between physicians and their patients since he first went to Columbia as a child seeking lifesaving treatment. Though there are now more medical centers that offer specialized care, he showed me that quantity over quality—economics over outcomes—has sadly become the new norm. Even more importantly, Gilbert warned that what should be the bedrock of medicine—the alliance between patients and their physicians—is in serious jeopardy. His message calls us now to change direction and return this ship back to the original course where this alliance guided us. Here we find a brighter horizon.

The latest trends in US healthcare threaten to render physicians perpetually incompetent in this time-honored and hard-earned art of healing. For the past several years, I have witnessed the destructive effects of technology, economics, legal liability, and politics on my beloved profession. Today, nearly everyone—from physicians at the height of their careers to medical students eager to join the ranks—feels backed into a corner, powerless to affect any true beneficial impact on their patients' lives. Doctors have become disheartened technical cogs in the enormous wheel of healthcare bureaucracy. Doctors need to be both caretakers and healers. We need to know our patients and let them know us. The impersonal model of bogged-down doctors as uncommunicative, distanced medical authorities does not work.

During his life, Gilbert warned that this trend has to stop—for the sake of both physicians and their patients.

I believe that the fundamentals of a good patient-physician interaction are so important that I have made them central to the questions at the heart of this book. What is it that we as Americans truly expect and desire from our physicians and our healthcare system? Do we feel that the current system is the best we can do? If not, how do we improve it?

To best answer these questions, we need to step back and take a long look at our current US healthcare system. Gilbert Tremain's life story runs through the remainder of the book, weaving the moral story of our exceptional American healthcare system with all of its achievements and failures. Like the proverbial voice in our heads, he advocates for honesty and integrity between patient and physician as the pillars supporting all medical technological advancements.

Through the lens of my personal experiences as an academic physician on the front lines, I will walk you through the history of our unique and often exceptional US health institutions. I invite you into my world so that you can better understand how our system evolved since its noble foundation. I share my own professional journey in the more recent decades as I stepped away from the urban base of New York City to the outlying suburban communities of my childhood, where I continue to base my medical practice.

With the pride and love I have for my profession, and in respect to the lessons that patients and mentors like Gilbert taught me, I will analyze and criticize our current course. I will highlight my concerns and sincere beliefs that many aspects of our current path threaten the honor and potential of American healthcare.

Then, I will return to my optimism regarding America's unique healthcare system by emphasizing the particular strengths of our profession, again best epitomized through the poignant stories of several of my other patients. I will address the relevance and urgency of the healthcare reform that have been so prevalent in our political debates and come into sharp focus during the COVID-19 pandemic. I urge physician leaders to return to their historic role as champions of America's well-being, picking up the mantle laid down by the generations before us that made my relationship with Gilbert Tremain possible.

PART I

MY JOURNEY

CHAPTER 1

LESSONS LEARNED FROM ONE MAN'S JOURNEY TO REPAIR A BROKEN HEART

In December 1950, the doctors at Columbia wanted to perform a procedure on my patient Gilbert Tremain called a catheterization. Born in Roscoe, New York, Gilbert considered himself a country hillbilly. To travel to a big city and a big hospital to be prodded, poked, and x-rayed and then put to sleep for a procedure was a lot for him to handle. He was terrified. During the catheterization, his veins collapsed, and his doctors could not continue. They eventually gave up and let him return home for Christmas. Before the New Year, his family received a call, and Gilbert went back down to the city. He was always a very curious child, and the doctor knew it. He asked Gilbert to take a walk with him to his office, and when they got there, the biggest Santa Claus lollipop Gilbert had ever seen sat on his desk. The doctor gave it to him.

While enjoying the lollipop, the doctor explained the catheterization procedure: "We put a tube in your arm and slide it up the vein to your heart. We then take blood samples from each of the chambers of your heart. I don't think you liked us putting you to sleep the last time, so I'll make a deal with you. You let us do this, and I'll let you watch."

Two days later, Gilbert came back for the procedure. After getting the local anesthesia to numb the pain, the doctor slid the long, hollow, wire-like catheters into the large artery and veins in the bend of his right arm. The screen to view the procedure was directly on top of Gilbert and thus out of his view. So the doctor had a nurse hold up a mirror. Gilbert was probably one of the first people to see the blood pumping in his own heart. He was amazed, yet scared. His curiosity had definitely gotten the best of him this time. It wouldn't be the last.

Gilbert was lucky that he was born at a time when procedures were being invented to help correct Tetralogy of Fallot. Before the unlikely trio of Dr. Alfred Blalock, Vivien Thomas, and Dr. Helen Taussig developed the surgical procedure known as the Blalock-Thomas-Taussing (BTT) shunt in 1944, there was no way to treat Tetralogy of Fallot. As portrayed in the movie *Something the Lord Made*, part of the problem in babies and children like Gilbert who are born with Tetralogy of Fallot is that the outlet of their right-sided pumping heart chamber, which pushes the entire body's oxygen-depleted venous blood into the lungs to receive new oxygen, is blocked to varying degrees. This condition is known as pulmonary stenosis. In the 1940s, if this blockage was mild, you might have survived for a few years. This was Gilbert's situation. If it was severe, you likely never survived for more than a few days after birth. The shunt bearing the doctors' names was actually a short portion of the nearby oxygen-rich subclavian artery, which they cleverly diverted away from one of the patient's arms to connect directly to the pulmonary artery just beyond the level of blockage into the lungs. They thus devised a way to bypass the pulmonary stenosis.

The problem with the BTT shunt was that it did not last for more than a few years in the patients, as they were now able to grow well beyond infancy. As toddlers and preschool-aged children, they soon needed even more blood flow into their lungs. They became cyanotic again, losing energy, and too many eventually died. Sometime after the BTT shunt became the standard of care for Tetralogy patients, other surgeons solved this problem. One of them was Dr. George Humphreys at Columbia. He and his colleagues came up with a procedure in which they opened the pulmonary stenosis by cutting an X-shaped hole through the blockage that fortunately lay directly on the top of the heart, just beneath the patient's chest bones. Gilbert was Dr. Humphreys's eighth surgical patient.

When Gilbert was five years old, his younger brother Melvin, then just two-and-a-half years old, began to have convulsions. His parents took Melvin to local hospitals, but they eventually had to take him to Binghamton, New York, which had the major hospital in the area. As was then the standard practice for patients with seizures, Melvin was quarantined. For weeks, specialist doctors from all over observed him from behind a glass window, but they could not figure out what was wrong. One day, however, the door to Melvin's room was opened, and his mother could hold her young and frightened child for the first time in a very long while.

The doctors figured out the problem—Melvin had a brain tumor. They handed his parents papers to sign so that they could operate to remove the tumor. As an adult, Gilbert later recalled, in 1946, operating on a tumor was not what it is today. The doctors told Gilbert's parents that Melvin had a 50-50 chance of surviving the surgery. However, without the surgery, he would keep going into convulsions, and eventually, the tumor would crush his brain. His parents had no choice but to sign the consent papers. Melvin never made it off the operating table alive.

Four years after this tragedy, Dr. Humphreys at Columbia slid similar papers in front of Gilbert's father to perform the second operation on his heart. Gilbert's parents once again heard those same horrifying words. Gilbert had a 50-50 chance of surviving the surgery. Over 60 years later, Gilbert asked me to reflect on this moment.

"You have to stop and think what that must have meant to my father. Although he was 6'1" and over 300 pounds of pure muscle, he wasn't strong enough to lose another child. However, he knew that if they did not operate, his surviving son would be gone before he was 15 years old."

His father bravely signed the papers, and a date for the operation was set.

My patients have taught me more about being a doctor than any textbook or class in medical school. For the most part, all I've had to do is be a good listener—listening to their hearts with my stethoscope while also listening to their worries, fears, hopes, and dreams. From the moment I entered medical school at Columbia's College of Physicians & Surgeons in 1987, my teachers and mentors began filling my head with copious facts about the human body and disease. But what my patients taught me is how to harness these facts to best benefit those I care for as a physician. They've taught me to be a healer. Throughout this book, I weave their most memorable stories as they best illustrate the principles that have shaped my worldview as a physician-citizen.

No single individual shaped my view of how to be a doctor more than my patient, Gilbert Tremain. When he was born in 1942 with a life-threatening birth defect in his heart, the researchers who aspired to treat his heart condition were still experimenting on animals in their laboratory. The first successful operation by Dr. Blalock and Vivien Thomas for Tetralogy of Fallot would not take place for another two years. Even then, their first patient lived for only a few more months. Fortunately, Gilbert was born at just the right time, lived in just the right place, and had loving and proactive parents. By the time his parents were offered his first BTT shunt surgery at Columbia, many of the procedural kinks had been worked out.

Gilbert's mother understandably wanted to protect him because she saw his heart as fragile. His father believed that even a child born with a bad heart and a shortened lifespan should be given the opportunity to live well and be happy. This approach forever shaped Gilbert's own attitudes about life that made him a survivor. Just when he started to show the signs of becoming ill with increasingly frequent cyanotic spells during play, the dawn of human heart surgery entered his family's home. Together these doctors, researchers, and families such as Gilbert's laid the foundation for worldwide heart surgery from the halls of America's great medical institutions.

Sixty years after the initial surgery by the Johns Hopkins team, several British researchers looked specifically at the issue of quality of life in children born with congenital heart defects. Their study reaffirmed many of the lessons that Gilbert and his family emphasized so poignantly in their approach to his cardiac care. The researchers summarized their work by writing:

> [E]vidence suggests that children's views are reliable and can differ greatly from the views of their parents or education and health professionals... Quality of life measures focus on daily life experiences and outcomes during childhood and adolescence and facilitate the development of interventions to support families and promote resilience, or positive adaptation, in long-term survivors with chronic disorders... A child-centered approach is fundamental to communication between children, families, and health and education professionals about individual care, as well as to promoting good coping strategies and social inclusion to enhance the lives of children with congenital heart defects (CHD) for whom long-term survival in adulthood is now a realistic expectation.[6]

Gilbert would have laughed respectfully but openly at the notion of any presumed need for such research. His family never required a study to tell them what they already implicitly knew. They just needed their doctors to fully include them in the assessment of his health status

6 Knowles, R.L., Day, T., Wade, A., et al., "Patient-Reported Quality of Life Outcomes for Children with Serious Congenital Heart Defects," *Archives of Disease in Childhood,* 2014; 99:413-419, https://www.ncbi.nlm.nih.gov/pmc/articles/PMC3995241/.

over the years and to make decisions only after conferring with Gilbert directly. This included addressing Gilbert honestly in an age-appropriate fashion that would empower him to always maintain possession of his own health. This was the way their doctors had treated them from the start. Why would anyone take a different approach when this worked so well?

The British researchers went on to state:

> Experiencing recent or frequent health interventions may increase awareness of CHD as an ongoing health burden, with a consequent negative impact on quality of life. Greater attention may therefore need to be paid to the cumulative burden of interventions and medical care experienced by young patients. It is conceivable that some children with CHD who participate fully in school and sports rate their psychosocial quality of life high despite scoring their physical functioning lower, because they understand implicitly that they are 'successfully' negotiating the physical limitations of their condition.[7]

This conclusion echoed the sentiments that Gilbert drilled into my psyche as he repeatedly told me, "Doc, my heart has taken me this far, and I have done well. I already beat the odds and surpassed what anyone expected. Don't just mess around with my heart because you feel that you have to do something if you are not sure that it is really broken. You just might end up making things worse. Let's just agree to keep an eye on things together, and we'll see."

Gilbert would be puzzled and frustrated by such studies. I can imagine him asking why it became necessary for research to tell us what we should already understand as common sense. If doctors truly want to help their patients, all they need to do is talk and listen to them as equal partners in care.

7 Ibid.

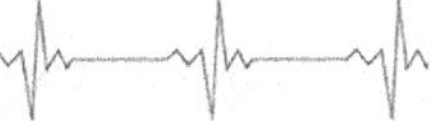

It is noteworthy that the three medical professionals at Johns Hopkins who made Gilbert's heart surgery possible were themselves viewed as defective or broken in some way prior to their success with this procedure. Alfred Blalock had such an impression of himself. Initially, he failed academically to attain his dream position as a surgical resident under his idol, Dr. William Halsted, at Johns Hopkins. Since he could not study at Johns Hopkins, he now believed that he could never be capable of becoming a truly great surgeon. He had not met his own expectations and aspirations. Heartbroken and shaken, he resigned himself to study surgery at the less prestigious Vanderbilt University in Tennessee, where he ultimately found his true calling as the researcher and surgeon to whom Vivien Thomas was later assigned as his personal lab assistant.

Vivien Thomas was a black carpenter working at Vanderbilt University who aspired to become a physician at a time when Jim Crow still ruled the American south. Society then believed that a black man could never have the intellectual capabilities to become a physician, especially one who could treat a white person. His slim chances of becoming a physician were fully derailed by the Great Depression and World War II.

In 1927, Dr. Helen Taussig was turned away from Harvard. It was decreed by the male leadership that a woman could never meet the intellectual and physical challenges required to be a physician. She eventually was accepted to Johns Hopkins, where she resigned herself to becoming a pediatrician and cardiologist, rather than following her initial desire to practice internal medicine. This gender discrimination was compounded by a physical deficit when she became completely deaf in adulthood due to the lasting ravages of a childhood infection.

Dr. Blalock, along with Thomas, repeatedly revolutionized the medical field by making vital discoveries, such as the causes and treatments of shock, just in time to save many lives during World War II. In response to his successes, Dr. Blalock was invited back to Johns Hopkins in 1941 as chief of surgery and insisted that Thomas accompany him. Because structural racism and the associated economic restrictions did not allow him to pursue a formal medical education, Vivien Thomas stayed with Dr. Alfred Blalock as his assistant.

Years after Dr. Blalock passed away, Vivien continued to research and teach at Johns Hopkins, where he was ultimately awarded an honorary doctorate in 1976. Dr. Helen Taussig became famous for putting down her stethoscope and using her sense of touch to examine her patients' hearts, instead of allowing the perceived handicap of deafness to interfere with her work with children. She is recognized as one of the founders of the then-fledgling field of pediatric cardiology.

In pursuing their work to treat patients with Tetralogy of Fallot, this odd trio was vehemently told by the medical field leaders that religious edict dictated that humans should not intervene in the ways of God by operating on anyone's heart, including that of a child. In response to this, Dr. Blalock famously raised up his hands for all to see and asked, "Didn't God make these as well?" They did not accept that they were inferior to anyone else in the eyes of their God and openly denied the degrading proclamations of their human leaders. They displayed the full and glorious diversity of American exceptionalism.

The professional success of these three pioneers with the surgical repair of Tetralogy of Fallot was in no small part due to their strength of will to overcome the many obstacles they encountered. They had been deemed incapable or intrinsically broken by those around them but refused to let this keep them down. Merit in their society was based on the American ideal of individual achievements. The transformative power of their work remains their recognition and incorporation of each other's gifts and abilities brought to bear on their medical discoveries.

If they could tackle these artificial barriers individually, together they could achieve the unthinkable. They could even repair the faulty heart of a child so that it would never be seen as broken again. To do so, they had to overcome the racial, gender, and religious biases of America. Their dramatic collaborative struggle is the stuff of medical legend.

The story of their pursuits to treat children with congenital heart defects exemplifies the essence of the American values that were incorporated into our early healthcare system. They achieved superior results because, despite the superficial differences and labels of inferiority attributed to them, they shared a common conviction to heed a higher call—that each life is precious. They in turn passed this philosophy on to generations of American physicians who would repeatedly shatter the ceiling of limitations for medicine and surgery, specifically. This trio was both a product of American values and an outstanding model of what was possible if we maintained these values together. Americans like Gilbert lived and became healthy under their care. This is why Gilbert never wanted me to forget the values they still represent as visionaries for our American healthcare system.

Gilbert was referred to me by a colleague, a local cardiologist who did not understand how to evaluate and treat patients with Tetralogy of Fallot. On a crisp fall day in 2005, Gilbert entered my life. He was a larger-than-life, strongly opinionated, intelligent personality with an intense will to survive wrapped in the body of a handsomely mustached 60-year-old man with a midline surgical scar running the length of his entire chest.

We bonded immediately. I looked forward to our sessions together—a mixture of medical care and philosophical discussion—until the day he died in 2018 at the age of 76 years old.

Gilbert had an astonishing life and indelibly shaped my sense of what remains invaluable and vital as our nation struggles with healthcare reform. A little boy with a heart defect so severe that his parents were told he might not survive his childhood, Gilbert went on to have a successful career and become a great-grandfather. His life experience calls us back to refocus on the priorities of our patients and our people, rather than get lost in the quagmire of impersonal technology and economics. Partnering with Gilbert to provide him the best possible care left me with a much clearer sense of what our uniquely American healthcare system can achieve if we do not wander too far from our intended path. His words remain the strongest voice admonishing me as a physician to stay on this path and call others back to join us on the quest for exceptional healthcare that we embarked upon as a young nation. Gilbert never overlooked the power of this goal that literally allowed his physicians to save his life. Through his eyes, I continued to care for my other patients and families and teach many of the next generation of nurses and doctors to seek what really matters to the people for which we care.

Gilbert lived a long life despite being born with a broken heart because of science and technology. He lived a full life because together he and I agreed that a life filled with meaning was more important than extending time without happiness and purpose. His legacy is a testament to all the people who became a part of his life journey because they shared a common belief in the inherent value of every human life. This philosophy does not place a higher value on one life compared to another but seeks to maximize the full potential of each life. Because this approach strives to remain free of judgment of relative worth, it also has no preordained expectations or demands. It is nothing less than unconditional love brought to bear in each patient-physician relationship.

I have learned that the rewards of this type of caring are great and filled with the many miracles, large and small, that arise when least expected. I think of the bear hug of a 10-year-old boy with Down's Syndrome giggling with excitement to see me just months after heart surgery. One of my patients, who received a heart transplant after I resuscitated her as a girl—now a young lady, filled with her own dreams of becoming a physician—returned to ask me through tears of joy if she could work with me for the summer before starting college. These are just two of hundreds of examples of my most cherished memories.

In repairing Gilbert's broken heart, he survived. In striving to heal Gilbert's repaired heart, he lived well. His story remains a testament to the value of a philosophy that I strive to incorporate into every patient encounter—no heart is too broken to try to fix. When we heal our patients, we also heal ourselves. The lifeblood of this book is to educate and empower readers to engage in America's much-needed healthcare reform. This book is dedicated to all the Gilberts of the world, whose hearts may have started out broken but ended up strong enough to allow the hearts of all of us to come together through our efforts to heal our nation.

I too have experienced my share of professional failures as I navigated through the halls of academia and community institutions. Each time I get knocked down, my drive to succeed initially weakens. I begin to question my choices and purpose. It is my patients that give me the will to get back up and carry on. When I think back to my first night on call in training year one of three as a pediatric cardiology fellow, it is a wonder that I persisted in becoming a pediatric cardiologist at all. I could have so easily chosen to pursue a lifelong career in general pediatrics after just completing a combined three years of internship and residency in May 1994.

Both Viyada and I took a step back for one year as a family to spend more time with our one-year-old first son, Daniel, who was talking up a storm. The first year of his life consisted of a tag-team effort between Viyada, myself, and her newly retired UNICEF diplomat father. On occasional weekends, when we were either on call or post-call, Viyada's mother, a full-time neurosurgical New York City-based nurse, and my parents would also help. Eventually, after our active second son, Christopher, arrived, we caved and needed to fill the schedule with a professional nanny, an energetic, wavy-haired, blonde woman in her early 40s with a heart wrapped in gold, whom our boys call Naan to this day.

Now a solid inquisitive toddler needed to see more of his parents. We thus both took part-time day and night shifts in the Columbia and Westchester emergency rooms. I further complemented this with a part-time position at an upcoming and very busy general pediatric practice with offices in the immigrant-rich Washington Heights neighborhood of upper Manhattan and Jackson Heights, Queens.

This very important year as a family flew by all too fast. Then just crossing into our 30s, we both began our postponed subspecialty training at Columbia—Viyada's fellowship in adult gastroenterology and mine in pediatric cardiology. One evening in July 1995, I found myself again walking the wards of Columbia all decked out in blue scrubs under a brisk, starched-white, long coat. My senior colleague left the hospital after we had gone over a detailed medical update of the approximately 40 pediatric cardiology patients then on the hospital wards or waiting in the emergency room. In retrospect, I should have been more nervous, but my year of independent practice as a young attending physician made me more confident in recognizing my clinical strengths and weaknesses. Upon this experiential base, I was excited to begin in a new field.

When I received the page at 10 p.m. that night to come to the obstetric delivery room, I was pumped to tackle my first pediatric cardiology case. I respectfully introduced myself to my counterpart in Obstetrics, a clear-speaking woman in her early twenties who wore the marks of a very busy night. She brushed long strands of straight, dark brown hair away from her lightly sweating forehead in her now-wrinkled scrubs with the sleeves rolled up above her elbows.

I began, "Hey, Sarah. So what is going on with the baby you called me about?"

Sarah looked up from her clipboard while swallowing the last bites of a sandwich wrap. "Hey, Eric. Good to see you, but the truth is there isn't going to be much to do for this little one. Didn't they sign this one out to you? The mother is in that last part of natural labor, and the baby should be born within the hour."

"Nope. This family was not on our list for tonight. Guess the communication broke down a little. What's the baby's problem?" I asked with curious concern.

Sarah glanced back at her clipboard. "Not exactly sure. Just says here that the parents are aware that nothing can be done for the baby. After delivery, we are to keep the baby calm in the transitional nursery until he passes."

The matter-of-factness of her words hit me like a stone wall. I was determined to obtain more information before I accepted the full validity of this situation. "I'll go down to our department offices and see if I can find out more details."

As I ran down the nine flights of stairs, my mind was so distracted that I almost ran past the second floor door that led to my office. As I looked through the computers and the charts, I discovered that this baby was determined to have a life-threatening blockage of his main left-sided heart valve taking oxygenated blood to his body. This diagnosis was made by my senior professor, Dr. Lindsey Allan, a world-renowned specialist in prenatal evaluation of a fetus's heart. Dr. Gersony had only recently recruited her from Great Britain to Columbia. Dr. Allan's notes from the mother's last outpatient visit with her were very detailed. She indicated that the combination of the fetus's extremely small and blocked aortic valve with the accompanying relatively small, scarred, and weakened lower left heart chamber could not sustain life beyond a few hours after birth. Nothing was available to repair or palliate this situation in a newborn other than an immediate heart transplantation, which the parents elected not to pursue. The final big pill to swallow was that the parents decided to have a natural delivery but did not want to see the baby. He would die apart from his family in the back rooms of the delivery unit.

And that is exactly what happened three hours later as I watched this full-term, well-developed, and handsome baby take his last breath at 2 a.m. One of the nurses I truly enjoyed working with for years wrapped him up in a soft warm blanket and watched him breathe shallowly for over two hours. She now called me on my pager to ask if I could keep an eye on him while she and the neonatologists attended to an emergency C-section.

"No problem. I'll be right up," I replied sadly.

The nurse returned 20 minutes later to find me alone in the dimly lit room, saying a prayer over his still body. She startled me a bit as she came from behind to lay her firm hands on my shoulders and whispered respectfully, "You certainly chose a tough field, Eric. I'm sorry. What a way to start your first night."

Somehow I finished that first night on call. I talked it over with Viyada a dozen times. She and my colleagues advised me to tough it out with the consistent sentiment of, "You knew it wouldn't be easy, but you're made to be a pediatric cardiologist. Things will get better." With the support of open minds and hearts from my colleagues and family, it did indeed get better. Over the next five years, medical centers around the world increasingly performed lifesaving, catheter-based procedures in newborns to stretch open their critically narrowed aortic valves.

Over the next decade, leading centers such as Boston Children's Hospital would even apply this procedure to unborn and premature children, in the hopes of keeping them alive during pregnancy. Miraculously, several of their initially small and struggling left heart chambers would grow before and after birth to be part of a fully functional heart. Several such infants are now thriving young adults who later became my patients as I started my private practice just a few years after my first memorable night on call. This became just one of dozens of experiences in my field that taught me to never look back, only forward.

Before I knew that I would ever return to my hometown community to practice pediatric cardiology, I had a different career path in mind. I would become an academic physician teaching, researching, and caring for critically ill patients with congenital heart disease. I was particularly interested in the relatively new subfield of pediatric interventional catheterization. Unlike in Gilbert Tremain's case, when he underwent a catheterization in the 1950s simply to make and confirm his particular type of cardiac defect, I trained in the era in which a specialized, painless, and noninvasive ultrasound known as an echocardiogram could readily help make the diagnosis.

Catheterization during my training was therefore used only in complex cases where the detailed anatomy and dynamics of a patient's heart problems were not possible with the echocardiogram. Over the past four decades, the creation of plastics and other related materials also gave rise to new tools that could be attached to or inserted through the catheters themselves. Everything from miniature balloons, metal alloy plugs, small drills, and reinforcing stents were now deployed through catheterization techniques to perform mini-operations that could replace or avoid more invasive surgical approaches. Some of the original catheter-based tools to be used in the human heart or blood vessels were actually first used in children. There seemed to be no limits to what might be possible through this rapidly expanding field of interventional catheterization.

In no small part due to my experience with my first critically ill newborn patient, I spent the 18 months of my pediatric cardiology fellowship planning to become a catheter-based interventionist. I was well aware that, at that time in 1997, even Columbia, as the largest pediatric cardiology program in New York, did not have a full training program for catheter interventionists. All of the doctors in our program who performed catheterization did so on a part-time basis, mixed in with their other responsibilities. I would have to leave New York to study for a couple of years at a program with a full-time, dedicated catheter intervention program.

I set out to carve a small niche for myself as an interventionist with my eye on possibly remaining at Columbia or joining another large academic tertiary center when my training was complete. I wanted to be marketable. I therefore investigated the use of miniaturized ultrasound cameras that attached to catheters. These were mainly used by adult cardiologists to address the diseases of the smallest vessels of the heart that made up my adult colleagues' bread-and-butter work—atherosclerotic coronary artery disease. Some of the founders of the field of pediatric cardiac intervention began using these ultrasound catheters to guide their novel procedures. I wrote a full research proposal six months in advance of my last research year as a Columbia fellow to obtain the necessary ultrasound catheter equipment from a vendor. I then began several animal- and human-based research projects that ultimately carried me through my last year of training and for two more years as a junior attending physician. I never had to leave Columbia. Around this time, our department hired its first full-time pediatric interventionist, a young Harvard-trained physician with tremendous energy and a passion for teaching, Dr Robert Pass. This new colleague expressed an interest in my ultrasound catheter work, and I looked forward to working with him.

It looked like all my planning was going to work. I was now more confident and elated than ever. I would remain at Columbia as a full-time academic physician, specializing in interventional catheterization and carving out a role as the program's specialist in ultrasound catheter-guided procedures. The icing on the cake was that I had also been given the opportunity to set up a Columbia-owned private practice in my home community in New York. Through the offices of a new outreach-oriented administration, I was designated as a liaison from Columbia to this community in the Greater Hudson Valley, just one hour north of New York City. I was all set, or so I thought.

Just as I was completing my fellowship training at Columbia, our chairman, Dr. Welton Gersony, announced his imminent retirement. In a series of one-on-one meetings with him, he specifically reassured me that my career path was solid. He was not worried for me. The arduous task of finding Dr. Gersony's replacement, directed by the university, took our department through a series of temporary leaders. Finally, after two frustrating years of no clear direction, culminating in an outcry from many of our senior members, Dr. William Hellenbrand from Yale University was selected. He was a well-recognized pioneer in interventional catheterization, and I envisioned an even brighter future for my ultrasound catheter work under his supervision. Nothing could have been farther from the truth.

Dr. Hellenbrand wasted no time in telling us all that he did not foresee a prominent role for ultrasound-guided catheter procedures in our field or our specific program. He intended to bolster the catheterization program by recruiting more full-time members, such as Dr. Pass. Everyone who worked in some way in the catheterization facility suddenly felt the stress of uncertainty about their own roles in this venture. I was soon called upon less frequently to carry out ultrasound catheterizations as part of the cases we performed. Dr. Pass and some of my mentors continued to work with me for patient care and research, but Dr. Hellenbrand never called on me. I soon found myself spending much less time in catheter facilities and spending more of my efforts on the inpatient wards and outpatient clinics. Ultimately,

I drifted toward my community-based clinic as my patient volume began to grow. I also spent more time as a clinician and director in the community hospitals.

Finally, I sat down with Dr. Gersony, who was winding down his leadership efforts in the transition to Dr. Hellenbrand's reign. I was internally conflicted about my feelings as I respectfully sought his blessing to leave my full-time academic position at Columbia. I reviewed the events of the last year that took me away from the catheterization work and toward my own patients in the Hudson Valley. I proposed that I now become a part-time attending at Columbia to grow my outpatient practice and the local hospital services. I felt like I had failed in my academic pursuits. Dr. Gersony, on the other hand, supported my decision as noble and very worthwhile. He left the door open for me to return to my full-time position if I ever so chose. My heart felt broken that day.

One of my first experiences with professional rivalry occurred at Columbia in my last year of fellowship training to be a pediatric cardiologist. This was the first time in my recollection that I had been knocked down in the course of my tireless efforts to do a good job and the right thing on the behalf of a patient. One of my supervising junior attendings, who was only two years my senior, reported that I still had not demonstrated sufficient competency in my outpatient care skills. This report came after I questioned her directly in terms of a particular patient's management. I had been respectful but confident in my tone, just as we were all trained to be in this rigorous environment. Such questions were an intrinsic part of our learning, but this physician clearly felt threatened by my inquiries.

Somehow this interaction transformed into an assessment of my abilities as lagging behind where I should be at this point in my education. She made no qualms in forcefully telling me so in the public hallway with my back up against the wall as others walked by. I felt humiliated and immediately began doubting my own intentions and abilities. In a flash, I abruptly and subconsciously returned in my mind to my early days in college, when I still wondered if I could realistically ever become a doctor. She knocked me down, and I was emotionally on my knees.

I was on pins and needles when Dr. Gersony and my direct adviser, Dr. Daphne Hsu, called me into the conference room for an unscheduled review meeting that same day. I had been up all night caring for a very sick baby and tried to remain respectfully alert as they asked that I close the door behind me. I was vulnerable. They explained the matter at hand to me, even going as far as to identify the source of the complaint. To my relief, they did not evoke a sense of anger or disappointment. To the contrary, they explained that the physician who brought this negative report forward had recently been given the almost identical review—literally verbatim—by them.

Dr. Gersony explained, "I have seen this pattern many times before. It typically comes from someone who is somewhat insecure and threatened. Having just received a concerning report by us, your questions threatened her, so you were the likely target of her response."

They went on to explain that they were never personally concerned about my knowledge base or capabilities and were actually quite pleased with my performance to date. However, to display a sense of fairness and reverence to the seniority of the reporting physician, they had chosen very specific decisive corrective measures. I would spend extra time with Dr. Gersony in his outpatient clinic so that he could personally attest to my competencies. My punishment was actually a hidden reward in disguise, as time with the very busy and respected Dr. Gersony and his patients was a coveted commodity. By her body language, I could tell that my accuser was clearly very jealous and upset that her intentions backfired. She knew that she could not pursue the matter further. I was now more reassured that I could successfully complete my training. I was standing back up on my feet.

Dr. Gersony's requirement that I spend a full month, rather than the usual two weeks, in the clinic with him to portray that he was taking matters into his own hands was one of the best experiences that I have ever had. It was an honor to learn directly from him and spend so much concentrated time with him and his devoted patients. It was here that my outpatient skills were formed and finely tuned. To this day, I still attend to my patients in the same manner he demonstrated back then. Even the new office building I personally designed was modeled after the system that he practiced.

He was extremely organized and consistent in his approach, and I felt as if I were learning music from a master composer. He never made a patient feel rushed. Through his queries about their lives and interests, he made certain to establish a clear and strong relationship with each and every one of them. He was possessive of his patients to a fault, and they felt secure in his hands knowing this. I met many senior physicians whose years and stature would potentially imply that patients should be very fond of them. However, many of them reveal no true bond with their patients and consequently have no significant degree of true patient loyalty. Dr. Gersony's patients would rave about him to everyone and honestly loved him. He taught me how to legitimately earn that kind of love.

Because many pediatric cardiology patients are potentially very sick and require very risky and invasive procedures if they are to not only survive but flourish, they and their families need to know implicitly that the physician guiding them through all of these procedures is entirely dedicated to them. This may on the surface appear "old school." To my understanding, it is fundamental for our patients' successful therapeutic outcomes to this day. In his words and practice, Dr. Gersony gave witness to the fact that the patient-physician relationship should not be a dictatorship but rather a partnership in a battle against the serious and determined enemy we call disease. At times, a doctor needs to be ready to clearly step forward as a general in battle. In these situations, the family has to believe in their souls that this is the right person to follow. Any second-guessing can cause serious mistakes and bad outcomes that will forever be ingrained in the family's experiences.

He also clearly took pride in the fact that he started this academic pediatric cardiology division at Columbia himself years ago and therefore was intrinsically committed to its success. That meant that he cared dearly not only about each and every patient but also about those physicians that he trained to pass on his legacy. Amongst all of his achievements, both academic and clinical, the most important gift that he gave to his students—his disciples—was his determination to treat every patient as worthy and special. This did not have to be spelled out or enforced through some form of administrative process. He lived and breathed it every day, and thus this philosophy permeated our education like the permanent dye of a valuable cloth.

He applied this principle equally to all patients, regardless of their culture, race, or social status. I remember one day that left an iconic image burned forever into my memory. By the halfway point in our clinic month together, he entrusted me with starting the initial steps of the visit for some of his most prestigious patients. On this particular day, we had about three or four patients moving simultaneously through the clinic and diagnostic testing areas. I went hurriedly to update him on everyone's progress. Typically, he could be found in his administrative office if he was not with a clinic patient. He had already seen all the current patients, so I did not initially think to search the clinic.

I looked everywhere for him for about 20 minutes and could not find him, until I walked down the clinic hallway and looked into the farthest patient consult room. The doorway was slightly open. He did not see me there, but I could see and hear him clearly as the bright ceiling light revealed the scene. He sat on the floor across from a six-year-old African American child from the local Harlem community. The boy had come with his grandmother to discuss the details of the upcoming surgery to close a large hole in the wall dividing the two sides of the lower chambers of his heart. The grandmother apparently stepped out for a moment, and Dr. Gersony stayed behind to watch the boy.

While there, instead of sitting at the small consult room desk to fill in the typical paperwork in the chart, he took the opportunity to engage directly with this child. He and the boy sat, legs folded comfortably on the floor, directly across from each other, the imposing doctor's desk no longer between them. The boy seemed sad and somewhat scared as this doctor leaned in closer. I will never forget his powerfully simple words to this boy as he reached out and touched his arm.

"You know, young man, I was an orphan too. You are being raised by your grandmother. I was raised by my aunt after my mother died when I was eight, just a little older than you are now. I know how you must be feeling. It was also very hard for me at first. I believe that everything turned out alright for me, and I know that it will be fine for you too. We will get through this together."

The child leaned forward and smiled. He was already much better because of this verbal healing, and I was forever changed. The surgery was still to come, but the healing started then and there.

Howard Zucker was the energetic and exceedingly bright director of Columbia's pediatric intensive care unit while I was training and into my early years as a junior pediatric cardiologist. Newly arrived from Harvard, trained in multiple medical specialties, this Doogie Howser-appearing whiz kid with the unkempt Einstein-type hair was the consummate teacher. He constantly challenged all physicians, students, and seasoned physicians alike to meet the highest standards of clinical care possible. He expected no less from himself and demonstrated an internal drive the likes of which I have never seen since. Then and now, as the current Commissioner of Health for New York State, he places emphasis on clear communication amongst physicians as the best and most efficient way to care for our patients and society. Faced with the public health disaster of COVID-19, I can think of no better physician prepared to meet the challenge.

In my review of a recent TEDx talk by Dr. Zucker,[8] I realized that he believes that healthcare should be guided by a centering principle or force he refers to as the "social center of gravity." He explains that this force is analogous and just as essential to healthcare as the force of gravity is to physics. I strongly agree that we risk losing our entire healthcare system—if not our nation—if we remove this "social center of gravity" from the infrastructure of our system. Like the critical piece in a Jenga puzzle, its removal would break the whole structure as it comes crashing down upon us.

I would advocate that this force described by Dr. Zucker is sustained by an intense energy core sourced from the well of "common good," which is so fundamental to our American national identity. Our current cynicism threatens to undermine this force. Dr. Zucker contends that a perfect storm defined by an intense mistrust in the pillars of society is brewing. This cynicism is understandable in the face of the ulterior and selfish motives of many in the media who align with powerful corporations and money brokers. It is exacerbated by the ubiquitous and instantaneous Internet-based social media platforms. This has led people away from sound and rational thought, no better exemplified than the medical profession's and scientific community's struggle for credibility during the COVID-19 pandemic.

---

8 Zucker, Howard, "From Einstein to 'Baby Sharks': Relativity in the Age of Virality," *TEDxCornellUniversity* (online), https://www.ted.com/talks/howard_zucker_from_einstein_to_baby_sharks_relativity_in_the_age_of_virality.

We no longer believe the press, who should ideally be in a position to present important information that would open our eyes to potential health threats. The politicians are also no longer viewed as unbiased in their formation of relevant policies to address these public health issues. This lack of fundamental trust further erodes our public health authorities' capacity to carry out these policies on our behalf.

Science alone cannot bear the weight of this lack of faith in our institutions. It cannot hold back the onslaught of social-media-derived misinformation that Zucker paints in frighteningly vivid strokes as a viral plague of its own. Unlike the SARS-CoV-2 coronavirus that causes COVID-19, this social media virus preys on the sentiments and emotions of a public that the disseminators of this technological virus wish to frighten and control. They use this biotechnical weapon to toss aside any semblance of rational scientific thought. This negates science and directly threatens our public health. This intentional disturbance of the mindset of human beings incapacitates the amazing potential for technologies like the Internet to disseminate sound evidence-based data *en masse* for the scientific and public health benefit. With his typical subtly cynical tone, he warns us that there are those who benefit from the chaos created by this virally induced misinformation or lack of information. He coins this cover-up scheme, "technologic virality." He invites us to see through this smoke screen.

Like the best clinicians, he does not stop at identifying the culprit pathogen causing the disease. He provides a potential treatment and cure for this virality. He boldly suggests that we turn the weapon back against the perpetrators. He advises that social media itself needs to be the vehicle to counteract virality through concentrated efforts to deliver relevant and sound scientific knowledge in the form of regular targeted public education. He postulates that only in this way can we begin once again to think for ourselves and regain trust in our vital institutions. We must dispel mass misinformation and fearmongering in favor of clear and empowering explanations.

Dr. Zucker's therapeutic challenge is by no means a new concept, but today's media is seen as less likely to work alongside or on behalf of our public institutions than in the past. I still maintain a poignant childhood memory of the landmark government-sponsored televised public health campaign about the rubella virus vaccine of the late 1960s and early 1970s. When I was only six years old, a *New York Times* article from June 14, 1970 claimed that "Dr. Vincent Guinee has sold New Yorkers on the new vaccine for rubella (German measles) in the same way that American advertising sells breakfast cereals and toys—to the parents through their children." Through the black-and-white television commercials I viewed from our family living room, the image of a white umbrella with red spots—the "rubella umbrella"—was burned into my cerebral cortex. Children bought into this approach and bugged their parents so much that this campaign helped to virtually eradicate the main risk of rubella—life-threatening or altering neurologic and cardiac damage to unborn children of expectant mothers.[9]

Knowledge is power, especially when it is grounded on the strong common foundation, like Dr. Zucker's "social center of gravity," directed to those we love and cherish—our children. If I know anything about Dr. Zucker, he will not leave the bedside, he will not rest, until he knows that this therapy cures America's broken faith in each other.

No one would be faulted for coming to the conclusion that America is in serious trouble on many fronts. Even before the pandemic, there existed the notion that something deep in the fabric of American society was broken or, at the least, beginning to crack. The expanding heroin epidemic literally changed the way that our police and emergency medical technicians are trained. Gun violence is spreading from the already excessive individual assaults and murders to almost numbingly frequent mass shootings. The resurrection and expansion of race-based

---

9 Brody, Jane E., "City's Rubella Drive on TV 'Sells" Children on Need for Shots," *The New York Times*, June 14, 1970; p. 60, https://www.nytimes.com/1970/06/14/archives/citys-rubella-drive-on-tv-sells-children-on-need-for-shots.html.

assaults are opening wounds that have never been allowed to fully heal. Political divisions have become entrenched and characterized by even wider chasms between now completely opposed sides. There is an unbridled poisoning of our once-sacred environment in favor of industrial progress and liberties. The rising costs of medical care correspond with ever-worsening healthcare standards compared to other economically comparable nations. These are just a few of the grave problems we face.

Just when we think this is all too much to bear, COVID-19 decisively blows up everything. The perceived cracks are now gaping holes with barely any visible solid surrounding structures to define them. We are relegated back to our individual domains, if we are even fortunate enough to have a place to call home. We are stunned and in such severe shock that even the fluid resuscitation discovered by Dr. Blalock and Vivien Thomas does not appear to revive us. There is no lingering doubt. More than any other nation on earth, the heart and soul of America is seriously broken.

The question now at hand is will we get back up? Once we find the willpower to do so, we are in no position to simply return to the way things were before the pandemic. To do so would also make no sense. There is no room for controversy and doubt that the preexisting problems made us critically susceptible and vulnerable to the scourges of COVID-19 or any other natural disaster for that matter. To continue to debate this issue only lessens our chance of recovery. We are experiencing a societal illness of such great magnitude that all efforts need to focus on recovering the patient, our nation, if we are to survive at all.

Will we be able to learn from our failures and mistakes? I believe so. This will take tremendous efforts and self-analysis, a process which has already begun with the historic level of protest marches and the 2020 presidential debates. Healthcare reform must be a part of any lasting healing process. We all need to engage in and commit to this reformation—this reimagination of the way we deliver medical care—if we want to succeed.

Gilbert would say that we are paying the stiff price for allowing our medical profession to wander off course. The answer to him would be glaringly simple. Return to the value of cherishing every single human life that we Americans profess to hold dear. Do we now once and for all lay complete and all-inclusive claim to this birthright of every American and individual who touches our soil, drinks our water, and breathes our air? This is the philosophy that allowed his childhood generation of doctors to believe that anything was possible in this nation. These healers cry out from this not-too-distant past for us to reclaim that legacy for ourselves and our children. They are extending us a lifeline for resuscitation and rebirth. Are we listening?

Over the past two decades, I suffered my portion of setbacks and disappointments. My own heart has gone through repeated bouts of aching. As I recount in later chapters, each of these experiences ultimately made me stronger. Initially, as with my choice to abandon my plans to become a pediatric cardiac interventionist and remain a full-time academic physician, it took quite a while for me to find my bearings and feel solid ground under my feet. Later, even when the politics and power struggles of the academic centers and community medical systems became more prominent, I recovered more quickly. With the wisdom that comes from years of practice and many arrows in my back, I learned to hold onto my deep-rooted values as my anchor. My family was always there and believed in me. The encouragement of my patients, staff, and students helped me cut through the BS and to question myself less in regards to my consistent endeavors to improve the healthcare of my patients and community. The reality before my eyes revealed a growing and thriving practice. We continued to make a positive difference.

I kept getting back up and moving forward. I am fully resigned to the likelihood that I will face other obstacles. The current COVID-19 pandemic is innately another trial in a series of events, and I am fortunate to have been toughened up by my mistakes and failures before it arrived. If I was still wet behind the ears, I have no doubt that I would not have professionally survived emotionally or economically intact in its wake. In many ways, this book was born out of both my best and worst experiences and is a testament to the efforts of all who joined me.

CHAPTER 2

THE LEGACY OF INSTITUTIONS

Gilbert was scared to death. Just prior to his second heart surgery at Columbia, he met a five-year-old kid who just had the same operation Gilbert anticipated. This boy was one of the more comforting individuals Gilbert met during his stay there because he clearly was doing well, running around the hospital as if he had no surgery at all. He was only five, and Gilbert was nine at the time, so he thought to himself, "Maybe I can make it out of the surgery alive too."

His grandmother lived with his family, but she could not visit him in the hospital because she was at home in upstate New York taking care of his two-year-old sister. His mother stayed with a friend of hers that lived across the river in Hackensack, New Jersey. It was just a bus ride over for her to come and see him. Soon after getting out of surgery, he was given a private room. Anesthesia then was not what it is now, so he kept drifting in and out of sleep for the bulk of the first two postoperative days. One of the times that he woke up, he decided to write a letter to his grandma to reassure her that he was all right. As he finished the letter, he fell asleep again, and when he woke up, he made sure to give his mother the correct date to put on the letter before it was placed in the envelope. Years later, he recalled that it was January 2, 1951. His mother was particularly amazed that, despite how groggy he had been, he was well aware of the correct date. Why wouldn't he? This was a very special occasion. He made it through the second of three operations, and he fully intended never to look back, only forward.

Because he was recovering well, he was transferred to the regular ward just three days after surgery. After spending two more days there, he suddenly felt very sick. The doctors explained that he came down with either the common cold or the flu. During one of our conversations, he remarked introspectively, "I wish I could find the hospital files of my stay during that time because I think I received a blood transfusion. This was during the time that people in New York City sold their blood to buy booze. I think the person whose blood I received had hepatitis B because, later on in my life, I found out that I had it." Coincidentally, as a young adult, Gilbert worked for several years in a large blood bank. It was a requirement that every employee get the hepatitis B shots before they were allowed to handle the samples. "My titers were not taken before getting those shots, so I cannot be certain, but I have a feeling that I was exposed to it when I was in the hospital following my second surgery," he recalled matter-of-factly with a tinge of nostalgia.

Before this second surgery, his father made a deal with Dr. Humphreys. The surgery would be limited to just placing a patch over the X-shaped incision that would expand the pulmonary artery so that blood could easily flow into this artery and out into the lungs. There still remained a large hole in the wall separating the right and left bottom pumping chambers of his heart, known as a ventricular septal defect. Closing this opening would be more complicated than the first two operations, which did not require the doctors to open his heart.

The defect was inside the heart. Placing a patch to fully seal off the hole would require a brand-new technology that could stop his heart for several minutes while keeping the blood flowing to the rest of his body's vital organs. This bypass machine was still investigational at Columbia, so Gilbert's family and their doctors agreed that this last procedure would be left for a future operation. The patch would keep him alive until another surgeon, Dr. James Malm, could finish his current work on developing one of the first heart-lung bypass machines.

Gilbert informed me that "If they had the technology, they would have done everything in one surgery, which is how it is done today. But the machine was not ready yet, so Dr. Humphreys would have to do what he could in the three-minute window that my heart stopped. My father said that unless there was a major change in my condition and the third surgery absolutely had to be done, he would not personally sign the papers again. They would have to wait until I was old enough to sign my own papers for the third and final surgery. My father made sure that Dr. Humphreys put that in my chart."

A BRIEF HISTORY OF AMERICAN HEALTHCARE

Just as I was about to formally accept and start a coveted new position at another prominent academic medical institution—Albany Medical Center—Dr. Gersony contacted me on behalf of the administrative leadership to offer me an alternative and potentially more innovative career path.

I began my professional career at the onset of a new era of American healthcare reform, which involved both the organizational and, in large part, economic restructuring of healthcare delivery. I conducted my medical training in New York City in the last two decades of the 20th century. At that time, there were many different large and small hospitals within the five boroughs of the city. Some of these institutions were private or community-based without any overt academic tendencies or affiliations. Others were large institutions with a relatively longstanding history of clinical and academic prowess. Historically, the larger institutions were staffed by the best and brightest minds and benefited from secure, strong economic support, thus allowing them to lead the way in the advancement of medical care. Through research and the implementation of their discoveries, these institutions had all the components necessary to establish themselves as the pioneers of American healthcare.

As with the arts, medical science flourishes if the proper environment is established through strong leadership and civic support. This was the type of productive environment that then existed in New York City, as well as several other major metropolitan areas. New York was fortunate to have had a head start. The first medical school in the American colonies[10] was actually The College of Philadelphia—later known as the University of Pennsylvania—established in Philadelphia in 1765. In 1767, prior to the American Revolution, New York started another medical school at King's College[11] under a charter granted by King George II of England. This was the foundation or the first academic medical center in the American colonies[12] to grant a degree of bachelor of medicine in 1770. After the American Revolution, the college reopened as Columbia College and by 1912 became Columbia University. It was around this time that this academic medical center aligned itself with The Presbyterian Hospital, a well-recognized, large, urban hospital. By the early 1920s, Columbia and The Presbyterian Hospital purchased property on the original site of the Yankees baseball team stadium. There they built a new medical center, Columbia-Presbyterian Medical Center, which is located there to this day.

The merger between medical facilities such as The Presbyterian Hospital and academic university centers such as Columbia University in the eighteenth century ushered in a revolutionary era in American healthcare. Before we were even a nation, they combined their resources

---

10 Fee, Elizabeth, "The First American Medical School: The Formative Years," *The Lancet.* May 16, 2015, **365** (9981) 1940-1941, https://www.thelancet.com/journals/lancet/article/PIIS0140-6736(15)60950-3/fulltext.

11 "The History of Columbia University," Columbia University in the City of New York (online), https://www.columbia.edu/content/history.

12 Humphrey, D (1975). "The King's College Medical School and the Professionalization of Medicine in Pre-Revolutionary New York," *Bulletin of the History of Medicine,* 49(2), 206-234.

to establish standards to the medical field that would remain the benchmark of legitimacy and authority for the next two centuries. In my field of pediatrics, this model promoted the establishment in 1887 of the first hospital in New York City to be dedicated to children,[13] The Babies Hospital, which formally affiliated with Columbia in 1900. It is this legacy, supported by many years devoted to the service of others, that I came to believe is the actual definition or essence of a term that is too often carelessly thrown around—"Institution." This embodiment of Institution represents the tradition I was fully immersed in during my medical education. It is therefore no wonder that I believe that, if there ever was a place in New York that fit the Merriam Webster's definition of an institution (*"A significant practice, relationship or organization in a society or culture; an established organization or corporation (such as a bank or university) especially of a public character"*),[14] it was Columbia-Presbyterian Medical Center.

The combination of institutions of higher education where students learn to become doctors with clinical facilities and experienced doctors constantly practice medicine proved highly successful through both world wars and into the post-Vietnam War era. After the Columbia-Presbyterian Medical Center was established, institutions around the country followed suit, several within the boundaries of New York City itself. As I finished my subspecialty training at Columbia, there were signs in the air that these larger institutions would soon be sought after to support the many smaller ones and eventually begin working together. If they all were to survive financially and with their reputations intact into the next phase of their respective journeys, they needed to recognize and embrace the mutually beneficial symbiosis of their combined resources.

---

13 "Morgan Stanley Children's Hospital," Wikipedia (online), https://en.wikipedia.org/wiki/Morgan_Stanley_Children%27s_Hospital.

14 "Institution," Merriam-Webster.com, https://www.merriam-webster.com/dictionary/institution.

As the twenty-first century began, additional factors entered the healthcare arena to stir the waters. Medical insurance companies began to decrease the level of reimbursements for medical care under the guise of their own inevitable economic restructuring. Americans had seen this before. Every generation or so, this phenomenon of third-party payors changing the ways medical services were paid for was almost expected. In addition, the advent of extreme growth and dissemination in technological capabilities, such as CT scans and robotic surgeries, changed the healthcare landscape in unanticipated ways. The increased public demand for these technologies became the norm and was guiding the healthcare market. Patients expected to be provided with the latest and best medical tools that existed, even if cheaper alternatives were just as good or even better.

Every time a patient bumped their heads, the emergency room was expected to order a CT scan of the brain, even though the less costly standard of care—the doctor's neurologic exam of the person and observation for several hours—remained normal. If someone needed their blocked and inflamed gallbladder removed, it was deemed necessary to use the newest robotic surgery machines that a hospital just purchased, even if the surgeon was equally or even more skilled without using them. With the dissemination of these technologies, the larger medical institutions therefore no longer held a definitive advantage over the smaller ones. Technology allowed access to information and procedures, particularly in combination with private industry, that leveled the playing field. Some of the smaller institutions were now able to compete successfully to provide patient services with outcomes that were as good as some of the larger institutions. However, these newer technologies came at an increased cost just as the insurance companies threatened to reduce reimbursements for the procedures incorporating these tools. Together, the small and large institutions levied more bargaining power to negotiate for better payments from these payors than they could on their own.

Many of the medical students and trainees I graduated with at Columbia and from other renowned training centers began to establish clinical programs at the smaller institutions in the city and the surrounding suburbs, where their specialized medical or surgical skills had never been available. With this influx of new intellectual property, many of the smaller facilities could actually provide good care more economically and efficiently than the larger institutions that now found themselves somewhat bogged down culturally by a philosophy that was prone to digging in their heels to maintain the old ways and standards. The old ones were no longer as potent or nimble as in the decades before.

In the first decade of the twenty-first century, these symbiotic relationships between the larger institutions and their smaller counterparts provided a mutually advantageous situation because it kept the patients within their combined network. It also allowed a constant stream of newly trained physicians and nurses to be extended from the larger academic mothership. These partnerships seemed initially successful, but the larger institutions soon found themselves fighting for even broader-ranging networks as the third-party payors continued to threaten reduced financial reimbursements for medical care. These financial constraints hindered the autonomy of these networks and became the motivation for the next step in this evolution of healthcare reorganization. The larger institutions now considered the benefits and the feasibility of working together to establish increased economic leverage when negotiating reimbursement contracts with the insurance companies.

The combination of the need of larger academic medical centers to increase their financial solvency and the realization that such medical institutions would be more powerful if they joined forces was just coming to the forefront during the last year of my fellowship training at Columbia. In 1998, the first year after I completed my training—just as I shed the worn-out, light blue scrubs that symbolized my fellowship status to start my career as a pediatric cardiologist—Columbia and Cornell Universities officially combined their medical institutions. The conglomeration of Cornell's NewYork Hospital and Columbia's Presbyterian Hospital, founded in 1771 and 1868, respectively, became The NewYork-Presbyterian Hospital (NYPH). This was the first full asset merger of two world-class academic hospitals in America. This new entity allowed the institutions to maintain their clinical, academic, and financial prowess and remains to this day one of the most successful mergers of its type in the United States and worldwide.

As I donned my uniform of a formal button-down shirt and tie to signify my new status as an attending physician, I soon became aware that many hospitals implemented different models to remain competitive. Outside of New York, several private industries known as healthcare corporations were established. Elsewhere, private hospitals continued to expand medical services independently of academic institutions and started employing the physicians directly. All of these models have since been implemented in different parts of the country or regions of our states with varying degrees of success. Each model appeared to be more applicable to particular geographic areas or states than others. Some areas readily accepted the physician-as-employee model, whereas others only tolerated entirely physician-controlled operations.

MY FIRST STEPS BEYOND SCHOOL

Though I was only 25 years old when I essentially went out on my own, I was "old school" at heart. I was taught the age-old values of respecting physician leadership and hierarchy in my academic training. My worldview of healthcare was depicted by physicians at the helm of any medical system with physician ranking based on a combination of professional achievements and experience. This made sense to me because it was both the academic paradigm in which I trained and a proven means of sensible oversight to ensure that patients received a safe and comprehensive approach to their medical problems. My exposure was limited to a strong academic physician-driven model, which I accepted as a prerequisite for good healthcare delivery. Even though I wasn't yet an experienced doctor, it was also important to me that I never become stagnant intellectually. I remain convinced that this *modus operandi* of intellectually sound physician leadership fosters an open mind, a tendency to seek regular constructive dialogue with colleagues, a desire to base my clinical care on evidenced-based research, an attitude of endless patient-centered curiosity, and ultimately the maintenance of high standards of care.

In the third and final year of my pediatric cardiology fellowship, I instinctively sought any opportunity to work in an academic setting. There was no other career option even on my radar. I sent out many application letters and, in between my research and patient responsibilities, made telephone calls from the office I shared with eight other trainees. Eleven years had passed since I stepped onto the Princeton University campus, uncertain about my ability to become a physician. Now here I was, seeing the end of my subspecialty training in sight and seemingly endless possibilities ahead.

For the next several weeks, I felt both exhilarated and exhausted. I was ready to brave the future and scared to death to leave my comfort zone. I was also happy that I made it farther than my wildest expectations and yet sad to leave my friends and mentors. After only a few weeks of sending out applications, I was relieved and honored to receive an offer to join the academic practice at Albany Medical Center. This was a relatively small four-physician group that lost a senior colleague to retirement. Their pediatric cardiology program was expanding, to include the active recruitment of a recently graduated pediatric cardiac surgeon. They were seeking young blood.

My wife was simultaneously finishing her specialty training in adult gastroenterology at Columbia. Because there thankfully are many more adult patients with gastrointestinal issues than children with heart conditions, her job opportunities were more extensive than mine, and she felt assured she could find a job in the Albany area as well. Daniel, now five years old, was excited to move closer to his upstate New York cousins, and one-year-old Christopher was still oblivious to all the commotion. My mentors expressed support for this opportunity, and I accepted the Albany offer. I would soon officially end my training and become an attending physician. Everything was set, or so I thought.

Just as I was preparing to pack up my young family for the move to Albany, I received a call from my chairman at Columbia, Dr. Welton Gersony, to attend an *impromptu* meeting in his office after my morning patient rounds. Just three days after my acceptance of the Albany position, a newly formed outreach branch of the NYPH contacted Dr. Gersony with a proposal. They were committed to partnering with four community hospitals based just one hour north of Columbia. For many of the same economic reasons that the NYPH system was created, these much smaller community hospitals recently united to establish a regional medical enterprise, known as the Greater Hudson Valley Healthcare System (GHVHS). The NYPH administration had done some research and discovered that I grew up in the Hudson Valley, where my parents still lived in my childhood home in the town of Monroe. Still only 7:30 a.m., I quietly knocked before entering Dr. Gersony's office. The head of the NYPH network—a dynamic, middle-aged woman whose personal energy was contagious, if not, at times, overwhelming—Ms. Cynthia Spears, sat next to Dr. Gersony on his formal couch.

She wasted no time getting to the point as she stood up and firmly shook my hand. "It is a pleasure to meet you, young man. Dr. Gersony and I have been talking about you, and he is apparently quite confident in your abilities." Before I could respond, she continued without taking a breath. "How would you like to return to your hometown to start a brand-new pediatric cardiology practice and also be the first physician to formally represent Columbia and Cornell's new network in the Hudson Valley?" Dr. Gersony just smiled approvingly back at me.

My head was spinning. The chance to begin my career within the confines of my academic *alma mater,* with all its historic importance to our nation's health system, was extremely attractive to me. It would provide me with a sense of structure and familiarity as I ventured forth. My new ship, small as it was heading into uncharted waters, would still be anchored to the mothership. It allowed me a unique opportunity to step off with a strong foundation into a new venture in a community setting where pediatric cardiology services were not readily accessible. It was a personal added bonus that I would proudly return with my Columbia-learned skills back to the community in which I had been raised. I could actually make a difference there. With one foot on solid ground and the other on relatively uncertain territory, I was inclined to believe that this new proposal provided me with the best formula for possible success and the beginning of a meaningful career.

Was I up to the challenge? What would I tell the Albany team? I needed a few days to decide. Ms. Spears indicated that she would await my response, turned, and exited the room.

When I first started my medical training in the city, the perception of my colleagues was that my hometown was somewhere ambiguously far north in essentially another culture up in the woods. Now Columbia miraculously became interested in connecting with the Hudson Valley communities around my hometown. My home was finally officially recognized as "on the map."

I requested several subsequent formal meetings with the newly established NYPH administrators before I would decide to accept their offer. Ms. Spears explained in detail and with sincere reassurance that my position as an envoy from the NYPH network would be bolstered by the world-class status of the successful partnership between Columbia and Cornell. She recognized that this would be my first administrative position, so she would be right at my side for the first couple of years. Though there were some formal business details to be worked out between the NYPH and GHVHS teams in terms of their collaboration, it appeared to me that they had already agreed upon the essential components for future success.

Dr. Gersony—a man I admired and trusted immensely—also represented a generous heaping of added security. He settled my nerves over a cup of coffee in the local cafeteria. "I know that this latest offer was unexpected and that you have already given a commitment to Albany. If it helps, please rest assured that if your new community-based efforts on behalf of NYPH prove unsuccessful or unfavorable to you, your full-time position as an attending physician in our Pediatric Cardiology Division at Columbia will remain intact."

A subsequent phone call from the director of the Albany Medical Center group, Dr. Eric Spooner, also blessed my new venture and offered to graciously maintain their offer for one year if I ultimately chose to move farther northward. "You know, it's hard to find a good candidate nowadays. The team has met and agrees that you're worth waiting for. We will not fill your position for now. In the meantime, we wish you the best of luck."

There followed many late-night discussions with Viyada after the kids were fast asleep. She has always been the practical one and I the dreamer. As my boys said it years later, "Mom is the practical weight to your idealistic soaring balloon." For 11 years, we went through our entire medical training together. Every decision before was always fairly structured and predetermined. The only other time we had been so uncertain was when we decided to postpone our specialty training for one year to work part-time and spend quality family time during the first year of our oldest son's life. That proved to be one of our best decisions ever.

The NYPH offer meant that I would essentially hang up a shingle to start a new practice. We were well aware that this was a risky enterprise given the financial uncertainties of the healthcare market at the time. What did I know about how to start a practice and run a business? Nothing. On the other hand, I would be somewhat of a pioneer, and Viyada knew that this challenge appealed to me.

She weighed in with support. "If anyone can do it, you can. I'll get a regular job, and we will make it. Now's the time to give it a try." My parents would also love being close to their grandchildren.

I received some contractual assurance of initial baseline financial support from Columbia, backed by the NYPH network, while I set up shop. This satisfied the practical side of Viyada's brain. We took a deep breath, and I officially came aboard the NYPH network. I now found myself heading to a suburban community with no significant infrastructure to enable me to provide pediatric subspecialty care according to my training. Dr. Gersony indicated that he would always be a phone call away for intellectual support. Unlike in the past, though, when he had transiently been on site working side by side with his other trainees to establish several community-based practices closer to the city, his current responsibilities at Columbia and the geographic distance of my new venture would not allow him to physically join me. As I was welcomed by my new community-based colleagues and GHVHS administrators, I definitely felt a combination of both optimism and apprehension. Had I made the right choice?

OVER MY HEAD?

Like the merger of Cornell and Columbia, the Hudson Valley region's large healthcare partnership—the GHVHS—was also just a foundling venture. The local restructuring coalesced a significant portion of southern New York's population from a hodgepodge of four smaller local hospital communities into one streamlined and united healthcare system. The fact that the GHVHS now essentially cornered the market of the region's hospital-based patient population inevitably attracted the attention of my larger *alma mater.* The proposed collaboration between the city and community-based systems ultimately created the scenario that allowed me to return to my home town as a medical diplomat who represented both parties.

On a crisp fall morning in 1998, I arrived at the doors of Horton Hospital in Middletown, New York for my first day on the job. Everything seemed so small in comparison to the immense landscape of the NYPH, where I spent the last 11 years training. As a child, Horton Hospital seemed impressive to me, situated high on a hill overlooking the west side of the county. Today, I noticed the faded paint and the worn-out floor tiles. My heart rate sped up. Had I made a mistake?

I couldn't help worrying that this was not the right place from which to launch a new pediatric service. I walked into an aging, outdated facility with limited capacity to serve an ever-expanding community. As part of the negotiations between NYPH and GHVHS, I had been designated as the Director of Pediatric Specialty Services to the Hudson Valley region. I was therefore now ushered by a kind assistant to the administrative wing of the hospital. She welcomed me to my temporary, cinder-block-walled office—just slightly bigger than a closet—in which a small industrial desk with a black two-shelved metal file cabinet by its side occupied over half the floor area.

She smiled widely, cocked her head, and remarked, "You must indeed be important because the door behind your desk opens into the headquarters of the hospital's chief executive officer." Did she know that I just finished my clinical training and had no administrative experience at all?

Within 10 minutes of organizing my desk drawers, testing the phone lines, and finding some hospital letterhead, I was informed by the assistant that I had a meeting in 15 minutes with the full administrative team in the CEO's office. As I passed through the door behind me into my boss's office, I laid eyes on the three men who would become my local mentors for the next few years. These three amigos, as I came to fondly refer to them, insisted that I call them by their first names: Jeff, Jay, and Norm. They all had impressive pedigrees.

Jeff Hinds had a master's in health administration from Duke University. He became my mentor in all things administrative. His ability to navigate between strong tense negotiations at one moment and genuine friendly banter the next was disarming and impressive.

Jay Wilson, the System's Director of Contracts, had been the right-hand man of the former Dean of the Columbia-Presbyterian Medical Center. He was familiar with the politics and procedures of both the local hospitals and that of their partner, NYPH. He often bragged to me behind closed doors that he helped create many of the financial models at Columbia. Jay educated me about the business of medicine at all levels. I owe any of my astuteness in this area to the sound foundation he laid for me.

Norm Samuels, the medical director, was a retired pediatrician who trained at Yale, one of the nation's premier pediatric medical centers. He initially struck me as an outgoing and warm soul with a frenetic energy who made the art of multitasking look seamless. He opened my world to all the local pediatricians and obstetricians, including the internal politics and rivalries between the different groups. Through his consistent support, he facilitated my role as a practitioner and director in the community amongst the four hospitals.

In my first week, I do not believe I even sat down at my desk again. Norm had so many things for me to see and people to meet. He introduced me to his soft-spoken counterpart, Larry Epstein, the CEO of the county's east-side St. Luke's Hospital, which sat perched on the shores of the Hudson River overlooking the beautiful Beacon Bridge and the mountains beyond.

Norm made a concerted effort to connect me with my young counterpart in neonatology, Dr. Kay, who was based at St. Luke's Hospital as the director of the county's first neonatal intensive care unit. Like me, Dr. Kay recently finished his specialty training, and this was his first clinical and administrative experience. At our first introduction, with no patients or staff yet in the facility, Norm sat us down in the middle of a brand-new, high-tech nursery with monitors and fancy temperature-controlled cribs all neatly placed along the four walls of this 40-by-40-foot space with windows looking down on the rolling Hudson River.

He addressed us with pride. "You two young docs are the foundation of the GHVH system's efforts to keep more sick children in the local hospitals. From here on out, I urge you to work together as the system's only full-time, dedicated pediatric subspecialists. Along the way, I promise to give you my full support."

While walking the halls of the cardiology outpatient facilities in the Horton Hospital, I was greeted professionally by a physician that Norm somehow managed *not* to mention during his strikingly thorough tours. I soon learned that this omission was not an oversight.

"Hello, are you the new pediatric cardiologist from Columbia?" asked the clear voice from about 10 feet behind me. As I turned to look back, a middle-aged, clean-cut man with prominent eyeglasses, a focused gaze, and a clear demeanor of authority stood before me. He continued, "I am Dr. Michael Gewitz, the Director of the Pediatric Cardiology Department at Westchester Medical Center. We have been coming regularly to this hospital from our base in Valhalla, New York for years. We provide all the services they need when we come up. I do not think that you will have much work to do here."

In retrospect, I don't even know if I gave him my name or said anything that was semi-coherent. I was caught off guard and needed to reestablish my equilibrium. I immediately went to Norm's office to learn why I or Columbia were never told that Dr. Gewitz and his team had an established clinic within the walls of Horton Hospital.

Norm explained that the Westchester team came up only one or two days a month. He was sure that there was more than enough business for both his group and my practice. "So, you had the pleasure of meeting Michael," he reflected, revealing that they were on a first-name basis. "Our affiliation is now with Columbia, not Westchester. We are committed to supporting you, so do not worry about Dr. Gewitz's team. You will be here full-time and therefore have the competitive advantage. "

I was still naive and easily forthcoming with my trust. I initially did not give the matter a second thought and continued with my original enthusiasm. I had yet to learn the full implications of the "competition" Norm so flippantly mentioned. The arrows had not yet been fired in my direction or struck my back.

Within two weeks, I relocated to a newly renovated office space directly across the street from the Horton Hospital Emergency Room. For the first time, I now had my own reception area with 10 chairs, two exam rooms, and a relatively spacious private office. It was here that I placed my first shingle, recruited my first staff—a nurse and biller—and began regularly seeing patients. I proudly held my first open house event for my colleagues and family. It was in this space that I first felt like an independent physician. I often inconspicuously walked through the rooms, touched the furniture, and breathed in the experience.

At first, the whole situation felt very intimidating because so many expectations were now placed on my shoulders. I did not want to fail anyone—my mentors or my home community. My mind was soon set at ease. From day one, I sensed the constructive energy in the air. I became fully immersed in a combined academic and community-based venture focused on new ideas and opportunities. My own insecurities lay in my honest self-assessment that the administrative aspects of my new directorship position had not been part of my formal education. I soon realized that, though I had been trained in the art of medical care, I now embarked upon a real-life education in the subfield of healthcare delivery.

I had never read a book or attended a lecture on the distinction between medical care and healthcare. In a very hands-on way, I came to understand that these components of our health system are essentially two sides of a coin. I was confronted with the importance of understanding this distinction in my daily efforts to establish new pediatric subspecialty services in a community that historically always outsourced this type of medical care to the urban medical centers. Hundreds, if not thousands, of children were transferred away from the region for medical attention that could not be provided locally. My learning curve was steep and at times daunting.

Medical care, as I came to live and breathe it, is the intellectual and scientific ability of a society to address and fight disease. My Columbia ties sufficiently instilled in me an awareness that the United States is a leading force in the medical care side of the coin. Healthcare, on the other hand, is a much broader topic that encompasses the many ways that medical care is delivered to those who need it. The two are mutually interdependent.

Though we had one of the best medical systems in the world, I became powerfully aware that the United States was sorely behind many other nations and continued to slip downward in the healthcare ranking. In my directorship role, I faced the all-too-disappointing reality that too many of our community's patients had to fight for access to the best medical tests and treatments. The real world served as my classroom, and the lessons were at times harsh.

Here I learned about the numerous problems with our healthcare system. I faced the bureaucracy created by the insurance companies, the for-profit incentives which drove many of the hospital policies and decisions to exclude needed patient services, the economic need for quantity over quality of care, the high cost of medications and technology, and the growing encroachment of corporate forces into our medical profession. I found myself voraciously reading about these issues. I questioned how they could have been so absent in my medical education. We were sent forward without sufficient preparation to tackle the complexities of the healthcare system outside the ivory towers of academia. Did my educators actually believe that we could not fall victim to this overwhelming system? Had they just crossed their fingers and hoped we would survive?

As I saw it, my job boiled down to extending one of the world's highest-quality medical care resources based in Columbia and Cornell to the sick children in my suburban and rural community. I knew how to diagnose and treat a child's cardiac problem. What I did not yet know was how to reach the patient in the first place. Many did not even have a means of travel to my office. To get some of them to Columbia for treatment or surgery, I literally drove them myself for the one-hour trip—day or night, on sunny days or through snowstorms—down the New York Thruway or Palisades Parkway and over the George Washington Bridge. In emergency situations, I jumped into the back of the ambulance alongside the parent, not knowing how I would actually return home myself. When children were sent home from surgery, we soon realized that essential services, such as home nursing or feeding equipment for children, did not exist in our area. Even the local ambulances were hesitant to take responsibility for a sick child, so I waited for hours at my young patient's bedside for the city-based transport system to arrive.

I started teaching new pediatric skills to anyone who listened or showed an interest. I created a lecture series for the nurses in the newborn nurseries, worked with the ambulance teams to show them how to give certain medications in the field, and met with local adult home nursing agencies to expand their services to include children. This list of tasks seemed endless. But we were literally building the wheel, and we started to roll. I was motivated by the progress we made locally and envisioned creating a fully functional high-quality vehicle that could eventually drive itself. Little did I know then that I would spend the remainder of my professional career working to achieve this goal.

One brisk morning, in early March 1999, in the first year of my fledgling outpatient pediatric cardiology practice in New York's Hudson Valley, I received a call from a local obstetric group. I was 35 years old, clean-shaven except for a blond manicured mustache to match my still-full head of hair, and still enthusiastic with a self-motivated drive to give it my all whenever called upon.

"Dr. Fethke, you may not remember me, but we met briefly at a recent physician meeting at St. Luke's Hospital in Newburgh. My name is Clarise. I'm the blond, middle-aged, somewhat disheveled nurse practitioner from the community clinic's obstetric team. We were wondering if you would be able to evaluate the fetus of a young woman from our clinic for a suspected serious heart condition in your local office?" the soft-spoken nurse practitioner pleaded. She elaborated further that the baby's mother was a teenager named Tanya who had no personal means of traveling to the city for healthcare. Tanya was addicted to cocaine, and Clarise's community-oriented obstetric team was following her in their clinic.

We all feared the prophesized doom and gloom of the impending Y2K. Not all pediatric cardiologists at that time performed prenatal cardiac evaluations of unborn children, especially in community settings. Fortunately, during my last couple of years at Columbia, I had the opportunity to train with two of the founders of the prenatal approach to the assessment of heart problems known as fetal echocardiography.

"Of course," I answered the nurse without hesitating. I enthusiastically agreed to become involved in Tanya's case because this would be my very first prenatal cardiac evaluation in my community practice. I promptly arranged to meet Tanya with her social worker at the St. Luke's Hospital outpatient clinic the next day. Situated in the town of Newburgh, New York, St. Luke's demographics remain to this day surprisingly similar to those of the Washington Heights neighborhood in Manhattan where I trained at Columbia. Both neighborhoods pulsed with a mix of deep history and mixed-race cultures with rich and diverse arts and food, all violently and relentlessly clashing with the socioeconomic inequities brought on by decades of racism, corruption, and power struggles. While I grew up in the Hudson Valley, Newburgh was considered dangerous—a down-and-out town of 28,000 inhabitants where drugs, rape, robberies, gang stabbings, and shootings ranked it amongst the top 10 list of urban murder rates.

As Tanya entered my clinic, I could not stop thinking that she was an innocent kid, just entering her teenage years. I could barely see her face because she kept her head down and avoided contact with her subdued, deep brown eyes. Only her bare forearms and hands revealed her café-au-lait-colored skin. She barely spoke, whispering only a quiet "hello" in response to my greeting.

After she somewhat hesitantly agreed to lie back on the uncomfortable exam table, my nurse and I began an ultrasonic evaluation of Tanya's 26-week-old fetus. To help her, we needed to capture enough images to fully determine the formation and workings of her baby's heart. Were there any parts missing? Was the heart strong or weak? Were the blood flow patterns normal without leaks, holes, or blockages? The going was rough because the echocardiogram machine was out of date, the cinder-block room of the clinic was small and dimly lit, and the air felt close with the familiar smell of human sweat.

As we proceeded slowly and methodically, I realized that Tanya was not only an extremely young 16-year-old, but she was also very detached from the situation. She did not ask any questions regarding my own background or anything about the baby as I performed the study. Within moments, it was very clear that her unborn baby boy had a complex and life-threatening congenital heart defect. The right side of his heart had not fully formed, and the baby would require surgery as an infant. Because all the oxygen-rich and oxygen-depleted blood would mix together in his one remaining left-sided lower heart chamber, but he had no serious blockages out to his lungs, I concluded that he would have somewhat lower oxygen levels than normal at birth. He would not be in any immediate danger. If I was correct, he actually should be quite stable in the newborn period and could go home without immediate surgery.

Still, it would take at least two open-heart surgeries in the next couple of years to ultimately correct his heart condition and allow him to live beyond the first three to five years of life. Using hand-drawn, multicolored illustrations on a small whiteboard, which would become the hallmark of my practice style, I calmly and clearly explained everything to Tanya. I put my hand on her shoulder to make some form of personal contact given the seriousness of her baby's situation, but she only nodded, never raising her eyes. I remained somewhat perplexed and bothered by her stoicism. Did she truly understand the information we learned? I felt a deep sense of sadness and helplessness from her and somehow knew that troubled times lay ahead. She left the room escorted by her social worker. I then used my Blackberry to call the referring obstetrician with an update.

Clarise indicated that, given the complexity of Tanya's baby's heart defects, her obstetric colleagues were hesitant to deliver the baby at their community hospital. She explained in a serious tone, "Please don't shoot the messenger. We all stayed late last night to review the situation. Though Dr. Kay's neonatal intensive care unit at St. Luke's is doing very well, it is still in its first year. Eventually, Dr. Kay and his staff should be able to handle such difficult cases, but they have never managed even a simple heart case yet. It just seems too early for us yet. Our gut response tells us that the baby should be born in the city at one of the high-level pediatric centers."

I must admit that her comments unsettled me. I had just completed several years of training at Columbia, the most recognized of the premier institutions to which her colleagues were referring. I was specifically recruited to the Hudson Valley to identify and manage children with heart conditions so that they could be appropriately kept at home or transferred urgently as needed. Now faced with my first complex heart situation, willing to bring all my training to the front lines, I faced an impasse that I did not foresee—fear of professional risk and liability.

The next morning on the landline in my new office, in a forced but good-natured tone, I forwarded my best argument for keeping Tanya and the baby home to deliver. "I feel certain that my training allows me to evaluate and manage this patient locally. It is my understanding that I was specifically recruited to practice pediatric cardiology in this community to reduce the number of patients that have to be sent away. I am confident that between myself and Dr. Kay, Tanya's baby will be in capable hands and do fine." Remembering my impressions of Tanya during our visit, I added, "Furthermore, I am also concerned that Tanya does not have the resources to travel back and forth over one hour to the city for several prenatal evaluations. It will be extremely hard for her to make it down to Columbia some 35 miles away if she goes into premature labor."

My obstetric colleagues remained unconvinced. It was unclear whether they were more interested in protecting themselves or Tanya. I could not change their opinion. The self-identified senior physician of the group spoke up, kindly but undeterred. "Eric, I have no doubt that you are well trained and that your intentions are excellent. I suggest that we meet you halfway in this first complex case. In addition to your comprehensive and detailed medical consultation report in the patient chart, would you be willing to write a signed letter indicating that you take sole and full medico-legal responsibility for the outcome of this baby at birth, thereby dismissing all liability for any of the other physicians involved in the case if the baby does not do well?"

I thought this was a peculiar response and approach. At that time, though, I was totally focused on my ability to help Tanya and her baby. I believed with every fiber in my body that it was important for Tanya and her baby to receive care in their own community. I further rationalized that there would be plenty of trips to the city when her son got older. So it was without hesitation that I wrote and signed such a legal letter and placed it in the medical record.

I saw Tanya every two to four weeks as her pregnancy progressed. Her fetus continued to appear strong and thriving. I felt especially confident because I successfully enlisted the support of Dr. Kay in my efforts to keep Tanya and her baby close to home. He offered to remain available at any time to support the well-being of this baby once it was born. Even more encouraging was that Tanya's shyness started to dissipate. She came out of her emotional shell and communicated with us more freely with each visit. She appeared hopeful and excited about the baby. Each visit ended with my congratulations and a handshake. We all looked forward to her having this baby. Everything was in place as we approached the third trimester of Tanya's pregnancy. My initial sense of foreboding lifted.

However, my celebration was premature. In the 36th week of her pregnancy, I received a distress call from Clarise. "Tanya has just been found lying on the side of a street in the freezing rain. She must have been there for hours after apparently overdosing on cocaine. She is now in active labor on a street corner a mile from the hospital."

An emergency three-way phone call ensued. Both the obstetric team and my neonatal colleague now urged me to help transfer her care immediately to Columbia. They were all clearly very apprehensive about delivering this baby locally, given the combination of active substance abuse, prematurity, and his heart condition. Given the current circumstances, I lost the fight to keep Tanya home. Emotionally, I reluctantly agreed with the transfer plan. Professionally, I knew it was the right decision.

The ambulance team who picked Tanya up from the cold, wet ditch, their engine running, waited for our final decision. I directed them to transport her directly to Columbia. I couldn't help but feel that this was the very situation that we all worked so hard to avoid. Just before the emergency medical technicians raced down to the city with my patient, I called ahead to my Columbia colleagues to give them advance notice regarding the circumstances. Because I worked at the Pediatric Hospital of Columbia as an attending physician, I was comforted by the fact that I could still closely follow this baby down in the city. I hoped that I could bring this small family back home very soon.

As I hung up the phone with the ambulance driver, the sirens blaring loudly in the background, I crossed my fingers, with doubt and disappointment creeping in my subconscious. I suddenly experienced a rush of mixed thoughts and concerns. Should I have written that letter and taken all the risk on my own shoulders? Had my lack of any legal sophistication or apprehension regarding my own liability blunted my clinical judgment? Today, any of the lawyers I worked with over the past several years would likely experience an emotional breakdown or stroke if I blindly repeated this pattern with other patients. Mostly, I solemnly hoped and prayed that I was correct in my assessments and that the baby would do well. But I knew that Tanya's baby's heart was already fragile, and now he had been exposed to what could be a potentially lethal dose of cocaine. Would he be able to overcome these odds? Had I been overconfident or naive? Had I endangered Tanya and her baby?

It was now six months since arriving in the Hudson Valley. I found myself working in a very vibrant and constructive environment. Most rewarding was the sense that I was actually helping to make a significant positive difference in the lives of the children of my home community. However, as the demands of the community-based healthcare work steadily increased, time became my most vulnerable commodity. I essentially performed three jobs—a physician seeing patients and covering local hospitals 24-7, a health system administrator, and a full-time position as an academic physician caring for patients and teaching students at Columbia.

As the first year of my community efforts came to a close, it became more difficult to effectively juggle all these demands. When I considered regular nights and weekends on call locally and in the city, I found myself working 60 to 70 hours per week. I was seriously concerned about not being able to deliver my best work in all these venues simultaneously. Thankfully, due to our successful ventures locally, I no longer needed to take frequent ambulance rides with my newborn patients to Columbia. The local ambulance teams were now more capable and proactive in transporting infants and children who were otherwise stable. Even more encouraging was that the local hospitals were less likely to reflexively transfer a potentially sick child without first attempting to evaluate and stabilize them on site. More sick children were staying close to home than ever before.

The collaboration between the GHVHS and NYPH carried me through the next 12 years of my professional career. As time went on, both my academic and private practice careers grew. I also assumed increasingly administrative responsibilities as we recruited other pediatric subspecialists, including perinatal high-risk physicians known as perinatologists and additional neonatologists to work with Dr. Kay. I was involved in the local education of nursing and hospital staff as well as other general pediatric colleagues in the community.

With the sense that the GHVHS's administration had proven to be truly supportive and that Dr. Kay and I laid a solid foundation upon which to expand, I then recruited other pediatric subspecialists from Columbia-Cornell to join us. I literally knocked on the doors of the directors of every pediatric department at NYPH. I soon had representatives from several pediatric specialties, including hematology-oncology, gastroenterology, and neurology, visit my private practice office to attend to patients. Together, we set out to establish a strong multidisciplinary medical and technical team based upon the tried-and-true partnership between nurses, physicians, and medical technicians. We were actively creating new, local, pediatric medical and healthcare services.

CHANGE OF PLANS

The continuation of this progress in the Hudson Valley required that I make a crucial choice about where to expend my energy. After several sleepless nights and long conversations with anyone willing to engage with me on my options, I knew what I had to do. I therefore had one of the most serious and life-altering conversations of my professional career with Dr. Gersony. If I could obtain his intellectual and moral support, I would make the heart-wrenching decision to step back from my dream of becoming a full-time academic attending physician and professor at Columbia-Cornell Universities. I was fully aware that this change in status meant that my salary support from Columbia would come to an end. I spent countless hours crunching the financial numbers over and over again. If my calculations were right, I could just barely make it on my own as a private practice.

Over one of our regular early afternoon coffee conversations at Babies Hospital, I humbly explained to Dr. Gersony, "I truly do not wish to offend your gracious support in establishing a full-time position for me in your department here at Columbia. However, we have made significant progress in the Hudson Valley, and I believe that, if I am to be successful in the task that you and the NYPH set before me, more of my attention will need to be dedicated to my community work. I cannot in all good conscience give Columbia my full attention, as you should reasonably expect." I went on to argue that this change in my academic status would not only benefit the local community, it would also expand NYPH's geographic reach to the surrounding communities and thereby increase the referral of more complex pediatric patient cases to Columbia and Cornell. After taking a deep breath, I finished, "I therefore now respectfully request a transition to a part-time academic position with you."

A brief but potent silence ensued before he spoke. "I can tell that this decision was not easy for you. Matters of this importance rarely are simple. I agree that your main focus should now be toward your community. It is time, and you would regret not having tried."

I fortunately already knew deep down that Dr. Gersony wholeheartedly believed in my proposal because I had learned it from his example. Since his arrival at Columbia in 1968, he established a large community-based network in towns closer to New York City and essentially built his academic department around this model. He trained the majority of the pediatric cardiologists himself and then sent them up and outward to a combination of private practice and academic positions over the next several decades. This outreach formula proved extremely successful and became the foundation for the most prestigious pediatric cardiology service in New York City. It was also a microcosm of the larger network between the academic medical center and the community-based healthcare system to which I had been sent as an ambassador. Dr. Gersony therefore supported my decision while reemphasizing his original reassuring offer that I could return to a full-time academic position at any time.

The legacy of Babies Hospital at Columbia can best be summarized in one of its earliest mission statements from the late nineteenth century. "The mission of Babies Hospital is to relieve mental and physical distress, and even though the death rate is increasing thereby, a case is never refused admission because it is hopeless."[15] The ethos of this credo was absorbed deep into the psyche of everyone who trained, worked, or was cared for in this institution. This philosophy traveled with the founders of Babies Hospital as it outgrew its original buildings on 55th Street and eventually established its current base on 165th Street on the site of the original Yankee baseball stadium in 1929. Here, Babies Hospital joined Columbia University, and the status of academia lent further credibility and authority to its founding principles. Years later, sensing the commonality in purpose between his medical team and that of Dr. Gersony's, even Dr. Blalock from Johns Hopkins considered coming to Babies Hospital with Vivien Thomas to continue their work.

The founders of Babies Hospital, and many other American institutions, understood the innate blessing of each sick child to society. It is not a fluke that such institutions arose from the depths of the darkest periods of our nation's health history. At the turn of the nineteenth century, the high rate of infant and childhood mortality was a stark reality. Any parent who has lost a child understands the agony—"the mental and physical distress"—that this event creates. Our leading pediatric institutions, often established by women, shone a light in the dark when we needed it most. Their mission was to never give up trying to save a child's life. To do so would relinquish hope to the realm of the impossible. Our early pediatric leaders demonstrated to the nation that the exceptionalism of American medicine resides in our full commitment to better the lives of each individual from the moment they are conceived to be part of society. They taught us that to accept despair as normal, to give up hope, cannot be in our DNA if we are to survive and prosper as a people. Simply stated, regardless of the outcome, when we set out to save a child's life, we end up saving ourselves.

---

15 "Morgan Stanley Children's Hospital," Wikipedia, September 27, 2023, https://en.wikipedia.org/wiki/Morgan_Stanley_Children%27s_Hospital.

Until the day I was faced with the prospect of even partially breaking my connections to Babies Hospital, I did not comprehend how deeply ingrained the philosophy of this institution—my mentors and colleagues—had become in my own professional and world view. I desperately did not want to let go of any part of what Babies Hospital meant to me. I would be adrift without a course to follow, and this concept was terrifying. I vowed that I would not let go until I was ready to set out on my own path.

As I drove northward home from my eventful meeting with Dr. Gersony—the shrinking reflection of the NewYork-Presbyterian Medical Center and the George Washington Bridge in my rearview mirror—I was well aware that another chapter in my life had just begun. My mind raced, and an internal voice kept telling me, "Great medical care is useless if those who need it most cannot access it."

My heart called me to be honest with myself. If I limited my community efforts to just transporting sick patients down to the city every time, I would definitely end up working fewer hours, but to what end? Every time a family's life would be rocked by a serious illness in their child, the added trauma of having to uproot all support networks and hunker down in unfamiliar surroundings was unacceptable to me. I was also aware that many underserved families had significantly fewer resources than others, and they were extremely vulnerable. A serious medical event would have chronic, life-altering repercussions for them. My views had been deeply shaped by my community experiences.

Halfway home, all these thoughts suddenly collided into one very clear vision: I had to focus on my own local community's health standards. I was determined to play a significant role in reversing the national trend of poor access to quality healthcare for the underserved so that they could benefit from the excellent medical care that young physicians like me were trained to provide. To do so, I would have to establish resources in the community to foster the philosophy of keeping children home as much as possible.

This mission would require a local army of pediatric-oriented professionals and laypeople—home-care nurses, social workers, medical technicians, diagnostic technicians, fundraisers, skilled transport personnel, professional associations, and family support groups. We would have to educate and employ the next generation of local technicians and clinicians ourselves so that they could become a proud resource within their own community. The level of local technology for testing in and outside the hospitals would have to significantly expand. The urban medical centers would have to establish trusting relationships with their community counterparts so that communication could foster smooth and efficient transitions between medical facilities. Most importantly, in the beginning, my own office would have to become the hub for all this activity. We would soon need more facility space.

This would be massive healthcare reform at a local level. We would potentially be laying the groundwork for our own local pediatric institution. We certainly had our work cut out for us. With the life of each child comes new hope, and I reassured myself that this hope would lead us forward. I rolled up my sleeves, ready and eager to get to work.

CHAPTER 3

A SHIFT IN PRIORITIES

After his second heart operation, Gilbert traveled to Columbia with one or both of his parents every six months to be checked by the doctors. Years went by, and there was no obvious change in his condition. Yet, on one particularly memorable visit accompanied only by his mother, a young surgery intern told him that his heart was getting sicker. The doctor instructed him that he urgently needed to bring both of his parents along next time because it was time for the third operation to close the remaining hole in the wall of his bottom heart chambers.

That evening, Gilbert told his father about the day's visit, and in a few weeks, they drove down to Columbia together. The intern took his father into one of the examining rooms, leaving Gilbert in the hallway to just barely make out the words of their muffled conversation. But Gilbert was not the type of young man that you excluded from matters so relevant to his own health. "They are talking about *my* heart, so they have to talk to me too," he thought as he stormed through the door five minutes into the visit.

By then, though, his father was fed up and done with talking to the intern. He glanced over at Gilbert and then shouted directly to the intern, "Young man, I may not be a doctor, but I am pretty sure that you don't have a clue about my son's heart situation. I insist that you get Dr. Humphreys down here right now. I don't care if he is now the head of heart surgery at Columbia. He's the only one that Gilbert and I will trust with his heart."

They sat waiting in the exam room for less than 10 minutes when they saw Dr. Humphreys strolling down the hall. Gilbert's father explained to him why they were there earlier than the usual scheduled appointment. Dr. Humphreys called the intern in and asked, "Where's the drastic change here? Do you see any drastic change in his health status? If you took the time to read about this patient, then you would know that if there is no drastic change, then we don't do anything. Now you're going to make him an appointment to come back in six months like he always does." Dr. Humphreys was such a soft-spoken, easygoing guy, and yet, for those few minutes, he was a stone-cold caveman with a club in his hand. Years later, Gilbert remarked that the intern had probably been a little worried since Dr. Humphreys was holding his entire career in his hand.

Gilbert always thought that Dr. Humphreys was an exceptional man. Not only was he incredibly intelligent, he also had a remarkable bedside manner. When he talked to his patients, he was never condescending. In fact, he never talked down to anybody, despite being in such a high position. Gilbert also always admired this great man's ability to be a friend to a kid like him. Gilbert explained, "A lot of people did not know how funny he was, but because I was his patient, I got to know him very well for over 15 years."

When Gilbert was a senior in high school, he was a hall patrol monitor. This position of responsibility foreshadowed his future careers in the fields of security and rescue. His final job until his 70s was as a school crossing guard, where I saw him each morning on my way to one of my satellite medical offices near his home town. Gilbert emphasized that only seniors in his school usually took on the role of hall patrol, stopping by each one of the classroom doors while the teachers stood in the doorway to supervise. Gilbert vividly remembered stopping in front of Mr. Button's classroom one day. Gilbert had been rushing, so he was breathing heavily. His heart beat much faster than usual. At that time, he was keenly aware that his heart still was not perfect. He still had a hole between the two chambers of his heart about the size of a quarter.

As he greeted Mr. Button, all of a sudden, he realized that his heart was not thumping anymore. "My heart stopped! I started to feel a tingling sensation, and my eyesight started closing in from both sides," he explained with an air of drama.

At that moment, he thought back to the time when Dr. Humphreys told him how he restarted his heart after his first surgery. "He did it by squeezing my heart with his own hands," he recalled admiringly. "So I naturally visualized myself reaching into my chest and squeezing my own heart." He tried to think of some way to start it again, and all he could think of was to use his lungs. He took about three long, deep, and powerful breaths in and out. As he did, it felt like somebody turned the pressure switch back on. "I thought that the blood was going to blow right through the top of my head."

While this happened, Mr. Button stood there, leaning against the door and staring in amazement. He proclaimed, "You just turned as gray as a ghost for a moment."

Gilbert nonchalantly and proudly replied, "Oh my heart just stopped, but I got it going again." Gilbert saw the teacher's knees buckle and thought for a moment that he might have to rescue him from passing out. "I guess he never forgot that experience until the day he died," Gilbert chuckled. Years later, Gilbert became a CPR instructor, and one of the lessons he proudly taught was the precordial thump technique to restart someone's heart if it suddenly stops. He told me that he regretted that the precordial thump is not taught as much anymore. "It was exactly what I needed that day—someone to punch me hard in the chest to get my heart going."

UNWITTING COMPETITORS

As I threw myself into my now independent and private medical practice, I learned a very basic and important life lesson—if one focuses all efforts on a particular venture instead of multitasking, the likelihood of success is significantly improved. I spent the next three years concentrating entirely on strengthening the availability and quality of my local pediatric cardiology services. With fewer responsibilities at Columbia, I now opened the office six days per week for patient hours and was now available to my patients and colleagues seven days a week, day or night. Within the first few months of increasing my local presence, the local physicians and hospitals clearly embraced my clinical services as an intrinsic part of the local healthcare network. The volume of calls for my consultations rose exponentially.

Whenever I was called by one of the pediatricians or family care physicians to see a patient with a known or possible heart condition, I made myself immediately available in the office or hospital. Years later, I would learn from my colleagues that my uniquely high level of "accessibility" at the beginning of my private practice was perhaps even more important for increasing my referral volumes than the actual quality of my clinical services. Referring clinicians explained that they were consistently concerned about the high risk associated with our young cardiac patients. They were often blatantly honest and transparent about wanting not only to help their patients as quickly as possible but also to minimize their risk of legal liability as practitioners or a hospital if a child should become sicker or even die while under their direct care.

Before my arrival, they minimized their risk by consistently shipping the patients at least one hour away to the larger urban pediatric institutions. As a local specialist, I essentially served as an immediate cushion to absorb this risk. If the child did not do well, they could now point to me and claim that they made the appropriate referral. They had done their part. I fully acknowledged this aspect of my role as a specialist. While I was at it, I even decided to take the opportunity to push the envelope one step further and embrace the original purpose of my recruitment to the region. I now openly made it my goal to significantly reduce the incidence of this stubborn, old, reflexive pattern of transferring potentially high-risk cardiac patients out of the regional communities—a phenomenon known as outmigration. To accomplish this, I had to prove myself trustworthy by consistently stepping up to the plate and taking full responsibility for a given child's care each and every time they were referred to me. Again, time became the most precious commodity as my hours of sleep steadily decreased.

Two years after I finished my cardiology training, now 36 years old, I was self-motivated and fully invested in the potential to increase the local volume and complexity of my pediatric cardiology services. However, to meet the growing demands and anticipate future growth, I needed to strengthen my own clinical team. For the first time, I became an employer of physicians. I hired a part-time, seasoned pediatric cardiology colleague from Columbia and recruited a young, full-time possible future physician partner. The nurse who I originally recruited now needed to increase both her clinical and administrative duties. Together, we supervised an increasingly large support staff, including medical assistants and a part-time diagnostic technician to perform our own cardiac ultrasounds, known as echocardiograms.

We soon found ourselves moving from our original 500-square-foot office space across from the Horton Hospital into a new 2,000-square-foot space that we were able to design to accommodate our needs and unique practice patterns. It was advantageous that this space was also owned and operated by the local Greater Hudson Valley Health System, our new landlord. I could have rented from other entities, but I was ever cognizant that this new and enhanced relationship with the GHVHS could maintain and strengthen my strong alliance with the local institutions early on during this critical time of expansion for our new private practice.

We soon found that not only were we establishing ourselves as a locally reliable resource for pediatric specialty care, we also unwittingly and unintentionally became a local threat to the Westchester pediatric cardiology team led by Dr. Gewitz. His team historically relied upon this northern geographic area for referrals back to their home base. For years, they sent a physician to our area to run a satellite clinic in the local hospitals—Horton and St. Luke's—one or two days per month. To compete with our full-time practice, they soon found themselves needing to increase the frequency of their clinic presence to one day per week. Eventually, they decided to establish their own local private outpatient office apart from the local hospitals.

Meanwhile, with Dr. Kay's hospital-based neonatal unit well underway, I had also begun to branch out beyond pediatric cardiology. I had recruited two other pediatric subspecialists from Columbia—one in neurology and the other in gastroenterology. This too proved to threaten the Westchester group because they had colleagues in these fields with established local clinics. Their stronghold and network in the area was challenged by our expansion.

I had never been informed by Norm or anyone else about the Westchester group's clinics. I was not intentionally targeting them as I focused on my original mission to expand pediatric services under the collaboration between the GHVHS and NYPH. I became increasingly sensitive to the fact that we had been pitted against each other from the beginning in the endeavor to expand the NYPH network with the GHVHS. Why hadn't anyone given me a heads-up about this? Were they concerned that, if I knew, I wouldn't have taken the job?

Thus began a decade of mutual competition in which we maintained the local advantage in cardiology because of our full-time availability to our referral base and patients. Word-of-mouth recommendations became our only advertisement. At the time, Westchester and our small practice were the only two groups providing such pediatric subspecialty care in the Hudson Valley. Our small

Columbia-founded group did its best to manage our patients' medical conditions in the outpatient office or local hospitals. Only if they were seriously ill did we transfer them to the city. Therefore, many of the pediatric patients with cardiology, gastrointestinal, or neurology problems who historically were transferred to the city or Westchester now stayed in the community for their care. Westchester tried to adjust for the pace of our growth in cardiology, but they could not. They lost a significant amount of their market share to us over the years.

This fierce competition was never my direct professional objective nor an intentional economic strategy but rather a byproduct of my focus on raising the availability and scope of pediatric cardiology care locally. I do not deny that I am competitive at heart. What motivates me professionally is academic achievement, quality, and outcomes in patient care, not finances. I am not unrealistic, however. As a private practitioner and administrator, I learned early on that we cannot provide high-quality care for free.

Deep down, I have always had an aversion to the public mixing of money and medicine and never saw them as equal components to good healthcare. Money should serve healthcare, not the other way around. Advertising, for example, does not seem appropriate or respectful in a field that I consider honorable. Perhaps I am romantic or naive, but I strive to be successful as a physician before I reap any financial benefits. As in the movie, *Field of Dreams*, I believe in the philosophy of "build it and they will come." Our success in the early years of my private practice was due to our accessibility and the high quality of our care. This meant that we treated our referring colleagues and patients with the utmost compassion and respect. We wanted to be partners in care, not dictators. My nurse manager colleague proudly summarized this concept in one beautiful phrase that she regularly reinforced with all the staff—"We shine."

In the middle of our busy lives, the world changed in an instant ball of flames. On September 11, 2001, al-Qaeda committed the single deadliest terrorist attack in human history as they drove four of our own planes into the heart of our economic and military institutions, crashing into the Twin Towers in New York City and the Pentagon in Washington, D.C. Like many others that day, I will always remember where I was at that moment.

It was early morning. I just finished my rounds in St. Luke's Hospital ninth floor neonatal intensive care unit. I reviewed the patients with Dr. Kay and stepped onto the elevator to travel to the first floor. The doors opened, and as I walked out of the elevator, I saw a very large crowd squeezed into a small waiting room, all mesmerized by the wall-mounted flatscreen television. Instinctively, I joined them and was forever traumatized by the images of black smoke spewing from the side of one the Twin Towers and the repeated slow-motion video of an airline plane flying directly into it.

I could not concentrate as I drove Route 84 westward across the county back to my Middletown office site. To this day, I do not even remember if I held office hours that afternoon or just drove straight to the county headquarters to volunteer to go to New York City and help in any way. About 20 other volunteers and I were driven to a local firehouse on standby to visit the site of the Twin Towers or the nearby St. Vincent's Hospital in lower Manhattan.

Nobody spoke, except to call family and loved ones to give an update on our status. Finally, hours later just past midnight, the fire chief joined our small band. "Good morning, everyone. Thank you for volunteering and waiting so patiently. We have been in touch with the New York City mayor's office. I regret to inform you that our services are not needed. The reality is that very few victims have come into the local hospitals from the crash site. They are lost below the rubble. It looks like almost everyone was killed at the site, and there are very few survivors. You are free to return home."

This tragic event, henceforth known as 9-11, changed everything. The hallowed ground of the now-collapsed Twin Towers—Ground Zero—became a site for salvage, not rescue. The city hospitals, with all their skills and experience, were initially helpless to change the situation. Months later, they became overwhelmed by the numerous sick first responders who suffered from the secondary debilitating and deadly health effects of breathing in the toxic air around Ground Zero. In a pattern that would eerily foreshadow the response to the COVID-19 pandemic of today, there was both an outmigration from the city and an increased reluctance of the suburbanites to go into the city if any service, including medical care, could be found closer to home. There soon followed a population surge in the Greater Hudson Valley. The need for local healthcare just received a sudden boost.

The Westchester pediatric program did not sit idly by. They responded aggressively by increasing their local services in other subspecialty areas of pediatrics. They focused their most intense efforts on the local newborn nurseries. Prior to my arrival in the area, the approximately half-dozen community hospital newborn nurseries provided only the most basic care. These "Level 1" facilities did not manage any newborn medical conditions more serious than mild dehydration or jaundice. There were no specialist newborn physicians (neonatologists) working in them. Only the local pediatricians and the hospital nurses cared for the babies in these nurseries.

If a baby had an unexplained fever or anything potentially more serious, they were automatically transferred to New York City or Westchester. It was not a circumstance that the regional network of newborn nurseries in New York were coordinated and regulated by leading neonatal physicians, including the directors from Westchester and Columbia. In their meeting rooms, they worked together as colleagues to designate which nurseries were Level 1 all the way through to their own sophisticated Level 3 neonatal intensive care units (NICUs). This made clinical sense in terms of ensuring a seamless path up and down the acuity levels of the nurseries. In the real world, these two directors were fierce competitors for the market share of sick newborn patients. Their basic objective was to control as many Level 1 and Level 2 nurseries to capture the downstream referrals to their Level 3 NICUs. Westchester had been in our community years before Columbia, but now their Level 3 nurseries were directly competing in our neighborhood.

The new nursery at St. Luke's Hospital, run by my neonatology colleague Dr. Kay, was designated a Level 2 NICU because of his training and full-time presence in the hospital. As with our pediatric cardiology practice, Dr. Kay made himself available full-time to assist all the local Level 1 nurseries in the care of mild to moderately ill or premature newborns. Initially, we worked in collaboration—as Directors Norm Samuels and Larry Epstein envisioned—so that newborns with possible cardiac problems could be managed locally.

I spent many hours training Dr. Kay's technical and nursing staff on the clinical management of sick cardiac babies. Eventually, I even recruited a highly sought-after intensive-care pediatric nurse from Columbia to complement his Level 2 NICU with increased pediatric services for older infants and children at St. Luke's Hospital. This combination of newborn and pediatric services at St. Luke's Hospital proved to be very successful and, within several months, was adopted by the county's medical and lay community as the new standard of local pediatric care.

Westchester did not back down on their efforts to maintain a local presence within this evolving regional pediatric healthcare dynamic. They soon took advantage of what we should have seen as an obvious Achilles' heel in our local neonatal services based at St. Luke's Hospital. Dr. Kay had actually been trained at Westchester and, similar to me, was beholden to and fond of the institution and teachers who taught him his craft. With Columbia as the official partner of Dr. Kay's NICU, the critically ill newborns were diverted to Columbia and away from their historic referral pattern to Westchester Medical Center's Level 3 NICU.

His own *alma mater* thus reasserted their efforts by initiating negotiations with the GHVHS to establish themselves as the rightful academic tertiary institutional partner to support Dr. Kay and his fledgling neonatal intensive care unit. I later realized that, behind closed doors, the Westchester administration was advancing many enticing financial and political offers to Larry Epstein to enhance their claims in this regard. They were understandably motivated to sway Dr. Kay back to their side.

During this era, barely three years into my administrative post and still a relatively naive young administrator, I was first blindsided by the business and politics of healthcare. When Larry and Dr. Kay respectfully informed me that Westchester was courting them again, I reflexively contacted my administrative team at NYPH-Columbia to inform their network of this turn of events. Over the three years since I was first approached by the NYPH system, they significantly extended their network of surrounding community hospitals and thus expanded their administrative staff.

One of the new physician administrators happened to be a well-recognized world-class general surgeon. This bald, athletic-appearing, 60-something man with the energy of a 25-year-old was a force to be reckoned with—I'll call him Dr. Spinwell. The last time I worked with him, I was a young resident rotating through his department. He had historically been an internal political competitor with the director of my own pediatric cardiology division at Columbia, Dr. Gersony. For years, they vied like two titans for a portion of the annual budget, facilities, and personnel resources at Babies Hospital. Like Dr. Gersony, he successfully established several outposts of his clinical pediatric surgical services. As was typical of many of these high-powered and rightfully respected physicians, he had a significant ego. He was assigned to the Greater Hudson Valley region by the NYPH network under the direct authority of the administrator, Cynthia Spears, who specifically recruited me to expand their influence to my home community.

On one occasion, when I was seeing patients at the Columbia clinic, I arranged to meet Dr. Spinwell in his administrative office on the first floor of Babies Hospital. As we sat across from each other at his desk, I informed him of my concerns regarding Westchester's attempts to make their own contractual negotiations within the GHVHS and consequently interrupt the local neonatal service established and then run by Columbia-Cornell. Within five minutes and in the middle of one of my sentences, he abruptly cut me off and indicated that he would take it from here. The meeting was adjourned.

Our subsequent interactions became increasingly tense. I was never fully satisfied that he had a full grasp of the political landscape around the GHVHS. Over the next few weeks, I tried to complete the curtailed first meeting with him. Finally, I resorted to emailing him a comprehensive account of our achievements since I had been recruited to the area. I respectfully reminded Dr. Spinwell verbally and in multiple emails that I had established a strong relationship with the key players in the GHVHS and therefore was an asset to the local discussions regarding neonatology. He never demonstrated any respect for my position as the community's Director of Pediatric Services, which included neonatology. It was as if he had forgotten that I was specifically designated as the outreach physician from his own tertiary center. I earnestly requested that he meet with me to review the regional political dynamics before he met Larry Epstein and that he include me in any meetings with the local hospital administrators of the GHVHS. I received a curt response that this would not be necessary.

Though my instinctive and now more experienced guard was up, I fell back upon my educational upbringing and respectfully acquiesced to his clinical seniority in this matter. During my training, the culture at Columbia instilled in me a strong sense of hierarchy, and Dr. Spinwell was and always would legitimately be my clinical superior. Administratively in the NYPH network and specifically in the GHVHS, I was much closer to his administrative level than I would ever be to his clinical status. I was deeply concerned that he was blind to the political dynamics around Dr. Kay and St. Luke's NICU and that we could therefore lose our affiliation with this valuable asset in our network. All the same, I did not assert my administrative clout in deference to his clinical superiority within our academic institution.

I now realize that my naive mistake was to confuse respect for a clinical superior with my need to assert myself as a local administrator. Dr. Spinwell's mistake was not to take advantage of my expertise and locally hard-earned respect. One of my colleagues—the then-future celebrity, Dr. Mehmet Oz—taught me the important lesson of confusing the objectives of the large tertiary centers with those of their local community partners.

Columbia had also worked with the GHVHS to establish an affiliation in adult cardiology. In many ways, the groundwork for this started even before I was sent to the Valley but had progressed very slowly. Dr. Oz was a more distant ambassador to the region than me, but his obvious intelligence and charisma somewhat made up for this lack of proximity. We worked together during our training at Columbia when I was a student under his then-general surgery residency and again later when I was a pediatric cardiology fellow under his junior attending status. He was always easy to talk to, and I enjoyed bouncing ideas off him.

As we sat together in a back room of the Horton Hospital in Middletown one late Friday afternoon, Mehmet vented some of his own frustrations about his administrative network activities. "Eric, I am concerned that my colleagues and I at Columbia may have made a critical mistake in our negotiations with this local region. Their cardiology leaders have been asking us to provide them with some of our latest balloon pump devices, which, as you know, can stabilize a person whose heart has been seriously weakened by a sudden heart attack. They want to be able to provide this service to the community and tout it as a competitive advantage compared to the other local hospitals."

I casually responded, "Sounds reasonable. What's the problem?"

He continued, "Our ego, that's the problem. We have been leveraging our ability to provide them this balloon pump service to get them to agree to send all of their patients to us, instead of the other centers that they have been using. That's a mistake, and I feel it. We should earn their referrals by extending them this service in good faith and showing that we are a good partner. This will create a more trusting and long-lasting relationship. It is not right to throw our clinical and political weight at them. "

I reached out. "Is there anything I can do to help as a local representative?"

"No," he said quietly, looking down. "It is too late for us. Only time will tell if we have been wrong. I only want you to promise not to repeat our mistakes and always remember that we must approach each other as equals in the service to our communities. We earn the right to care for patients by our actions, not our positions."

The young Mehmet Oz was right on all counts. I wonder today how many of the lessons he learned from these experiences translated to his later successes in working with so many people. The GHVHS broke its affiliation with Columbia adult cardiology within weeks after this discussion. They never fully trusted Columbia again.

Two years later, Dr. Spinwell's approach to St. Luke's neonatal service suffered from the same ego-related deficits. He assumed that his title and position at the academic center intrinsically granted him equal and full respect locally. In the end, St. Luke's Hospital and the GHVHS administration met with him briefly for one or two visits over the next month. I was never included in these meetings nor kept abreast of the discussions. My local colleagues even asked me why I had not joined them. I made some flimsy excuses about getting caught up with a patient.

Within two months, St. Luke's Hospital ended its relationship with NYPH-Columbia and signed a new contract with Westchester. St. Luke's Hospital thus relinquished its control of the NICU that I helped Dr. Kay to establish. Dr. Kay and his neonatal colleagues became full-time Westchester employees. They never trusted Columbia again.

This fracturing of the NYPH's relationship with the main NICU of the GHVHS set a series of dominos falling in my pediatric services. Four months later, now emboldened by their success with the neonatal services, Westchester also increased their local presence in pediatric neurology and gastroenterology. My two new young colleagues, who had worked fervently with me in my new west-side outpatient office across from Horton Hospital and who until then saw their patient volumes grow exponentially, soon noted that fewer patients came to see them.

After six months of my colleagues' patience while I unsuccessfully urged the NYPH-GHVHS network to help boost their local support of our pediatric subspecialty services through marketing and local outreach efforts, they ended their full-time commitment to the community. The neurologist was ordered by her department to return to Columbia to focus exclusively on her tertiary-center work. There would not be a full-time pediatric neurology service locally until 15 years later.

The gastroenterologist decided to split her time between her own local office and a practice in New Jersey. She never was fully accepted by the local Hudson Valley region. Twenty years later, Westchester aggressively increased its own presence in pediatric gastroenterology, effectively eliminating her chances of ever reestablishing the first full-time practice in the region that she began so many years before.

The reaction of the community referral base of physicians was unexpected and forever meaningful. They openly expressed a sense of abandonment. They held me accountable as the representative to NYPH. They had come to trust us as a reliable clinical service, which raised the bar on the local availability and standard of care. We were keeping the children home more than ever. Now what was going to happen? Would we all eventually just return to the city and give up on our community-based mission? Would we prove that they were wrong to trust us then and in the future?

Though my gastroenterology colleague would try for years to create a full-time local presence, this toxic period during which we continued to combine our gastroenterology and cardiology services under one practice entity would haunt her in some form for over two decades. Even though my full-time pediatric cardiology services remained intact, I too was affected transiently by the community's understandable sense of abandonment.

Because I was publicly portrayed as officially responsible for administering the expansion of pediatric services locally, and even though I played no direct part in the neonatal or neurology decisions, I became psychologically attached to their departure from the community. It took me over one year to reassure my local referral base and regain their confidence that I too would not soon abandon and leave the community to return back to Columbia. There ensued a longstanding, very strong distrust of Columbia and its networks amongst the pediatric medical community, and Columbia has never been able, to this day, to send another full-time pediatric subspecialist to the region.

What happened? In just three years, my professional sense of purpose was soundly challenged. There appeared to be a perfect storm all around me, but I could not fully make sense of all the intertwined components. Like the images of a disturbing dream, elements of internal politics, ego, power struggles, and profits all tangled in a dense bureaucracy, invading my waking and sleeping hours. I questioned whether this was a sign. Faced with the opportunity to accept Dr. Gersony's offer to return full-time to Columbia, I struggled privately for several weeks with the temptation to abandon my local practice efforts and professed commitment to the community.

As the next few weeks passed, I buried myself into my patient care. I found solace and was revitalized by the smiles and positive feedback from my patients and their families. As the storm began to break up, I regained perspective. Though I felt personally threatened, this was not about me. I started to focus on "why" things were being done, rather than on "what" was happening.

My pediatric services were everything to me, but they represented just a small cog in the large wheel of regional dynamics that were in turn influenced by the even larger shifts in our national healthcare system. The NYPH network, GHVHS, and Westchester had to deal with the larger scope of all medical services, not just pediatrics. I began to appreciate that everyone was just doing their best to compete and stay viable in this new world being shaped by strong outside forces directed at broad healthcare reform.

I promptly decided that I could no longer hide behind Columbia's walls because they too were obviously responding in their own way to the national policy shifts. Even if I returned to Columbia, I would ultimately still have to deal with these issues in some fashion. After several powwows at home with my always clear-minded and farseeing wife, in a moment of calm, I reaffirmed to myself a dedication to persist in my local pediatric endeavors. From here on out, I would answer only to my patients and myself. Hopefully, I could regain the local trust by doing so.

CUTTING TIES WITH MY INSTITUTIONAL ROOTS

The rivalries amongst the tertiary medical partners in our region were not confined to pediatrics. The adult medical services increasingly faced their own version of this battle for control of the patient-referral patterns. As Westchester and NYPH sparred for access to the GHVHS network, there appeared signs of stress and strain amongst the four local partner hospitals.

At the beginning of this tumultuous time period, I stepped back from my administrative responsibilities in the now-fractured GHVHS. I was spiritually and emotionally exhausted and no longer wished to be caught up in the political windstorm of the local hospitals. I sensed that I could do far better for my patients and community if I focused my full attention on improving and expanding my local outpatient practice.

This shift led me to make a profession-changing decision. For the foreseeable future, I would not align myself exclusively with any one medical entity within the community or with a single outside tertiary medical center. I wanted to be seen by my community as neutral and fully committed to the care of the local children. I promised myself that I would never again be vulnerable or beholden to any local politics that would distract me from my patient care. I would continue to run my practice as a private business, even though there were already signs regionally and nationally that the new trend appeared to be the amalgamation of smaller practices into larger entities.

Within five years, the GHVHS network split in half, essentially dividing the communities into east and west sides of the county. Over the next dozen years beginning in 2002, these two local sides would find themselves in heavy competition with each other regionally. Each side changed tertiary partners as frequently as every two or three years to enhance esteem amongst the local community and maximize profits by leveraging the negotiating power of the tertiary centers with the health insurance companies.

By 2003, just five years since I was sent out from Columbia, I became completely independent, standing on my own two feet. My success or failure would depend upon my own medical team and the support of my family. These two pillars were my foundation.

Now that I was fully on my own—administratively and economically—I was faced with the harsh reality that my medical education at Columbia never prepared me or my colleagues for the practical side of running a medical practice. This glaring exclusion seemed to be intentional, as if mentioning the business or economic aspects of healthcare during our training was somehow unethical. To the contrary, I now realized that this education deficit left me ignorant about practice management and threatened the very existence of my independent practice. I now saw it as educational neglect.

The little I understood about the operational side of a medical practice, including working with the insurance companies and medical billing, I gleaned from my interactions with the first hospital administrators who took me under their wing when I came to the area almost five years prior. The rest I put together with the input of my manager, personal accountant, and extensive reading, combined with a dash of stubborn common sense. I saw the business side of the practice as necessary to enable me to provide high-quality patient care. I remained realistic and idealistic enough to recognize that the business served the patient care, not the other way around.

I was also quite fortunate that my family was very supportive while I literally hung my entrepreneur shingle. Viyada was now more professionally and financially secure as a junior partner in the second gastroenterology practice she joined. She had been wooed to this well-respected and established five-person private practice by a former Columbia colleague. After several late-night discussions together, she decided that this was the time to adjust her hours for our now 10-year-old and six-year-old boys' sake. The current partners agreed to bring her aboard as a three-quarters partner with hours that allowed her to drive Dan and Chris to school and be home soon after they returned on the school bus. It didn't hurt that their office was closer to our home than her first group.

An added bonus was that her parents had moved up from New York City into a new home just four miles from our house. We were now a solidly suburban extended family and well-integrated into our local community. We made a "home," not just a house to live in. We felt blessed. This family arrangement allowed me to take a big chance on my new practice venture. It felt right because we did it together as a family. I routinely brought the boys to my office or on hospital rounds so they could see where I worked. In this way, the practice became part of their lives too.

Many of my brightest Columbia colleagues remarked that they were impressed by this entrepreneurial undertaking. One late night, while I was on call at Columbia, a colleague just three years my senior remarked, "I heard what you are doing up north. People rarely start practices from scratch anymore. I don't know if I could ever make such a bold move. I have no clue as to the first step to even start a practice, yet alone keep it going. I wish you the best." This type of support felt like validation of my efforts and provided further encouragement to spur me onward.

My career would likely have continued on this path unchanged for many years—running my private practice and serving as a part-time academic attending at Columbia. I thrived intellectually with my patient care and teaching at Columbia, where I rotated in a regular schedule with my pediatric cardiology colleagues to cover the complex hospital patients. We met regularly as a team to collaborate on the care of our mutual patients. About a dozen of us shared the experience of working in suburban practices in New York or New Jersey. Only three others besides myself remained financially independent from the university, and they had started their practices a decade earlier.

Despite the east-west split of the local GHVHS network, my practice blossomed. The word of mouth amongst colleagues and patients and my regular presence at the local physician meetings paid off. I now had a consistent patient volume that rivaled any of the other Columbia-affiliated pediatric cardiology practices established decades before. I covered my overhead costs and generated a small salary for myself. As long as I remained neutral to the politics and focused on delivering local care, the patients kept coming.

Yet even the best situations could be deterred or ruined by the one-two punch of a change in leadership and a loss of any true objective. Over 10 years into my private practice career and five years after I successfully stepped back from a full-time academic position, Dr. Hellenbrand experienced a new phenomenon back at Columbia. A new administration threatened to disturb my professional arrangement, which synergistically balanced academia with private practice.

My academic colleagues and I should have foreseen the shakeup of our ideal professional existence coming from miles away. However, we had been lulled into a false sense of security while still sheltered under the shadow of Dr. Gersony's legacy. We did not recognize the warning signs, as the significant financial strains at the medical center at large clashed with a lack of our new leadership's clear vision for the future course of our entire pediatrics program. Pediatrics historically was never a huge moneymaker for the institution compared to other fields, such as adult surgery and cardiology. Therefore, pediatrics always took the brunt of any economic cuts when finances were tight, especially when no influential representatives from our pediatric leadership sat at the negotiating table. The coming decisions would directly and adversely impact the status of our network between tertiary and community pediatric care.

Ten years into the partnership of Columbia and Cornell, their affiliate medical center, NYPH, became increasingly concerned about regional competition in healthcare and the possibility of losing its leading position amongst the other large medical institutions. With ever-increasing operational costs and lower reimbursements, they could ill afford any decrease in their market share of patients. The more patients a hospital institution covered, the greater their leverage in negotiating reimbursement contracts with the large health insurance providers. Competition amongst the big city hospitals to hold onto patients became fierce.

These financial constraints greatly strained the dialogue between our two oldest colleagues—the Columbia-Cornell Universities and the NYPH itself. Ever since the university-teaching hospital relationship was established almost 80 years prior and culminated in the formation of the Columbia-Presbyterian Medical Center, the university provided some of the best-trained clinicians in the country to work within the hospital. This symbiotic arrangement, which provided a constant, reliable, world-class pool of physicians to the hospital, had always been somewhat awkward at best.

There was an in-house joke that many Columbia College students had likely written their graduate theses on how this outwardly dysfunctional relationship somehow still proved to be successful. The university's trainees and medical faculty provided a relatively cheap source of labor, but the hospital always held the purse strings and the control over the facilities. The administrations of the universities and the hospital were caught in a perpetual tug-of-war over personnel and material resources.

"I am still fighting to get our division a portion of the technical revenue generated by the testing we do in the hospital's operating rooms and intensive care units," Dr. Gersony confided to us with a sigh of exasperation while he still led our weekly faculty meetings.

"We do the work, and the hospital reaps the benefit," was a typical response from one of the more senior faculty doctors.

I experienced the downstream consequences of the dysfunctional relationship between the hospital and the university as I embarked on my private practice venture. The university's two main sources of income were funds from the teaching hospital and a portion of the revenue generated by the academic faculty doctors' work caring for patients in the outpatient offices. Like many other universities in the 1970s and 1980s, Columbia elected to levy a significant tax on the revenue generated by the physicians in their outpatient faculty practices—the controversial "Dean's Tax"—to operate their medical schools and support the salaries of their academic staff.

As insurance reimbursements for physician outpatient services and research grant monies continued to decline, and the hospitals laid ever-increasing claims to the monies generated by the physician-guided medical tests, the Dean's Tax became more necessary to continue academic faculty operations. However, independent physicians like myself were trying to make ends meet in the outpatient practices we ran. In 1998, when I started my Columbia-based private practice, the Dean's Tax was 10 percent of all my gross earnings. As of 2003, this tax had become such a financial burden that it threatened the solvency of my growing practice. The tax thus became an additional impetus for my decision to separate my medical practice from the university's faculty practice model.

At this same moment, Columbia was actually battling in court[16] with two ophthalmology physicians over the legalities of this tax. I was aware that ending my faculty practice relationship would result in a loss of revenue for my division at Columbia, but I had no choice if my practice was to survive. In the end, freeing myself from the Dean's Tax allowed my practice volumes to grow large enough that I could support the universities and the NYPH better than ever by sending many patients to them for high-level tests and surgeries.

By 2005, the economic stresses in healthcare widened the existing fissures between the university medical school and the teaching hospital.

16 Yates, James A., "Odrich v. Columbia Univ.," Supreme Court, New York County, 193 Misc.2d 120 (2002), https://www.leagle.com/decision/2002313193misc2d1201299.

In response, the latest academic leadership placed an increasing and onerous emphasis on physician productivity. Within months, this had the detrimental effect of eroding the quality of care provided by the physicians and their teams. Truth be told, there was no one at Columbia or Cornell who believed that "everything was perfect" or that there was no room for improvement in terms of efficiencies or productivity. There was indeed some degree of fat to be trimmed when faced with financial realities. Many physicians were in the habit of spending hours reviewing just one diagnostic study, while others toiled away at a much higher volume. Others left the emergency rooms backed up with patients as they sluggishly rounded on the intensive care and inpatient wards. Not everyone carried the weight of their clinical responsibilities equally, but those who did not often made up for this through research or teaching.

In this new economically stressed environment, a pure focus on finances with less consideration of the quality of healthcare seemed to be the mantra of the day. On the one side, improved technologies such as the implementation of electronic medical records made sense. A shared electronic platform across the entire medical center, including immediate access to test results and images, eliminated the long-standing need to wander all over the hospital to obtain such relevant information. Such data sharing provided the potential to improve communication between clinicians, avoid medical errors, and create better patient health outcomes. With such efficiencies, the patients could potentially return home sooner.

On the other hand, a constant whipping of the medical team to be more productive and efficient in terms of patient and procedural volumes did not account for the high acuity and complexity of our patients. Compared to the patient populations of hospitals that referred patients to Columbia and Cornell, our medical center's patients were often much sicker. Over the decades, a handful of institutions established themselves as "centers of excellence." With this came the burden of more complex, sicker, and chronically ill patients. Some patients just needed more resources than others. To even try and make one size fit all was fraught with the potential to neglect or hurt our most vulnerable patients.

Years prior, our directors addressed the issue of patient complexity in our pediatric cardiology division by establishing a working hierarchy amongst the different attending physicians. The mainly outpatient-based doctors like myself rotated regularly throughout the different service areas our division provided, including exercise testing, echocardiography imaging, and other noninvasive medical tests. This well-oiled system not only provided additional personnel to reduce the regular full-time academic physicians' inpatient responsibilities, it also often allowed part-time doctors to see the less complex cases, which could be attended to in relatively shorter times. Therefore, some doctors could provide a high volume of patient visits and testing for less complex patients, while others concentrated on more complex patients at lower volumes.

Essentially, this allowed each patient to receive the appropriate level of attention for their medical situation. No physician was forced to worry about productivity over quality of care. We all understood and accepted that if a full-time physician needed to focus on one very sick patient to get them through surgery or keep them alive in the intensive care unit, the rest of us picked up the slack for the benefit of the whole operation. Such a symbiotic relationship between the physicians was of mutual benefit to all of us, especially our patients. Whenever I sent a complex patient to the hospital, I knew—thanks to this model—that my patient would receive the best care. The philosophy was simple but powerful. The patients belonged to all of us as a team. I came in once or twice per week and took the volume load off of my colleagues so that they could be free to care for my own and other colleagues' sicker patients. It was because of this highly collaborative system that our division achieved and maintained the highest standards in the city in the first place.

However, the new university and hospital leadership in the first years of the new millennium did not appear to understand or appreciate the value of our particular division's cooperative-care model. They also did not seem to appreciate that the paradigms for children's and babies' healthcare are intrinsically different from those of adults. They demanded that the full-time academic physicians increase their volume productivity in an essentially quota-type system. At this time, I also was first exposed to the terminology and concept of relative value units (RVUs), the latest method used to track physician productivity. In an RVU-driven environment, every work task that a physician conducts—from reading an isolated test like an ECG to providing direct patient care—creates some form of score that is then quantified and tracked.

The outrageous nature of this approach to our clinical care came to its highest fruition at a dinner meeting held by Dr. Gersony's successor, Dr. William Hellenbrand. I vividly remember this event. A large, dimly lit, private room with a long table that could just barely seat us all was reserved in the back of a New Jersey restaurant just over the George Washington Bridge. It was a weeknight, so many of us changed into more semiformal attire after our long day on the patient wards. This was an all-business meeting—no spouses and no fun.

All of our approximately one dozen part-time physician colleagues were invited to receive a very important announcement by this new director. This was the first forum that I can remember in which our complete group of exclusively outpatient part-time academic colleagues came together in any official capacity without our approximately 20 other full-time colleagues. Typically, in the event of any important clinical or business matters, the entire physician staff attended. Our other senior leadership was also not present. Why were we now being addressed in isolation from the rest of our team?

In a mildly shaken tone of voice, Dr. Hellenbrand preempted his comments by saying, "What I am about to tell you is coming directly from the new dean of the university. I want you all to know that I personally do not agree at all with this message. In fact, I feel so strongly that his directives in this matter are wrong for our division that, this very morning, I myself indicated to the leadership that I would rather step down from my position than carry out this plan. They did not accept my resignation and insisted that I must meet with you all as soon as possible."

This was not an auspicious beginning. I caught the eye of one of my colleagues, who shrugged, indicating that he was just as confused as me. Despite Dr. Hellenbrand's preamble to feign an excuse for what he was about to tell us, here he was as the university dean's envoy to carry out the orders. He went on to relay the ultimate culmination—the chopping off of our limbs—of our tried-and-true efficiency model of care. He cut to the chase. "In a nutshell, we are all now being told that the focus of the division's work should shift the burden of productivity completely to the full-time physicians. Your positions as part-timers within the division are no longer necessary or appreciated." He further explained that the dean decided there were enough full-time faculty physicians to do the work at hand. Our part-time presence just encouraged them to be less productive. We were directed to turn our full attention to our outpatient offices and not return to the division unless we became full-time academic physicians. The final emphasis of the message was that we should of course continue to refer patients back to the medical center just as before.

In one fell swoop, we were relieved of our clinical roles at NYPH and our academic position and responsibilities at the university. It was as if an army sergeant lured an entire battalion that the generals no longer wished to keep into a trap and efficiently eliminated them. No one else witnessed the event. In this backdoor termination, there was no conceptual understanding or acknowledgment of the important role that part-time academic physicians, such as myself, always played within the whole system. We were simply portrayed as medical personnel who prevented our lazy full-time academic physicians from being more productive. This scenario was deemed not to be cost-effective and was no longer acceptable to the university or hospital. The end.

I looked around the windowless room, which felt even more darkly lit than when we first arrived. My colleagues were as stunned as I was. I could see it on their expressionless and tired faces. No one spoke, but I noted significant body language and discomfort amongst my colleagues, many of whom had been my teachers. What was even more surprising to me was that, though they appeared disgruntled, there was very little, if any, verbal rebuttal originating amongst them. There was no clear and quick consensus that we should refuse to accept the dean's message or any proposal to strongly unite in opposition to this detrimental course.

It was suddenly clear to me that the insecurities and defensive mechanisms of each individual were stronger than the forces that bound us together. After waiting at least 15 minutes for any reasonable response from the team that never came, I quietly stood up and excused myself from the dinner. I was disgusted with the emphasis on money over mission with no attempt to provide a counterproposal. I had not even finished my now-cold meal.

"Why are you going?" several of my colleagues seated next to me asked as if in a daze.

I replied, "Because as far as I can tell, the meeting is over. Our silence seems to indicate that we are accepting this message without defending everything we have built. Unless you disagree, it is over."

They remained silent. I left.

The evening of the dinner, as I drove northward back to my home 60 minutes away, I began the process of physically and emotionally distancing myself from the academic center that had always been my professional foundation. The implications of the dean's message left me with a full-body-numbing sting. I barely remember exiting off the Palisades Parkway, merging onto the New York Thruway, and taking Exit 16 into my town. The engine idled in my driveway as I sat in the car for some length of time. My colleagues and I were rejected from the team that we had been so dedicated to without any opportunity to be involved in the decision or make alternative suggestions. Even worse, despite all the years together, my second family had not stood up for each other. I now fully realized that my allegiances were better directed elsewhere—to my own family and my community practice.

Over the next few weeks, I held several practical and moral discussions with Dr. Gersony, who still worked clinically and academically at Columbia. He was very supportive of my concerns about the future of the division. He shared many of them himself. We met for our traditional coffee at the hospital pastry shop in the lobby of the new children's hospital, which was funded through the generosity and efforts of a father of one of his patients and completed two years prior in 2003.

As we sat across from each other on a tiny circular table, he looked up from his hot coffee cup, waited a moment, and then spoke calmly and reassuringly. "I know that this turn of events has upset your sense of this institution. This is understandable, as I too am not pleased with the direction the current leadership is taking. Though I may not agree with all their decisions, it is time for others to take us into the future."

I held my cup between my two hands, trying to hold back my frustration and disappointment. "Yes, it must be hard for you to let go of control of the thing you created and built for so many years. I have been training, teaching, and working here for almost 20 years. This has always been my second home. I still don't quite understand the purpose of this decision. We have come so far on the foundation you laid for us."

"I know you care deeply about this place, but I am not worried about your future. Nor should you be," he interjected. "You have established a strong foundation in your upstate community over the past several years. I believe that you will remain professionally secure and successful even if you decide to ultimately break all official ties with this medical center and university." He looked down and spoke more quietly. "I'm actually more concerned about the eventual outcome of some of your other colleagues and how they will survive this new norm."

As he had stated before, he indicated he would always remain available for guidance and support through whatever capacity he maintained in the division. "I am not finished with my work yet. You can always reach out to me if I can help in any way."

"I appreciate that very much. Since I was a medical student, you have always been there when I was in need of support or advice."

"Remember," he spoke with pride and the experience of a successful career, "the foundation for success is not an institution or the walls of the buildings around us. It is the people themselves who are dedicated to a common cause, in this case, to the care for sick children." He explained that, for most of us, he was confident that we had been well trained and would be happy and successful at any institution that appreciated the high standards he instilled in us. "If any one of you I trained ever has to leave Columbia," he emphasized, "please rest assured that, as long as you continue to follow and emulate the standards I taught you wherever you go, you will always have my full support."

Cutting the umbilical cord was not easy, but I slowly weaned myself from my *alma mater*. One late fall night, a brisk wind coming off the nearby Hudson River, I found myself walking slowly and reluctantly back to my car. I was keenly aware that I just completed my last of several hundred on-call rounds at Columbia. From 1987, when I started medical school, to this moment over 20 years later, these buildings and streets had been the foundation of my professional identity. As I meandered aimlessly across the Columbia campus one final time as an official member of this institution, I passed the medical school dormitory where I first met my wife, crossed under the overpass to the newest hospital building where I and hundreds of staff helped manually transport very sick patients from the original old 1920s facility into this modern flagship facility, and finally came back to the building where my two sons were born.

While reminiscing during these ghostly rounds, several chills of uncertainty passed through my core. I wondered whether or not I could be successful without remaining a part of this place. The month prior, I had given my formal notice to my division and institutional leadership that I would be leaving the medical center to focus entirely on my private practice and my local hospitals. Weeks later, through my still-open communication pipeline to the division, I heard that my decision to leave might have made a small impact, but perhaps for the wrong reasons. The leadership, including the current chairman, Dr. Hellenbrand, who made the initial announcements to us all on behalf of the dean, reportedly was openly complaining that I would potentially send fewer patients to the hospital after I left. Nowhere in this reported response of his was there any mention of the loss of the quality of my clinical services—only the *quantity* of my referrals.

When I heard about Dr. Hellenbrand's reaction from my close nursing colleagues, I was even more despondent. I knew wholeheartedly that I made the right decision, but this could not temper my disappointment about how far quantity over quality had become the goal. As I continued to listen from afar over the next several months, bumping into my former physician colleagues at large, continuing-education medical conferences, or Columbia nurses who commuted from my local community at social gatherings, I was not surprised to hear that the interpersonal dynamics between the full-time physicians and a handful of remaining part-time colleagues became increasingly toxic.

The full-time medical staff also began to burn out. The collaborative clinical model that worked for decades was now completely broken. I could hear the strain in my former colleagues' voices when I called them at Columbia in regard to a patient. I felt frustrated and angry that this dysfunctional status infiltrated our professional home. I was particularly worried about the mental health of several of the physicians when I saw their tired faces at city-based professional meetings.

I wondered about the future of the division since hearing that Dr. Hellenbrand was officially moving back to Yale, leaving behind a stressed-out medical team. Something had to give, and I now understood how physicians could become disillusioned and even so depressed that too many in our country were taking their own lives. Thanks to a renewed focus on my home community's healthcare, Dr. Gersony's voice in my mind came through stronger than ever, reassuring me that I would not have to worry like the colleagues I left behind. My home base was now my solid foundation.

A year after I ended my official professional relationship with Columbia, I started feeling like a baseball player simultaneously recruited by several teams. Some of these teams were other tertiary centers. Local hospitals and private practices also started calling. I received job offers left and right. Many of these interactions were very distasteful, focusing mainly on who would control the practice and the economics. Rarely did the quality of clinical care make its way into the discussions. I met with several academic division leaders, the CEOs of three local large multidisciplinary medical practices and four of the community hospitals. Over and over again, with administrators, lawyers, and accountants in tow, I found myself sitting at large conference tables listening and hashing out details of business proposals. I eventually became a more astute negotiator and learned to discriminate between frivolous offers and potentially more reasonable ones.

Though initially, I was not inclined to look actively for these outside merger opportunities, I felt it was my responsibility as the leader of the practice to keep my mind and eyes open for anything that could benefit the practice, specifically anything that would allow us to maintain some stability within the healthcare environment given the forecast of rough waters ahead. During the days, I focused on seeing my patients in the office and the local hospitals. I received referrals from a wide geographic area that covered at least six counties. Occasionally, patients came from New Jersey and New York City. I had one part-time and one full-time physician colleagues in the practice. During the early morning hours and late evenings, I dedicated time to administering the functions of the practice, to include working with my staff, outreach to local hospitals and other clinicians, paying bills, and meeting with potential business partners.

I found myself working 12-hour to 15-hour days, coming home after everyone ate dinner and just in time to help put the boys to bed. I was both exhausted and exhilarated. There did not seem to be enough time in a day to get everything done. I was an independent entrepreneur feeling my way through a combination of extensive reading, advice from colleagues, and a heavy dose of common sense laced with dogged determination.

Over the next five years, I continued to engage in several business negotiations to consider merging with a larger medical group or hospital. I never was fully satisfied with the offers presented to me by their leadership, nor convinced that a particular deal was truly mutually beneficial to both parties. The bottom line often boiled down to the fact that our professional cultures were so different that they were not compatible. These negotiations took an increasingly emotional and financial toll on me and my family and required more and more of my time outside of patient care and the running of my practice.

As much as possible, I tried to shield my medical colleagues and non-administrative staff from these forays into the dark world of medical business. I rationalized that if too many of us got caught up in these business ventures, we risked distracting our attentions away from our primary main focus on patient care. Any time that I received a significant offer or update, I informed my team so that they were not kept in the dark. However, I did not want anyone else to be dragged down by the details or burdens of the merger process. Most notably, no one besides myself and my family took any financial responsibility for the hefty costs incurred for the legal and accountant fees associated with these negotiations. I began to question my logic for seeking another business alliance, instead of remaining independent.

Thinking back, I realize I made some mistakes. I was overprotective. I should have shared some of the financial burdens with the physicians who I employed. They would be the direct beneficiaries of any future partnerships, so why shouldn't they have contributed financially to the process? This would not only have alleviated some of the financial burden on me but perhaps also would have enabled these doctors to have more "skin in the game." As it was, any decisions or input they made only added to the complexity of the process but did not affect them directly or personally. Because they were always sheltered economically, they understandably often felt at liberty to advise that we accept nothing but the best offer when it came to any particular aspect of the discussions.

To my chagrin, the process for the best of four prospects dragged on for months. During one of my group's regular update meetings after patient hours, a physician remarked in a defiant tone, "We deserve a better deal. We are not new to the field and should be offered more vacation time and fewer hospital responsibilities."

I calmly interjected, "In any new partnership, we would have to do like the others in the large group. If we were given special privileges, then everyone else would demand the same. The ripple effect would create chaos. I think what they are asking is a minimal price to pay for the generous retirement and other benefits they offer. I could never provide you or our dedicated staff this coverage if we remain a small group."

After the meeting, the other doctor caught me in the hallway and contributed his thoughts. "I am not sure I will stay around for any deal. You should ignore any input from us and just do what is right for you and the staff." At the next week's meeting, his remarks took a 180-degree turn. "I think we should ask for more money and a bonus. Also, either we all come together, or none of us go. What do you think?"

My head was spinning with all the feedback. Though my intentions to protect my two physicians from some of the stresses of the business negotiations was an idealistic, respectful, and understandable position to take to keep their focus on patient care, it was not based in reality. I was often left standing alone—time and money having been spent by me—to counter a reasonable offer with more demands simply because my colleagues felt it was not completely perfect. At least one or two of the best offers were ultimately rejected because of this logic.

In 2009, I finally agreed to accept an offer with another tertiary institution, The Children's Hospital at Montefiore (CHAM). I had become savvier, so I negotiated a contract with CHAM to initially maintain full control of the day-to-day operations of my private practice. Because of the political and emotional unrest that recently occurred under the new leadership at Columbia, many of the Columbia clinicians followed one of my senior role models from NYPH, Dr. Daphne Hsu, to CHAM after she was successfully recruited to become the new Pediatric Cardiology Director there.

Her objective was to rebuild the CHAM Pediatric Cardiology Division, which had gradually dwindled to only a handful of doctors and was also in need of a bolstered heart surgery program. As per Dr. Gersony's advice, my decision to join the new team at CHAM was based on the high quality and character of the people who emigrated from our Columbia program, not necessarily the bricks and mortar or reputation of the institution. In her typical efficient fashion, during her first year as the new chief, Dr. Hsu brought over some of the brightest and most reputable physicians from Columbia-Cornell with her. She had been at the helm for three years when she and I embarked on productive discussions that resulted in my practice entering into a formal collaboration with her division and institution.

The final agreement with Montefiore was all-encompassing. It allowed me to continue to operate my private practice as a separate entity, maintain an academic position at their affiliated medical school, the Albert Einstein College of Medicine, and enter into a formal, legally compliant service relationship that guided my physicians' work at CHAM. After several months of negotiations, as well as personal time and expense, my small three-physician crew successfully integrated with Dr. Hsu's approximately dozen-physician team at the newly rejuvenated CHAM Division of Pediatric Cardiology. We soon developed a comfortable routine. Each of my three doctors traveled down to the Bronx once or twice a week to see patients, read echocardiogram studies at CHAM, and participate in weekly meetings where we all collaborated on our patients' care. Everything felt right again.

For the next five years, all went well. We maintained a wonderful balance of academics and hands-on clinical work that was reminiscent of our earlier days at Columbia. Our minds were once again stimulated with a focus on patient care and the latest therapies. Gradually, most of my sicker patients were referred mainly to Montefiore, where we once again played a more significant and proactive role in their care.

Because the patient volume of my private practice was now quite high, under Dr. Hsu's sound guidance, my practice played a significant role in promoting the growth and development of the CHAM Pediatric Cardiology Division. When she successfully recruited a new senior world-class heart surgeon for children to join the young surgeon who had also transferred from Columbia, the first patients with complex heart problems came from my practice. Over the next several years, many of my physician colleagues from CHAM regularly came up to our office to provide very specialized evaluations for children needing treatment for heartbeat abnormalities, blockages of valves and blood vessels, and surgery. Our local children were the beneficiaries of high-quality care in their own local community. We raised the local standard of pediatric heart care higher than ever. Montefiore's pediatric heart program saw more and more patients. The whole arrangement was a win-win for all involved, especially the children. I once again felt fulfilled by my career choices.

Around this time, my family took the biggest leap of faith and fully dedicated financial investment in the private practice. Over several dinner meetings, my wife and our two young sons diligently weighed in on my vision of highly specialized pediatric care for our local community in the future.

"Children won't have to leave to go to the city every time they are more than just a little sick or for a special medical test," I explained over burgers cooking on the grill during my weekly night to cook.

"Can we afford it?" my ever-practical wife asked.

"Can we afford not to if the city medical centers become my main competition?" I responded. "I need to provide something unique and special that the big centers don't have and that the community will come to rely on. Otherwise, I may not survive when times get more difficult for small private practices such as mine."

After several weeks of research, we decided to invest personally in a brand-new facility that would embody my ideal of a holistic, therapeutic environment dedicated to outpatient children's subspecialty services. I had been recruited to the region 12 years prior. No other medical group or hospital at either a local or regional level showed any inclination to invest in such a dedicated subspecialty pediatric outpatient facility. I wholeheartedly believed that it was the right time to create such a resource.

My clinical team and I fleshed out the concept of our ideal facility during regular early morning and late evening meetings over bagels and coffee. Paper sketches were strewn over and piled up across my desk at work and home. Gradually, these drawings transitioned from cold blocks of space to detailed designs of a warm, functional, and inviting place for even the most stressed families facing the serious illness of their child to find solace. We knew that we needed to both expand beyond our current tightly packed 1,400-square-foot rental space while maintaining the proper flow of patients in a calm and state-of-the-art environment. We also sought to preserve the essence of what we had achieved so far and could take along with us several years into the future—a safe haven that the families and children could rely on in even the most crucial times of illness.

Everything started coming together. I raced home from work one early spring afternoon to tell my wife that I noticed a very special property for sale. In anticipation of a proposed high-tech hospital, which would combine the two longstanding smaller hospitals, many new outpatient medical facilities were popping up along the main corridor of the town where my rental office was located. I also learned that the county and state envisioned a new offramp from the main highway into this corridor, which would make it easier for everyone to gain access to the future hospital.

Thrown into the middle of all these prospects was an enticing discussion about possibly using one of the old hospitals as the site of a new medical school. As I drove home one evening, I caught a for-sale sign on two acres of a wooded lot at the far end of this proposed medical corridor. I took several pictures of the property on my new iPhone and dragged my whole family to walk through the entire muddy land one Saturday morning. Convinced that this was a promising opportunity, my wife and I decided to buy the land using our own home equity. We rationalized two good options as built-in failsafes. Should circumstances continue to look promising, we would proceed with our own facility. If not, we could sell the land for a possible profit. This project progressively became so personal to my family—our greatest financial investment together and hard evidence of our dedication to our community—that we even created a real estate corporation named after our children.

I sat on the empty property for the next two years. My practice continued to thrive as the main pediatric cardiology service in the region and remained satisfactorily aligned with Montefiore. One mile down the road from our property, the newest hospital in New York broke ground and started to physically take shape. To my dismay, through the chain of local news and my regular discussions with other local conglomerate private medical practices, I soon learned that my vision might face serious competition. The largest of the local medical groups was apparently keen on establishing a comprehensive pediatric outpatient facility of their own right next to my property. My only consoling thought was that I knew the director of this large conglomerate medical practice was financially conservative and extremely practical.

I was instantly on fire as I made a strategic move forward. If I beat them to it and built my pediatric subspecialty center first, I was confident that their director would not challenge us. In fact, transiently, I entered into discussions with him about a mutual venture, but once again, it would be an understatement to say that our visions did not align.

"I want every child in the area to come exclusively to our practice. Your subspecialty team can become part of us, and no one will be able to compete," he affirmed as confidently as a general going to war.

"But as pediatric subspecialists, we need to remain neutral to the economics and political conflicts if we are to serve the whole community. Because children are far less likely to be sick than adults, we cannot afford to alienate our crucial, well-established, geographically wide referral base," I calmly explained and elaborated.

"We just will not have enough patients from your group alone to justify our presence in such a community setting." He seemed not to hear any other voices but those in his own mind as he continued outlining his campaign and completely ignored my concerns. After a couple of such meetings, I remained even more convinced that my practice would be more secure if we could sustain our independence. I politely declined his offer.

Finally, two years after we purchased the property, on an early winter Saturday morning highlighted by the season's first light snowfall, I sat down with an architect to turn our conceptual amateur drawings into an actual building. Just two months later, like a kid with special news that I was excited to share, I revealed the architect's sketches of the building to our new tertiary partners at Montefiore. Within a week, their administration made me a proposal to buy the building, based on the paper drawings alone. We hadn't even broken ground.

This offer confirmed that we were onto something special and made me feel more convinced and secure than ever that we needed to carry out this project on our own. Dr. Hsu read my heart, and she and her new Pediatric Chairman politely stepped in and admonished the Montefiore administrators not to be too aggressive. These physician leaders understood that this was my personal dream and vision, and they did not want to risk coming across as insensitive just as we were all now comfortably settling into our working relationship.

"Give him time to enjoy what he has built," Dr. Hsu cautioned her administrative colleagues at a formal meeting in my small office conference room. We met eye to eye as she continued, "If our alliance continues to flourish and proves to be conducive to moving in the direction of the hospital owning Dr. Fethke's facility, then we can always readdress this merger and facility purchase at a later time."

As the architectural drawings took form, the project took on a life of its own. With these designs, I could now determine the actual cost of undertaking such a building process. The property we purchased two years prior, during the height of the real estate market boom in 2007, had increased significantly in value. With the property as a down payment, a local bank agreed to a building loan and eventual mortgage. In retrospect, if we had waited just three months more, we would have found ourselves right in the midst of the housing-related market crash. We would never have gotten the project off the ground.

In just under two years, the building was completed and inaugurated. It was now an impressive 10,000-square-foot, one-floor facility designed to draw the attention of those driving by with its welcoming lighthouse-themed sign clearly visible on the main street and the sprawling, unique, blue-tiled roof mimicking ocean waves. The whole design, from the inviting outside to the open interior spaces, invoked a balance between the whimsical for children and more serious nautical motifs.

At the insistence of our boys, the whole family became certified scuba divers just three years earlier. From the moment we descended from the ocean surface into the magical marine world of the Caribbean, we became instant converts to this sport that we could share as a family. The main architectural theme of the facility was centered on our family's beloved pastime of scuba diving.

Along the long open corridors, built-in aquariums housed live fish, photos of sea life taken by my oldest son, and life-sized portraits of children from around the world—places we had visited as a family. In one hallway depicting a sandy shore, I even purposefully laid out a beach scene with a not-too-subtle message, a semipermanent editorial comment as an inside joke. Just above the chair rail, about one-third up from the floor, I positioned wall sculptures of several sandpipers busily searching for food on the beach. The same wall above these smaller birds depicted seagulls in flight fighting over a large captured golden fish. The contented and busy sandpipers represented our own pediatric endeavors on the ground level, now embodied by our new facility. Here we would work unencumbered by the larger institutional entities around us—faceless corporations continually fighting over the larger market share of adult medicine—seagulls and their fish.

We also had an indoor glass window overlooking the main patient waiting room. This was donated by the family of one of my first critically ill patients—a fair-haired, rosy-cheeked, adorable toddler named Kristen. Five years earlier, Kristen suffered from persistent inflammation of her heart muscle, known as myocarditis, likely brought on by a strong virus. This life-threatening illness is rare in children—occurring in approximately one to two out of 100,000, mainly infants and older children annually—and particularly unusual in toddlers.

To this day, there is no specific treatment for myocarditis. The medications provided attempt to support or boost the patient's immune system, reduce the immune system's inflammatory response, and strengthen the heart while their own body's defenses kick in. Lately, specific antiviral medications can also be given. Many children recover fully, while others continue with inflammation or suffer permanent scarring damage to the heart muscle. Kristen came to my office once or twice a week so I could closely monitor her medications and the progress of her disease. After several weeks, I became more optimistic because she appeared to stabilize. She was once again alert and the constantly smiling child her parents knew.

One late summer morning, I received a frantic phone call from the emergency room at St. Luke's Hospital on the other side of the county. Kristen was scheduled to see me in the office that very morning, but her breathing suddenly became labored, and her mother had driven her to the nearest emergency room. Just after she arrived, Kristen collapsed. The emergency room team tried desperately to resuscitate her. I directed my staff to reschedule my morning patients as I dashed across Route 84 heading east. I cut the half hour drive to just 15 minutes, and I ran through the emergency room double doors. The voices and commotion behind a drawn curtain in the ER led me to my patient. Kristen's mother stood there, white-faced, frightened, and powerless to help her daughter. Before I crossed the threshold, I acknowledged her with a brief touch to her shoulder.

As I approached Kristen's bedside, I noted the familiar pediatric intensive care nurse who had been recruited from Columbia several years after me. He led the arrest code at the head of the bed while manually delivering breaths to Kristen by regularly squeezing an oxygen-inflated bag attached to a small face mask. They had been trying to bring her back to a point where she could sustain her own breathing and heartbeats for at least 20 minutes with no improvement. With a nod to my nurse colleague, I stepped in to take over, ordering another round of medications and resuscitation. I held the mask firmly over Kristen's mouth. Her cheeks were now mottled and cool. The oxygen wasn't helping, and her own heartbeats had not returned. As I looked up across the crowd of medical personnel, Kristen's mother and I connected eye to eye from over 30 feet apart. She nodded, tears streaming down her cheeks. We both knew that it was time to let her go.

As I looked down at Kristen's lifeless face staring back up at me, tears rolled down my face. My nurse colleague's hand rested lightly on my shoulder. I leaned over and kissed Kristen goodbye on the cheeks. I called her mother to the bedside and then helped the nurses place a white sheet over her body.

"I am so sorry," I whispered to her mother while squeezing her hand tightly.

She wrapped her arm around me and said, "I know you tried your best. Thank you."

Kristen's parents and I have remained in touch for over a decade since. They are among the most remarkable people I have ever met. Though I lay awake many a night fretting about what I might have done differently, Kristen's parents never expressed any anger or bitterness toward our team. To the contrary, they opened up their hearts to other children in need.

Within months of Kristen's passing, they sponsored a support group for families of children with cardiac disease. They donated colorful bags caringly filled with toiletries and other necessities for parents and stuffed animals for the children who were admitted to the urban tertiary medical centers for surgery or serious illness. When we told them about our new office, they immediately became excited and wanted to see the building plans and tour the facility. During a phone call, they graciously insisted that they be allowed to donate a large, indoor, glass window sketched with a beautiful representation of toddler Kristen playing on a beach. Every day, we are all able to see her image there as she looks across the ocean with the eternal optimism of a child.

On October 16, 2010, I invited my teachers and mentors from Columbia-Cornell as well as my new colleagues from Montefiore for the opening day of our new building. My whole immediate family came—my younger sister with her husband and my two teenage nieces and nephew, my physician brother-in-law and his pediatric dentist wife from the city, and my parents and in-laws. Many dear friends, former teachers, professors, local colleagues, and patients also came. My Columbia mentor, Dr. Welton Gersony, and a healthy Gilbert Tremain sat together in deep conversation, recollecting about the original days of the Columbia pediatric cardiology program when Gilbert had all of his surgeries. I could barely separate them when it was time to formally inaugurate the building with a cake and champagne toast.

We named our main conference room the Welton M. Gersony Library. He stated that though he had many significant achievements and his name was associated with many research papers and academic ventures, this was the first physical facility named in his honor. Months earlier, I had proposed the idea to him during a phone call. He confirmed that he was truly emotionally touched by the initial gesture and even prouder when all the day's guests welcomed him with warm applause into the grand room named in his honor. Ten years later, Dr. Gersony told me that he held onto the copy of his portrait with the words honoring his career that I gave him that day—the original forever engraved on a bronze plaque at the double-door entrance to his library.

This official opening day was a celebratory culmination of all that I learned and experienced to this point, and I wanted to share this moment with all of those people who made it possible. From here on out, we planned to continue to do many great things in their honor for the sake of the community's children. I was filled with pride at all we had accomplished in the prior 12 years. Deep down, I wondered somewhat anxiously about what lay ahead, but in that moment, I basked in the laughter, love, and support of all those around me.

It was also during this time around the opening of our new office that I was able to take the clinical services provided in my private practice to the next level. Through several in-person negotiations and letters to the administration of my new tertiary institution, Montefiore, I laid out my priorities and clearly defined my objectives and expectations. I indicated that I simply wanted to increase the availability of the local clinical services for my patients and thus avoid the inherent tendency to create another model for transferring children away from their community. I remained true to the vision that was the impetus for my presence ever since Columbia-Cornell sent me out here over a decade before. I specifically and successfully negotiated for some of my Montefiore colleagues—specialists in heart surgery and interventional procedures—to come up to my office on a regular basis to attend to our local patients. I argued that if they wanted the existing referral patterns to now change toward their services, they had to "earn it" the old-fashioned way. They needed to meet the patients and their families in person, in their own community.

Many of my adult cardiology colleagues in the community had already begun to establish such specialty service clinical models to create a competitive edge for their practices. To my knowledge, this routine presence of children's heart surgeons or other cardiac interventionalists was never successfully pursued in pediatric cardiology in our region of the state. This approach quickly proved highly successful for both the doctors and the patients.

After meeting the heart surgeon or the highly specialized heart rhythm or catheter-based treatment doctors on their own turf, in my office, my patients felt comfortable following the doctor back to the tertiary center for highly complex and specialized procedures. These specialized colleagues of mine also found it personally rewarding to see patients in the more relaxed environment our office provided. It required extra travel time on the part of these visiting physicians, but this arrangement was a win-win for everyone. Competitors from other tertiary institutions in the region could not keep up with our expanded level of local pediatric cardiology care. Their relatively more long-distance and impersonal model turned patients away, and they gradually began to lose a portion of their market share. This level of service became the new norm in the practice and the region. We were now shining even more brightly.

CHAPTER 4

FOCUS ONCE AGAIN ON LOCAL INSTITUTIONS

Less than a month after the opening of the new building, I first met a child who would become one of my most memorable patients. It was as if everything we created came together just in time for her to enter our lives at that very moment. In the middle of a routine day, a tall, slender 13-year-girl with deep hazel eyes and long, straight, dirty-blonde hair leaned against her mother as they held hands tightly. I greeted her in the hallway outside one of the exam room doors as we were both entering the room together.

She nervously glanced up at me and quietly asked, "Am I going to die?"

These first words would stick in my mind forever. Somewhat taken aback by this brutally honest greeting, I looked at her calmly and replied, "Of course not, dear. What makes you think such thoughts? What's your name?"

"Brittany," she answered flatly. "And I was just wondering."

I reviewed Brittany's case. She had been referred to us because her pediatrician recently noted a consistent, mildly fast heart rate on several routine examinations. A normal 13-year-old's heart beats about 80 to 90 times every minute when awake and calm. Though there is some normal variation in heart rate amongst different people, Brittany's heart was clearly beating too fast for her age, at about 140 beats per minute.

I was immediately concerned and curious about why her heart was racing. I needed to determine if she was just nervous or if there was an abnormal source of her heartbeats. Our first order of business was to give her an electrocardiogram—a painless test which uses electrode stickers placed on a person's chest, arms, and legs and connects by wires to a machine to reveal the heartbeat patterns on a screen or paper. Her electrocardiogram revealed that the main source of most of her heartbeats was not the normal location at the top right of the heart known as the sinus node. The majority of her beats originated from a single spot in her lower heart chambers or ventricles. Brittany otherwise appeared to be well and had no specific complaints or symptoms.

I ended our first visit by looking at her directly to reassure her that I did not believe she was in any imminent danger. I explained that I wanted her to undergo some non-painful and noninvasive tests in the next few days. As I began to draw out the details of my findings and plans on the whiteboard in the exam room for the family, Brittany politely excused herself. "I don't want to hear any details because I don't want to be scared," she explained as she exited into the hallway.

I explained to her mother that I was ordering a heart monitor that Brittany would wear under her clothes for 48 hours so we could get a better sense of her daily heart rhythms. She also needed an echocardiogram—a sonogram which reveals all the parts of a moving heart and the blood flow in and out of the heart—so that I could specifically evaluate the health of her heart muscles from which the rapid beats originated. Finally, I wanted her to do an exercise stress test on a treadmill in our office to see what happened to her heartbeats as she started running.

Her mom spoke with a sense of apprehension reminiscent of her daughter's timidness. "Brittany has always been extremely active for her age. She always appears to be totally healthy and normal. Can she continue to play and exercise?"

I took in a gentle deep breath before responding deliberately and honestly. "Probably in the near future, but I just want to be safe and complete these tests done first. Then we can answer that question together with more information to support this decision and our next steps."

Within a handful of days, we compiled all the test results. The only finding of significance was the atypical ventricular source of the overwhelming majority of her heartbeats. There were no other obvious abnormalities or evidence of immediate concern. Brittany consistently excused herself from the exam room as I discussed the details and implications of the testing results with her mother.

I summarized by saying, "Let's continue to monitor Brittany closely, but I am not going to advise any medications or activity limitations at this time. She should go about her days in an age-appropriate normal fashion." Her mother was relieved but hesitant.

I followed Brittany as an outpatient, and she continued to be remarkably well over the next few weeks. I also collaborated in her care with two of my regularly visiting colleagues from Montefiore who specialized in children's abnormal heart rhythms—a field known as electrophysiology. The presence of these electrophysiologists was immensely helpful and fortunate for Brittany's case in particular. Just a few months prior, she would have been required to repeatedly travel down to the Bronx to see these specialists. This was particularly advantageous for Brittany given her apprehension, which would only have been heightened if she were to travel more frequently the greater distance to the big medical center. Each time she came into the office, she remained reticent about being involved in the detailed discussions regarding her heart. I soon learned to nonverbally indicate to her with a nod that she was free to leave the exam room so that her mother and I could talk.

She remained remarkably healthy and stable. Our regular visit routine lulled us all into a sense of optimism that she might remain well and that perhaps the extra beats were benign or would resolve spontaneously. Then reality entered abruptly. One day, Brittany began complaining of palpitations and dizziness while she sat in her classroom or tried to participate in gym class. With the onset of symptoms, our sense of security shattered. My colleagues and I knew we now had to reduce the abnormal heartbeats. It was time to start her on medications. My electrophysiology colleagues became even more active in her care. I also requested an evaluation of Brittany by some of my other colleagues who specialized in treating a group of childhood heart muscle diseases known as cardiomyopathy. Everyone was suspicious that there was truly some ominous heart muscle disease underlying her heart rhythm and symptoms.

The medication helped a little at first, though her abnormal heart rhythm continued to be the main source of her heartbeats. Then, the dizziness worsened, and she almost passed out at home. I was resigned to the fact that she needed to be hospitalized. I sent her to the Children's Hospital at Montefiore. This would be the first of her repeat trips to the Bronx. At least she was now familiar with the many faces of the doctors at this hospital because she had met them in our office. She underwent a full battery of tests, including a cardiac catheterization. She was so brave as the doctors passed a long, thin, hollow plastic tube—the catheter—up through the large blood vessels in her limbs directly into her heart. They diligently measured the pressures in all four heart chambers as well as all the vessels entering and leaving her heart. They also specifically located the source of the abnormal heartbeats. The results were devastating.

Her heart muscle was starting to become weak. The quandary was to determine which came first—the chicken or the egg. Was the persistent, abnormal, fast, ventricular heart rhythm causing the heart muscle to weaken, or was there a primary abnormality of the muscle—a cardiomyopathy—giving rise to these abnormal heartbeats? Brittany was discharged to go home with full exercise activity restrictions. She could no longer participate in gym, sports, or any other activity that could elevate her heart rate further. My colleagues gathered in the conference room to review her case. It was a somber discussion. Heart transplantation, we determined, was most likely the best and only therapeutic option she had. She was not sick enough for this step yet, but the timing of this transplant would prove critical.

Brittany's life changed dramatically. She was terrified. Her baseline cautiousness progressed to full-blown anxiety. Her mother was also distraught. I did my best to be supportive and encouraging, but I too was on constant guard when we spoke. I did not want them to give up hope, but I also could not paint an unrealistically rosy picture of her grave situation.

On Christmas Eve 2010, just shy of two months since I first met her, I received the call from her mother that I had been dreading. Hanging out at home with her family for the holiday, Brittany suddenly collapsed with full loss of consciousness 15 minutes before. She had recovered spontaneously.

"She's just resting on the couch with her cousins," her mother explained.

I felt a wave of shuddering flow through my body. I could hear the change in my voice as I went into full doctor control mode. "Call an ambulance, now, to take her to the local emergency room. Immediately. I'll call ahead and meet you guys there."

Though the mother sounded scared, she replied, "I would rather keep a close eye on her at home because it's Christmas, and all her family is here."

I patiently stressed my concerns. "The fact that she fainted with her heart so weak makes it dangerous to be away from medical care if she has another episode. She may not wake up by herself if this happens."

She tried to reassure me. "I think she will be fine. I promise to call if anything happens." We hung up.

For the next two hours, I called back to check on her several times. Just as the midnight hour approached and Christmas began, her mother called me back frantically. "Brittany passed out again, and she is lying unconscious on the couch. I cannot wake her!" She screamed and cried.

"It's OK. You need to calm down and start CPR right now. You know what to do." I tried to reassure her. "I'm hanging up now to call an ambulance. Keep doing CPR until they get there." I contacted the emergency ambulance services. I instructed the driver to take her immediately to the local emergency room. I urged them not to delay in any way and reassured them that I would call ahead to the ER team and meet them there.

I arrived just as they wheeled her stretcher from the ambulance and entered the sliding doors to the ER. We took her into a trauma bay room, and I took over to continue the full CPR arrest routine. I don't remember specifically when and how I took over chest compressions and ordered several rounds of adrenaline. As in my residency days, my training came back almost instinctively while we proceeded with this full arrest code. At one point, I inadvertently looked through the curtain and caught a glimpse of her frantic mother out in the hallway. We met eye to eye for no more than two seconds, but that moment of communication would be burned lifelong into our memories.

I remembered Kristen, whose happy voice now urged me to persist. The minutes felt like hours. Finally, the pattern on the monitor screen literally jumped to life. We were able to regain a steadier heartbeat and a low but stable blood pressure.

But Brittany had still not awoken. She remained unarousable. I was very concerned that Brittany sustained a serious lack of blood supply to her brain and vital organs. I was worried that I may have overdone it. What if I had been so aggressive in trying to save her life, only for her to end up neurologically devastated? I contacted my colleagues at Montefiore where she had been admitted and evaluated after her first fainting episode several months before. They arranged for Brittany to be directly admitted to the intensive care unit upon arrival. Her mother was almost catatonic as she boarded the ambulance to accompany her unconscious daughter on the ride to the city with our local ambulance crew.

On Christmas morning, my electrophysiology colleague, who had been collaborating in her care all along, sent me a text that I will never forget. "I am so sorry about Brittany. I know that you were dreading that this situation would arise before she could receive a heart transplant. She remains unconscious in the ICU, and her situation does not look good. I will keep you updated. You gave it your best. Again, so sorry, man."

That Christmas morning, I was exhausted. I hugged my two boys tighter than ever as we exchanged gifts, and I tried to remain outwardly cheerful. My wife sensed my mood and made the whole morning much easier as she directed the opening of presents. I was grief-stricken for Brittany's mother. I knew that she blamed herself, and I did not want any of this nightmare to happen to her. I also kicked myself that I had not been more insistent about calling the ambulance after her first fainting episode. With Christmas came hope as I prayed for a miracle.

"We have already lost Kristen. Please do not let me lose Brittany too."

TEMPTED OVER AND OVER

As we focused our efforts on the expanded care model through our facility, within weeks of opening, we attracted the attention of a newly arrived hospital administrator, Sam Batson. He was recruited to lead the next phase of the merger between the two local west-side hospitals—formerly part of the four-hospital alliance which made up the GHVHS—as they broke ground on the new hospital just one mile down the road from my office. Through his research into the local dynamics, my community colleagues told him about my initial efforts several years prior to expand the area's pediatric services. He now formally invited me to meet with him to discuss my vision of the future of local pediatric care.

I experienced an intense sense of *déjà vu* when we first met. His temporary office was the now worn-out and dated room in the administrative wing of Horton Hospital where the first CEO, Jeff Hinds, greeted me my first day on the job. To my further surprise, in the little room connecting to Mr. Batson's office, my first desk and black two-door file cabinet were still in the same place I left them over 12 years earlier.

A tall, ex-football-player-looking, handsome, middle-aged man with slicked-back brown hair waved me into the room as he stood up from behind a well-used desk. As he pulled up a chair next to me, he wasted no time in getting to the point. "I am sincerely concerned about the existing arrangements that continue to promote the significant transfer of children and babies away from the local community," he said sternly. It became imminently clear that these transfers were particularly frustrating to him because the majority of them were directed to the same tertiary medical center, which was now aligned with his rival east-side hospitals.

He had my full attention. He spoke my language and harkened back to the local vision of the original four-hospital system that supported my recruitment to the area in the first place. He had me hook, line, and sinker by the heartstrings, and I felt convinced that he really cared about the health services for our community's children. In retrospect, I should have picked up on the subtle inconsistencies that made his sincerity questionable.

Unlike the unified approach that characterized the original philosophy of the four-hospital GHVHS in 1998, Mr. Batson now rejuvenated a strong east-versus-west competitiveness that had ultimately strained and broken up the original GHVHS. Palpably concerning to him was the fact that the Westchester-based pediatric tertiary medical center's full support of our county's successful, east-side, decade-old NICU at St. Luke's Hospital—still operating under the steady clinical hand of Dr. Kay—relegated Mr. Batson's west-side NICU at Horton to relative obscurity. I should have seen that he wanted more than equal recognition and support. He sought market share dominance over the hospital where I first met the pregnant Tanya. It did not help matters for him that both hospitals' NICUs were officially affiliated with the same tertiary Westchester-based institution.

Mr. Batson looked directly at me as he leaned forward in his chair. "I do not appreciate or agree with the current arrangement. The tertiary center both hospitals are partnered with has too much control over the local referral patterns for our county's newborn infants. We need to change this situation and secure more control of where and when these babies go or stay." He paused and then finally declared the main reason that he wanted to meet with me. "I understand that you once laid out a plan to control this outmigration of our community's infants and children. I would now like you to provide me with a written proposal outlining how we can take up this effort once again before our new hospital is built. You have my full support."

I was simultaneously excited and reluctant about his plan. Not wanting to seem ungrateful, I calmly responded, "I appreciate the opportunity to meet with you and share my ideas for a community-based neonatal service. However, I am hesitant to get too deeply involved once again because of my past discouraging experiences with the original GHVHS. My practice now calls for my full attention. I am also concerned that there remains an apparent lack of support by key players for a long-term vision of local healthcare for our children. You know, I have barely removed the last of the arrows from my back after the last go-round in this venture."

He sat back and chuckled.

I finished by emphasizing my main concern, instinctively attempting to address the counterproductive divisiveness I sensed. "I remain convinced that only a true and honest collaboration between all the west-side and east-side hospitals will ensure the success of any pediatric program in the area."

"I couldn't agree with you more," he countered. "I'll back you up." He emphasized that the current monopoly status of the pediatric tertiary center was the only true foil to creating a locally controlled program, and he would back an alliance with the east side to create a solid, community-based pediatric healthcare presence.

Over the next several weeks, I therefore found myself at the drawing board again—this time somewhat wiser than before. I returned to the task of outlining my comprehensive and collaboration-centered vision of regional pediatric healthcare for Mr. Batson. I tried to stay detached and analytical. I didn't want to be overly optimistic again about the potential opportunities for the local children.

"Be realistic, Eric," I told my reflection in the mirror as I shaved, repeating the admonishment while I buckled my seatbelt and again when I sat down at the computer to work. "Change is hard for people to accept. Too many people have their own agendas. Never forget—money talks. Children always take a second seat to more lucrative and less risky adult medical needs. This might not work."

While I worked on this proposal late one evening, several of my trusted local colleagues who knew about my meeting with Mr. Batson sent me text messages that revealed his true intentions. The news wasn't good. To my extreme dismay, while I was finalizing the last components of the task he had set for me—an east-west healthcare partnership focused on children—he was simultaneously leveraging the eventual realization of my proposal as a negotiation tool in public discussions with the very same tertiary center that he so passionately purported to me to be his only true tactical competitor.

My local colleagues reported to me that, at a recent regular hospital pediatric meeting, he officially announced that he intended to create his own local NICU to compete with the St. Luke's Hospital NICU. He had no intention of collaborating with them. He made sure to direct his remarks to representatives of the tertiary medical center who were in attendance at this meeting. He stated publicly that he was willing to pursue the creation of his own independent NICU unless they agreed to transfer the bulk of their efforts from their original NICU at St. Luke's Hospital to his new NICU in the hospital being built. Otherwise, he would no longer ensure his hospital's affiliation with them and enter into a period of open rivalry between them and the St. Luke's NICU they supported.

I fell for it. I thought he talked to me honestly, while he was playing medical politics. His goal was to maximize profits, at whatever cost. During a follow-up group phone conversation, I respectfully thanked my medical colleagues who had called me to fully explain all this. They sensed how discouraged I was as I hung up. I started to feel like there were no administrators who actually cared about clinically sound best practices. Stakeholders, sure. Maximum number of patients, yes. But the quality of care provided to those patients? The ease of local access to the best practitioners? A feeling of security in the midst of the chaos of cardiac or other serious health problems? In their minds, what was truly best for the children was beside the point and secondary to the economic bottom line.

He was by no means bluffing. He knew that he had the upper hand because his west-side community patient population was more socioeconomically sound than the poorer east-side counterpart, which was dependent upon state-based Medicaid and Medicare. I laced up my running shoes, my mind racing as it hit me hard. My role in this process was simply to be used as a pawn in these negotiations with the tertiary center. He was never truly interested in running his own independent NICU locally.

As I huffed and puffed up the steepest hill in my neighborhood—a sort of self-flagellation for having been so gullible and stupid—I chastised myself. "How could you have been so naïve and duped this easily?" Mr. Batson now openly made it known that he would continue to outsource the operations of this new NICU facility to any tertiary center that met his demands and allowed him to maintain the competitive superiority over his east-side rivals. He was just gloating as he dangled the right of first refusal to the current tertiary-center partner. If they didn't grab the offer, others would in a heartbeat.

The Westchester-based tertiary pediatric center thus found themselves back in the tenuous position analogous to the time when they fought to obtain control of the St. Luke's NICU from Columbia years before. They were confident that St. Luke's Hospital was exclusively beholden to them and not in any position to enter into negotiations with another center at that time. However, they also feared potential regional competition from any of the other New York City tertiary pediatric centers that might grab at the chance to regain some referrals from the Greater Hudson Valley. Mr. Batson also maintained the potential to establish the locally based care model that I proposed. The Westchester program was in no position to turn down his offer. Mr. Batson had them in check. They thus made the only move left on the board. They diverted resources away from the St. Luke's community toward Mr. Batson's two west-side hospitals.

Dr. Kay and I felt betrayed. We talked ourselves down from our heightened emotions over several phone and in-person conversations. We had worked well together from the first day that Norm introduced us to each other. I vowed never to stick out my neck for any hospital administrations in the future. I would not risk getting my hopes dashed down ever again. Despite all the frustrations, from deep down in my psyche emerged a silver lining.

Working on the pediatric proposal had stimulated a new sense of my capabilities. After years of experience, I realized that I was no longer the new kid on the block. This whole event awakened my intrinsic constructive nature and commitment to my local community. I wanted to build something lasting for the children. My value system also became more solidified. I had become a doctor committed to honesty, integrity, constructive alliances, and kindness. I would seek out others who shared this perspective. My initial emotional response to withdraw back into the comfort zone of my practice would not last for long.

Brittany had barely survived a cardiac arrest on Christmas Eve. Now she lay unconscious in the pediatric intensive care unit of the Children's Hospital at Montefiore. I felt a bizarre combination of sadness and anger while I waited for her to show some signs of either improvement or deterioration. I tried to contact her mother, but she now maintained an understandably thick emotional wall between us. As the first snowfalls of New Year 2011 announced the start of a bitter winter, there was silence. I never met or heard from Brittany's father, and her mother never returned my calls. The sense of guilt she wore was evident in every interaction with the hospital team at Montefiore.

"She looks so scared and lonely. She always looks down and never looks anyone directly in the eyes when she talks. She is pale and barely eats," explained one of her more seasoned nurses during my daily phone calls.

On a later call, my colleague, Dr. Daphne Hsu, the Director of the Pediatric Heart Program, continued. "We are all very worried about what Mom might do if Brittany does not survive. I think we should call in psychiatry or the clergy. Maybe both?"

In a glass-enclosed isolation room, Brittany lay motionless on the intensive care bed, just barely covered by one thin, white sheet. Clear plastic tubes and wires came out of all parts of her body. Breathing tubes were taped to her mouth and attached to a consistently cycling respirator machine. Large-bore hoses filled with blood exited and entered her neck and groin vessels as they passed through a constantly turning bypass machine to temporarily replace her heart and let it rest. Everywhere and 24-7 around the clock, there were lights and beeps from the monitors and these machines. Her mother was a silent fixture sitting forward at her bedside, elbows on her knees, chin resting on her hands, as she kept vigil for any sign of hope. On the third day of this life support, Brittany showed the slightest evidence of improvement. By the fifth day, the intensive care team was able to wean back off the supporting medications, and she started to wake up.

My colleague, who initially expressed his condolences, called me with some degree of enthusiasm in his voice: "She's doing well enough that we can now officially list her as a legitimate candidate for a heart transplant." Within six months, just days before her 14th birthday, a donor heart was identified. Two weeks later, Brittany walked out the door of the hospital on her own, her mother at her side and a new heart in her chest.

Once again, I was amazed by the resilience of children. I was also sadly reminded that Kristen never got the chance to receive a new heart. Brittany fortunately made it to Montefiore, where Dr. Hsu brought her Columbia-based transplant skills and some team members from my training class who had all been taught by a great pioneer, Dr. Linda Addonizio. The first successful heart transplant for a child was conducted at Columbia in 1984 under the guidance of Dr. Addonizio and adult heart surgeon Dr. Eric Rose. The recipient was a four-year-old child, James Lovette, who had been born in Colorado with a severe heart defect in which he was completely missing one of two bottom pumping chambers. James went on to become a young adult and died suddenly in his sleep during his first week of medical school. Brittany was just one of the many beneficiaries of his legacy.

Over the next several years, Brittany's mom drove her to Montefiore to receive ongoing heart transplant therapy. The antirejection treatments that made organ transplantation possible had come a long way since they were first administered to children like James at leading centers like Columbia. I crossed paths with Brittany and her mother in the clinic or hospital lobby just three or four times over the next five years. Brittany waved to me excitedly. She told me she was doing well and back in school again. Though all of my prior heart transplant patients returned to receive care in my local office within one or two years after transplantation, Brittany's mother chose to continue commuting to the city. Each time we met, I gave Brittany a bear hug and the reassurance that I remained available if they ever needed local services. Her mother remained reserved.

When a road is blocked, you take a different path. Though the door to an expanded, locally controlled NICU service was closed, I still found myself feeling optimistic and open to the endless possibilities for enriching our community's pediatric services in the new hospital. On a brisk fall evening in 2011, the smell of fallen leaves in the air, the entire medical staff gathered impatiently in the large event room of the historic racetrack situated just across the street from the county's government center. This particular quarterly medical staff meeting had piqued everyone's interest because, for the first time, the administration planned to roll out the full details of the new hospital's proposed layout—floor by floor.

As the two-hour demonstration wrapped up and the discussion was opened to the audience's feedback and questions, the two dozen pediatricians in attendance collectively became visually enraged. One of the most vocal amongst them, a middle-aged, energetic woman with a clear voice, bellowed, "Are you guys kidding? Why is there no dedicated space for a children's ward?"

The medical director, Norm Samuels, timidly replied, "At this point, there are no actual plans to include a pediatric facility within the new building. Just like our current two smaller hospitals, we have decided to continue with the longstanding model of a mixed ward with children placed on the adult and surgical wards on an 'as-needed' basis. There will be no purely child-dedicated space in the new hospital."

With this final remark from the administration, the pediatricians stood up together and stormed out of the room. "You never really cared about the kids because they don't make money for the hospital," shouted an elderly, white-bearded gentleman, face red and fist raised up in anger, as he trailed his pediatric colleagues filing out the double doors into the cool night.

For the next few months, all my interactions with the community pediatricians found them grumbling amongst themselves about the unacceptable lack of attention to children's services by the administration. For my part, ever since the meeting, I felt strangely energized. I sensed that it was high time to turn the complaints and frustrations of the pediatricians and family practitioners into a concrete plan. I decided to push the limits by proposing a completely opposite scenario to the administration's half-hearted plans—a comprehensive hospital-based pediatric program.

For three weeks, I sat in the evenings at my home kitchen table drafting a detailed model of a pediatric service in the new hospital from inception through three phases of development over the first five years. The hook was the financial upside. I knew that the potential for making money would capture the interest of the administration. Years before many in the administration had even come to the region, as a child growing up in this community, I was aware that our local hospitals could only offer the most basic treatments for children. I argued that we were sending too many pediatric patients away to other hospitals over the past several decades. Two-thirds of these transfers were directed to the urban tertiary pediatric centers. The remaining third of our local babies and children were being cared for in other regional hospitals. I described this pattern as extremely illogical and costly. These other regional hospitals had the same or fewer pediatric services than those of our current two older facilities, which were slated to be absorbed under one roof in the new hospital.

I overlooked my personal sentiments. When I contacted Mr. Batson, I acted as if there had been no past issues. I wanted to give him an earful, but I bit my tongue hard enough to hurt. For his part, I couldn't even tell if he knew that I had found him out. Until now, we had never spoken to each other after our first meeting. It was as if this was our first encounter.

"Hello, Mr. Batson. This is Dr. Fethke. I would like to meet to discuss a proposal for a pediatric service in the new hospital that I believe will interest you in terms of potential hospital revenue. Since the new building is opening soon, I believe that time is of the essence."

"Sounds good," he pleasantly replied. "I will ask my business team members to join us as well."

I decided to present my current proposal without rehashing the past. I would simply propose pediatrics as a new and separate venture. To my pleasant surprise, after my 45-minute presentation, he agreed to move forward with my proposed pediatric program if, in his own words, I could "demonstrate a significant financial benefit to the new hospital."

The ability to create a crack in the façade of Mr. Batson and his administrative team was a calculated move on my part. During a recent meeting, Dr. Samuels earnestly addressed the staff. "The bank is asking for a very large down payment in the millions before we can receive a building loan and break ground on the new medical center. If anyone has contacts for donors, please inform our fundraising team. Ideally, we would love a generous donation from one or two sources to nail the deal." I then knew that they would be open to any potential new sources of business they called "product lines." This was our opportunity to get something more than the "mixed-ward" facility outlined in the fall meeting. Any potential revenue stream was open to exploration. Mr. Batson therefore put me directly in touch with the chief financial officer and the team responsible for all future hospital business ventures. I was given full access to the past three years of regional data pertaining to children and infants from our community who had been cared for in hospitals locally or elsewhere.

For the next three weeks, I barely slept. After my family went to bed, I spread out the many spreadsheets of regional pediatric patient data across my home office desk, the kitchen table, and my living room floor. I stayed up until two or three in the morning after busy days at the office combing through the data. I created tables on my computer to define three categories. The first comprised children who could have stayed in our community hospitals even before the new hospital. The second entailed those who could stay if the new hospital had just a few more services than currently existed, and the third were those who would always have to be transferred to city medical centers. After several weeks of review of my tables, the hospital business team agreed that my pediatric hospital-based proposal would keep a significantly greater number of children in the new hospital than in the past. They concurred that a dedicated hospital pediatric service would generate a significant new revenue stream that had been relegated elsewhere in the past. For me, it was about the patients. For the administration, it was about the money.

The administration gave their approval to proceed with the development and implementation of the pediatric program as long as we had the full backing of the pediatricians. To my relief, as the administration presented a brief outline of our now mutual vision at the next Pediatrics Department meeting, the pediatricians almost unanimously supported the proposal.

To my embarrassment, several of my colleagues stood up and, glancing over at me, spontaneously emphasized, "We are in favor of such a sweeping proposal because it is about time that the children get some attention around here. Though historically we do not have reason to trust the hospital's intentions, we will support this idea mainly because Dr. Fethke is involved and has earned our trust and commitment over the years."

This was the icing on the cake that we needed. I could never have intentionally coordinated a better response. The administration thus blessed the community's first hospital-based pediatric service with their full support, to include creating an official medical directorship position for me at the center. Though I felt relieved and excited, I also could not help but recognize the irony of the situation. Now in the spring of 2012, I found myself full circle in the original local hospital administrative position that I was initially recruited to fulfill through the alliance with NYPH-Columbia-Cornell when I first moved to the area.

Because of all the changes in the healthcare landscape, it had taken 14 years to get here, but I was now as committed as ever to building a lasting mother-and-child-based healthcare service locally. In retrospect, when it came to my understanding of the scope and details of such a complex venture, I was now obviously more prepared to do so than when I first arrived wet behind the ears. It was now time to dig in and build a team.

At this stage of my career, I was therefore not surprised to learn that, once again, several other entities were threatened by our endeavor to build a local pediatric program at the new hospital. Two entities in particular—the large Westchester-based tertiary pediatric center that had been awarded the new NICU service and the largest physician mega-group in the region—suddenly began aggressively vying to be a part of this new pediatric service. Though they never stepped forward to actively promote such a local hospital resource in the past, they were all too eager to participate.

This time, I was ready in advance. I expected the pushback and preemptively advised the hospital administration not to repeat past patterns and give into the pressures of these entities. At our first official organization meeting, the acting pediatric chairperson, the director of nursing, the hospital medical director, and I sat at a 25-foot mahogany conference table. I emphasized the point. "The very fact that these two formerly silent entities—and, I anticipate, soon several others—are now so interested in joining us means that we are indeed onto something very relevant and unique. I encourage us as a hospital team to maintain complete control of the destiny of this pediatric service and to not cave into the past tendencies to delegate this service to any other entities. Any efforts to outsource our responsibilities will be seen by the community as the hospital placing a lower priority on pediatrics, compared to other service lines." They agreed implicitly and were very supportive. However, I was consciously skeptical that this had been too easy.

It did not take long for watchful eyes to come out of the woodwork. The tertiary pediatric center that now ran both the west-side and east-side NICUs of the county was the first to approach us. They indicated that they were prepared to also staff our new hospital with their own hospital-based pediatricians, known as "hospitalists." These pediatric hospitalist positions—in 2012, quite commonplace in large academic tertiary medical centers—were a vital component of my program proposal, but the concept was fairly new to pediatric services in community hospitals. Almost simultaneously, the largest multidisciplinary private practice in the area, already supplying the existing local hospitals with adult hospitalists, also argued that they were the best entity to staff our new pediatric hospitalist service. We found ourselves in the enviable position of having too much to choose from—a virtual bidding war.

The hospital leadership decided to formally hear all proposals and then review the candidates thoroughly before we made our decision. I provocatively threw in a third party for consideration by suggesting that the new hospital itself should create their own pediatric hospitalist service. Unfortunately, against my better judgement, at the time, the administration was still uncertain about the future of this pediatric venture and found it more practical to outsource this hospitalist service.

To be thorough and all-encompassing, we also invited three other outside entities—private physician recruitment companies, also known as headhunters—to make their pitches for providing us with their pediatric hospitalist services. In the end, after two months of meetings and our review, it came down to the two original entities: the tertiary pediatric center and the large medical practice. Just as we were about to announce the candidate we chose, the administration received a surprising phone call.

The Westchester pediatric tertiary medical center indicated that they were officially pulling out of the process and would fully support the candidacy of the local mega-group practice. The decision had been made for us. We all admitted that we were taken by surprise with this response by the tertiary center and wished we were flies on the wall to whatever conversation occurred between these two entities that so quickly turned admitted adversaries into allies.

Thus began the official "building" phase of our new pediatric service just as the brick and mortar of the new hospital was drying. I began by establishing a neutral forum in the hospital for clinicians, administrators, and technicians to meet monthly with a focus on developing the new service. I was fully conscious that this would combine members of multiple disparate and competitive entities, including doctors from the Westchester tertiary pediatric center and the large local practice. By declaring this process as nonpartisan, I hoped to utilize the combined resources of all involved and lessen the historical tendency for everyone to constantly claim their own piece of the action. My message was clear without having to openly shove it down their throats. If you wanted a portion of the meal, then you had to sit at our local table and put your hunting tools down before you came into the room. We would now be hunting together.

I also juggled the responsibilities of seeing patients, running my own growing private practice, teaching, and being a landlord with the added directorship of the hospital-based pediatric program. Though the hours were long, all of my efforts seemed to be wonderfully symbiotic. Everything was interwoven and made cohesive sense. My work and discussions in outpatient care seamlessly led to enriching my views and decisions about the local inpatient care. My clinical work finally felt complete and less beholden to the outside urban medical centers.

My collaborative approach worked. We opened the area's first children's emergency room and added several facilities dedicated to the cardiac monitoring of children. We brought in pediatric urologists and expanded general surgery in conjunction with pediatric anesthesia so that basic operations like hernias and appendectomies could be performed. We revitalized and increased pediatric gastroenterology and neurology services. All of this required a pediatric-dedicated infrastructure and constant training of the nursing and any ancillary staff. The general mood of my staff was contagiously constructive.

Within two years, we established the region's premier level 2 pediatric hospital program. We had not done any formal marketing, but the word of mouth was spreading all the same. The patients told their friends and neighbors that they did not have to leave the community to receive good pediatric care. Doctors from surrounding counties called me to ask if they could send their patients to us instead of to the city. The administration brought in consultants to give us feedback and advice. These consultants consistently gave us the same rave reviews—by breaking new ground, we were doing better than most. They reassured us that there were no comparable community-based programs with our complement of services and resources.

Over the next year, between 2013 to 2014, the weekly mileage on my car increased significantly. I was once again reminded that, dating back to my high school and college days, I was most happy when my schedule was packed. I settled into a busy but satisfying routine that balanced my time between my private practice, seeing patients at four different local hospitals, my directorship at the new local medical center, and my work at Montefiore. One evening, after hours of sitting in the dark reading room reviewing and reporting on echocardiogram studies at Montefiore, I asked Dr. Hsu if I could meet with her before I left for the day.

"Sure, come on down. I will be in my office and leave the door open," she warmly replied.

As we sat down across from each other at the small conference table in her office, I began, "It's hard to realize, but are you aware that today makes five years since I came to Montefiore? Time has gone by so quickly."

She responded thoughtfully, "A testament to a great working relationship, wouldn't you agree?"

I nodded and continued deliberately. "I think it's time to consider the merger between my practice and Montefiore that we broached during our initial negotiations together. I truly appreciated your holding off the other administrators from gobbling me up at the time, even before we signed our original working agreement. As I hoped, our alliance to date has been truly satisfying. I now would be open to the possibility of taking the relationship to the next level."

She paused to take my words in. "Are you actually considering giving up some control and merging your private practice with Montefiore?"

I looked back at her with a silent determination that came from knowing someone for many years. "Yes, if the arrangement would allow me to spend more time with my patients." She agreed to take the matter to the higher-ups within a week.

As I looked around my community at the end of 2013, I realized that almost every one of the local pediatric practices in my area had merged with a larger entity, whether it was a big multi-specialty physician group, an academic center, or a corporate enterprise. I was the proverbial "last man standing." I also was now spending an exorbitant amount of time running the business of my practice.

Whenever my closest colleagues inquired how I even managed to balance the hours between my management and clinical duties, I explained matter-of-factly, "In the first five years after I freed myself from Columbia, my time was divided up with 80 percent clinical and 20 percent administrative responsibilities. Over the next 10 years, this became 50 percent clinical and 50 percent administrative work, and now I am up to 80 percent clinical and 80 percent administrative efforts."

I devoted a minimum of 10 hours per day, 80 to 90 hours per week, and several weekends a month to the practice. Given the circumstances, the option to possibly hand off some of my administrative responsibilities to Montefiore seemed like a "no-brainer." When, just five days after our meeting, Dr. Hsu came back with a green light to proceed, I entered into formal negotiations with Montefiore.

Initially, these discussions went smoothly and constructively. However, after several months, they slowed to a snail's pace. I soon learned that this was because history once again repeated itself. New administrative players arrived at Montefiore as part of an institution-wide goal of advancing the center's regional economic prowess by accessing the initiatives of the fledgling Affordable Care Act (aka Obamacare) of 2010. For the next decade after Columbia and Cornell aligned, several of the other tertiary medical centers in the city area, including Montefiore, followed suit to enhance their competitive edge in a very stressful economic environment by merging with another large center or absorbing multiple smaller medical centers.

By 2012, these combined entities, with their extensive multidisciplinary workforces and technologies, were now more prepared than their smaller counterparts to incorporate many of the often complex healthcare reforms of the ACA. These reforms encouraged the establishment of healthcare networks with smaller hospitals and regional medical practices under the administration of the larger parent entities. These networks created even more economic and efficiency advantages for the large medical entities, thus improving their "bottom line." Most importantly, the regulatory capacity of these networks had the potential to create more consistent and improved clinical standards, thus raising the quality of regional healthcare.

This focus on quality outcomes by the federal and state governments led them to create a new designation for these large networks—Accountable Care Organizations (ACOs). Any large medical entity that could meet the government's requirements and standards upon completion of a rigorous application process could become an ACO. The incentive of this ACO carrot dangled before these networks was the potential for significant financial rewards if they could demonstrate, as per the government's criteria, that their network had become more efficient and improved their patients' care across broader geographic regions. Montefiore's new administrative team was all business and intent on dominating the healthcare marketplace by becoming an ACO.

As I came to expect at most medical institutions, children's services took a backseat to those of adults because adult care generated more money. Montefiore's financial incentives for achieving ACO status were thus preferentially directed to adult medicine, not pediatrics. This attitude and preferential attention to adult versus pediatric services made my already dragged-out negotiations a low priority for Montefiore. Every time we interacted, the administration brought up more and more details, indicating clearly that they were no longer fully interested in the venture.

Then, over one year into my negotiations, the process took a toll on me. I experienced painful flashbacks to 15 years prior with my original tertiary partner, the NYPH. I started regretting the time and effort that I spent in these negotiations with Montefiore and, most notably, the fact that it distracted me from patient care. The whole process became emotionally and economically unbearable.

While I was still in the midst of negotiations with Montefiore in 2014, Dr. Hsu invited me and several of my academic pediatric cardiology colleagues to an elaborate fundraising event for Montefiore Children's Hospital at the grand Waldorf Astoria Hotel in Manhattan. The evening's fundraising campaign was centered on the pediatric heart transplant program established at Montefiore by Dr. Hsu's team. Everywhere I looked, immaculately coiffed women wore real diamond necklaces in dazzling, low-cut, sequined dresses. Men in impeccable black tuxedos, sparkling cocktails in hand, peered down from the two floors of balconies encircling the packed 10,000-square-foot ballroom floor. All the Who's Who of New York's famous, wealthy, and charitable people were there to see and be seen. The place buzzed with conversation like a giant beehive filled to the full 1,500-person capacity, soft music barely audible in the background.

After the cocktail reception, while standing near the back of the ballroom, something familiar caught my eye. I glanced upward to the front stage, my head cocked back to take in the full view. I was confused at first, but then I understood. Projected on a large screen above the center stage was a photo of Brittany. I didn't know until that instant that she was the star of the night, her personal story the center of the fundraising campaign.

Moments later, within the elbow-to-elbow crowd, Brittany and I miraculously bumped into each other right as she and her mother were speaking to the hospital's president, Dr. Philip Ozuah. I gave her an embrace, trying not to ruffle her beautiful off-white gown. She leaned into my right ear to be heard over the background noise and explained that she was now a senior in high school and would be attending a prestigious university in the coming fall. Her mother and Dr. Ozuah came over to join us for a moment. She nervously exchanged some brief, nonspecific pleasantries with me, grabbed my arm in a warm hug, and then made her way into the crowd. I did not see her the rest of the night. Brittany, on the other hand, soon made her way up to the back balcony and with some friends had the spotlight aimed on her throughout dinner and the main presentation.

As Brittany's remarkable story unfolded on the video presentation, I relived her life-threatening arrest almost four years earlier at the end of 2010. Quietly, I became outwardly quite emotional. Though not specifically mentioned, her very survival represented the important role that my local practice had played toward the success of the Pediatric Center's outreach network and their advancing medical care abilities. My cardiology colleagues at our table knew that my practice was an intrinsic part of the growth of the Pediatric Cardiology program showcased by the Children's Hospital that evening.

On the other hand, despite the tacitly acknowledged important contributions of my practice to this program, standing up to applaud Brittany and Dr. Hsu's team, I could not silence all the nagging thoughts and feelings in my head. Why was I still struggling to complete my negotiations with the very same hospital leadership who now basked in the limelight of this fundraising event featuring my patient Brittany and taking full credit for saving her life? I was deeply conflicted. I was very proud of Brittany and the role my practice played in her life story.

Later that night, as I once again drove back home northward up the Palisades Parkway, I started to feel angry. A gnawing sense of the administration's lack of integrity crept into my subconscious. This was the proverbial "straw that broke the camel's back." By the next day, the fully conscious realization that I could no longer be a part of this hypocrisy and relive the history of my prior tertiary-center experience at Columbia was at the forefront of my convictions. I knew that Dr.

Hsu earnestly tried to facilitate and support my merger under the new administration, but to no avail. Within a week, almost two years after beginning formal discussions and seven years since I joined Dr. Hsu's team, in April 2016, I officially called off the negotiations with Montefiore. I planned, yet again, to redirect my full efforts to the directorship of my local hospital's pediatric program and my private practice. I tried to convince myself that I was done with academic tertiary medical centers. I knew better than to lie to myself. The honest truth would soon come out and tell another story.

News traveled fast. Over the next four months, after cutting official ties with Montefiore, I was once again a free agent. Several large practices and tertiary centers reached out to invite me to join them. I politely turned down their gracious offers. As I returned my undivided attention to my local patients, I initially felt a wave of fresh air. I was relieved to be free of the constant dealings with disingenuous administrators, institutional politics, and endless negotiations. My routine soon led me to be the last one still working many late evenings in the office. After patient hours, I switched my stethoscope for a checkbook to pay the operating expenses or some overalls to change the light bulbs and fix the plumbing. On weekends, I kept up with my financial spreadsheets to balance my bank accounts and prepare for taxes. As I watched my sons pass through their college years, I longed to recover some personal time with them. I again weighed the risk benefits of losing my autonomy over the practice with the potential to unload a significant portion of the financial and practice management burden to a larger and more secure entity. The highest priority remained the need to maintain control of the quality of my patient care. Was there any institution that could meet my needs?

Just as I was in the midst of reestablishing my personal and professional goals, an online social media article caught my attention. My only true competitor from the Westchester tertiary center had apparently just pulled off a major merger with the country's premier pediatric medical center, the Boston Children's Hospital of Harvard. They cleverly managed to cross state boundaries from New York into Massachusetts to establish a combined entity they named the Boston Children's Health Physicians (BCHP).

By focusing on the needs of the pediatric population of a region rather than state lines, together these institutions laid the foundation for a new frontier in organized healthcare that was consistent with the objectives of healthcare reform. This merger was also very relevant to me because Dr. Gersony had been trained at Boston Children's Hospital. In the late 1960s, he incorporated the philosophies and standards from this iconic Boston institution into my own alma mater's pediatric cardiology program. With this in mind, I felt strongly that my career could potentially, academically, come full circle in a very holistic fashion and be more secure in the future by anchoring my small boat to this iconic huge ship. I was admittedly weary of the constant competition with the Westchester group and open to the potential for us to finally align our commitments to the children of the region. I also could not ignore the potential benefits to my practice and the local hospital's pediatric program.

Still somewhat cautious, I first reached out to the acting director of the Boston Children's Pediatric Cardiology Division, Dr. James Lock. He readily recognized our common historical traditions through Dr. Gersony's legacy and was very supportive and receptive to the possibility of my joining the BCHP group in New York. He calmly explained, "Eric, your presence in the Hudson Valley for all these years has been an important asset to the regional pediatric cardiology care. We at Boston Children's have come to rely on your presence to comanage our complex patients who actually live closer to your facility. We trust you and your team and would not want our new partnership with Westchester to jeopardize all that you have built. Though I am soon stepping down from my leadership position, you have my full support to join us as we break new territory together." To say that his words meant the world to me would be the understatement of the century.

I was now pumped for my next step. I was ready to bury the hatchet. As soon as I hung up with Dr. Lock, I dialed the Chief of Pediatric Cardiology and one of the main masterminds behind the Boston merger, Dr. Michael Gewitz. For the next 20 minutes, we reflected on our mutual commitment to the region and the potential benefits of collaboration. I never even had to mention my conversation with Dr. Lock.

He warmly and graciously finished our conversation. "Eric, I agree. Perhaps it is time that we unite our services, especially in this very competitive market. I will be retiring soon enough. I am respectful of what you have created, and having you come aboard will definitely remove the concerns of us remaining in competition. I am open to moving forward."

Having gone through several of these negotiations in the past, I found myself much more sophisticated at this juncture. I indicated to BCHP that I could not tolerate another drawn-out process for personal and professional reasons. They agreed, and within four months, on October 1, 2016, we were officially part of this larger entity, thus ending my almost 20 years of private practice independence.

I had mixed feelings during this initial phase of working together, as if I somehow failed the practice entity I created so many years ago. My family supported me through this transition by reminding me that I should be optimistic about this step. After a late summer's day of scuba diving as a family in the Cayman Islands, while settling down to a fish dinner on the beach, they reassured me, "Dad, don't view this as an end to the original practice but rather as an evolution of the practice and an opportunity for a new phase of your story."

As the new BCHP signage went up around the office, my patients and their families, somewhat worried about the implications of this merger, repeatedly asked me, "Why are you joining with your prior competitors under Boston Children's Hospital? Are you going to leave us soon?"

I answered them honestly and confidently. "I have actually taken this step on behalf of all my present and future patients. I hope that this partnership will sustain us for years to come, not only by continuing to improve our capabilities and quality but also through the coming political and economic storms of healthcare reform. I promise you that I'm not leaving. To the contrary, we are stepping forward into a new era together."

A TANGLED WEB OF HIDDEN CONFLICTS OF INTEREST

By the beginning of 2017, after five years of sweat equity, the clinical capabilities of our local Hudson Valley hospital pediatric program expanded significantly. We had a new children's emergency room, an expanded pediatric inpatient floor, cardiac monitoring capabilities, child-appropriate radiology tests, and a full roster of pediatric subspecialty physicians, nurses, and ancillary staff. We were proud of our many original achievements, including the creation of the region's first community hospital-based child life programs.

The collaborative work environment I initiated with the monthly meetings was contagiously optimistic and productive. The urban tertiary centers were taking notice of our progress. For the first time, they began to take us seriously. Realizing that this community hospital's pediatric services were becoming more self-sufficient, they offered to collaborate like never before. These offers reinforced my convictions that we now had more leverage at the negotiation table. Everyone involved locally had a keen sense of an enhanced control of our own destiny. The bar for what was expected of us by others, and, most importantly, ourselves, had been raised. Sensing that I had finally begun to achieve the mission I had been assigned so many years before by Columbia, I let my guard down. I mistakenly gave my full trust to the hospital administration. Lulled by the constant enthusiasm of my colleagues into a false sense of security, I did not recognize the waning support and alternate agenda of the hospital leadership. By the fourth year of our program, many in the administration turned their attention elsewhere. They took the existence of our pediatric program and services for granted. Several of my clinical colleagues who had been present from the start became concerned that many of the newest administrators did not appreciate that the program was still in its infancy and very fragile. Little effort could intentionally or inadvertently dismantle our precious creation.

"Why do we need a separate group to meet anymore for the pediatric hospital program? Can't this just be absorbed into the regular general pediatric meetings as a line item? We don't need two pediatric meetings," offered one of the administrators.

Oblivious to the efforts of those part-time hospital staff who continued to work so diligently to build this unique service, another administrator piped in, "The hospital should now be able to run the pediatric services with their full-time staff. The part-timers can go back to their offices. We will keep them updated at the monthly meetings." Echoes of the comments from my Columbia departure meeting over five years earlier rang through my mind.

The administration's further forays into control over the pediatric program became painfully evident just one year later. Two new pediatric-dedicated general surgeons expressed an interest in joining our program. On the whole, the adult surgeons in our area were very reticent to operate on children in a consistent or reliable fashion. Only a handful regularly performed enough pediatric cases to consider themselves fully competent to still perform surgery for kids. None of them dared touch an infant with a scalpel. On any given day, it was a crapshoot as to whether the particular adult surgeon on call felt "comfortable" operating on a child for even basic illnesses like a straightforward appendicitis.

The pediatricians and emergency department never knew what response to expect from the covering surgeon when they needed a child professionally evaluated. This *status quo* led to many children having to be rushed away by ambulance to the tertiary pediatric centers. I saw this as a lack of dependability on our part. It was incongruous with our program's goals to meet the health needs of the community's youngest. It threatened to undermine the public's trust by sending mixed messages about our true pediatric emergency capabilities. We professed to families with children suffering from everything from acute abdominal pain to heart issues that we could now care for them in our own hospital. As long as this lack of reliable and consistent pediatric surgical services continued, it was unethical and misleading. So when I learned that there were two general pediatric surgeons willing and ready to come aboard our program to establish a full-time dedicated pediatric surgical service, I ran up the stairs to the second floor to tell the head nurse administrator, Kathy Teisler.

Excited and still winded from my climb, I informed her about these doctors' availability. "Kathy, I really think we should grab this opportunity by the horns. We may not get another chance like this for several years."

She agreed wholeheartedly and encouraged me to engage in an accelerated dialogue with the two pediatric surgeons to close the deal. "Bring me back a full detailed proposal, and I will take it up the ladder. Nice work!" she added.

It is never that easy because medical politics are never simple. Backroom deals happen in hospitals all the time. Other priorities and agendas dominate the landscape. Unbeknownst to Kathy and myself, some in the administration were already working with several adult surgeons on alternate plans that directly countered my efforts with the pediatric surgeons.

The hospital was constantly in confrontation with the largest local private physician mega-group—the very same one that mysteriously was awarded our local pediatric hospitalist service. Their sheer size gave them sufficient leverage to dictate many of the hospital's decisions. Mr. Batson and his team no longer wanted to be beholden to this group's every wish. In an effort to counterbalance this group's monopoly on the regional patient market share, the hospital began to create its own private medical practice. One of the key players in this new hospital-based private practice just happened to be an adult surgeon. He was determined to capture as much business as possible for their new hospital-supported venture. Like me, his goals also included a reduction in the number of pediatric surgical cases being sent away. Through his efforts, the administration directed him to establish pediatric surgery services under the purview of the adult surgery department. We were both working toward the same endpoint but ignorant of each other's presence as I diligently prepared my proposal with the two fully pediatric-trained surgeons.

Over the next few weeks, communications with Kathy became stilted. She and the administration seemed less interested in my pediatric surgical proposal. "Don't worry. We got it from here," she told me on a brief phone call. Having worked together from the beginning of the pediatric program, I trusted her. I told the two surgeons that we would get back to them shortly with an offer to bring them aboard. Along the way, I arranged for a couple of meetings for the pediatric surgeons with the upper administration to keep the coals hot on these prospects and officially demonstrate that we were still serious. After each of these meetings, a few details to solve were provided, and I quickly worked with the two doctors to address these issues.

To my dismay, the process appeared much more drawn out than I was comfortable with, and I was getting concerned that we would lose this valuable opportunity. None of the prior successful projects, which had become intrinsic components of our pediatric program under my watch as director, were so cumbersome. What was taking so long? What were the administrators talking about amongst themselves, and why was I not part of the conversation?

My guard was already up when I received the bad news. Kathy called me to her office. She was in a somber mood, so unlike her usual bubbly self. "Please sit down," she started. "The top echelons of the administration, many of whom are not very familiar with the history of our pediatric service, decided to not make any offer to the pediatric surgeons for this calendar year. They feel that our proposal is unclear and not ready to be part of the budget."

This smelled like a bureaucratic roadblock that made no sense. "I don't understand," I said calmly, fixing my gaze directly on her across the small circular table. "I have been working on this deal for almost six months. What went wrong? What more did they need?" Kathy was silent and apologetic but offered no substantive response to my obvious frustration. I walked out of the room, barely hiding my anger as I looked back. "Why wasn't I invited to the meeting?" Kathy remained silent.

As I left, I walked by Mr. Batson's office to request a meeting with him to discuss the matter further. He always had a fairly open-door policy with me on the very rare occasions I came around.

His very professional secretary returned from his office, closed his door, and politely informed me, "Mr. Batson advises that you set up a meeting with his new Chief Clinical Officer. He believes that she is the best person for you to talk to. I can make an appointment with her for you if you would like."

One week later, I met Dana Brodsky—a no-nonsense, obviously battle-tested, city-trained nurse—for the first time. I introduced myself, and we briefly entered into some small talk about our common backgrounds in the tough academic city hospitals.

"It's good to know that we have someone with your experience working on the pediatric program," she told me. "So what can I do for you today?"

I replied in a more serious tone, "What happened at the meeting last week that led you to reject the pediatric surgery proposal? I have been in serious conversations with the two pediatric surgeons for months. I need to know what to tell them now."

She politely but firmly responded, "Mr. Batson and I only recently became aware of this pediatric surgical venture. When we met with the administration, we concluded that their proposal for these new surgeons' services had not been fully or thoughtfully presented. It just wasn't ready yet to be included in the 2018 budget." I must have looked completely stunned as she raised her voice slightly to gain back my attention. She then asked me a few questions about my involvement and specifically questioned, "Why weren't you there?"

I sputtered back into the conversation. "I wasn't invited or even told when it was happening."

"That's a shame," she remarked. "Seeing that, within 10 minutes of our first meeting, you readily have sound and clear responses to all our questions that the others could not answer, we would have likely approved the proposal. Oh well, there's always next year." She reached out her hand as she stood up. "From here on out, you will work directly with me on such matters." With that, the meeting was adjourned.

I left Dana still not understanding why I had not been included in the presentation. I felt betrayed. Everyone knew how fortunate we were to have two highly sought-after and willing pediatric surgeons knocking at our door. The pediatric program was built in large part upon the trust that referring community physicians bestowed upon me. Why, several years into the pediatric program, was the administration not including me directly in such important meetings? How could I remain the trusted voice to the referring physicians, donors, and others who helped shape the program if I did not know what was happening behind closed doors? Was there another agenda?

Over the next week, I received several unsolicited apologies from my administrative colleagues about the failure to bring the two pediatric surgeons into our program. They advised me to try and keep the two surgeons' interest up for the coming year. They promised me that I would be fully involved in any other future pediatric program projects. I reached out to the two pediatric surgical colleagues on a group call. I was honest about what transpired, including my confusion about not being part of the presentation. To my surprise, they were not shaken.

"We have seen this many times before. This is par for the course with hospital administrators," remarked the most senior surgeon. "We know that this is not how you personally operate, and we have no resentment toward you at all."

I thanked them for being so gracious as I hung up. Despite their kind words, I sensed that I had let them down. I felt like a fool. After having come so far with many of the visionary hospital administrators, I did not want to become cynical. However, my years of experience made me aware that the pediatric program was still not safe and secure. We had created a novel, but fragile, high-quality pediatric medicine service in a community hospital. Without the supportive infrastructure of well-established tertiary medical institutions, it remained vulnerable to the ulterior motives of those less familiar with the nuances of children's healthcare. This stumble with my pediatric surgical colleagues was a warning shot across the bow, and I was not going to let them sink our ship. Too many children were already on board and depending on us.

In the last quarter of 2017, I made it a point to meet more regularly with the higher-ups and newcomers in the administration, who were now clearly stepping in to exert more control of the pediatric service, especially the economics. I was seriously concerned because they clearly knew so little about the idiosyncrasies of pediatrics. With some grey hair now on my head, I felt no reluctance to be direct with Kathy and Dana.

I started our first of several focus meetings by asking, "Is the pediatric program still a priority for the hospital?"

Caught somewhat off guard, Dana rallied. "Yes, of course. We just need to step back and take stock of the program in its present form to best decide where it should go in the future. We will soon be setting up a retreat to specifically address the Pediatric Program."

I responded bluntly, "Sounds reasonable. Will I and the other pediatric physician leaders remain in the driver's seat in regards to taking the program forward?"

Kathy remained silent as Dana replied, "We welcome your input and will let you know what we need from you when the time comes."

The current elected Pediatric Chairperson and I initially tried to be optimistic as we reassured the referring local pediatricians that we remained committed to working together with them to shape the next era of our young program. We started talking up the benefits of the retreat and inviting representatives from each group to join us. In collaboration with the physician leadership, I prepared a formal presentation to explain our history and visions to the administration. One week before the retreat, I provided the draft of this presentation to the administration to be incorporated into the agenda. Their response came out of left field.

On a phone call, Kathy informed us, "The retreat is going to be a four-hour meeting with the administration only. You and the Pediatric Chairperson will be the only pediatricians invited. You need to now uninvite the rest of the pediatricians. Furthermore, though we appreciate your efforts, you will not need to give a formal presentation. An outside consultant group has already been recruited to guide the meeting, and they already have an agenda. We will just incorporate some of your information into their materials."

I remained stunned and speechless on the other end of the line as I hung up. I couldn't wrap my mind around the proposed format to the retreat, especially the deliberate intention to not include the other pediatricians, who had so much stake in our program's future.

On an early dark and cold morning in December 2017, I entered the same boardroom where I made my first pitch for the program five years earlier. I tried to keep an open mind, but my cynical inner voice kept breaking through. The meeting was attended by over 40 administrators, including the CEO, Mr. Batson, the Chief Medical Officer, Dana, and Kathy, my nurse administrator colleague. Less than 5 percent of the attendees around the table were actively involved in the pediatric program. As I sat back and assessed their demeanor, for the most part, they appeared uninformed and somewhat disengaged. Very few raised any specific questions for the consultants. Other than some financial figures, they were basically being paid to tell everyone in attendance what we in the pediatric leadership already included in our rejected presentation.

Over an Internet connection projected onto a screen at the front end of the long table, like a talking head, the main consultant lauded our significant achievements to date. "Compared to other groups in your category, you have come a long way in a relatively short time." Her tinny voice continued, "Your bottom line and projected finances are also impressive for pediatrics. Most programs at your stage are in the red financially. You have surprisingly broken even."

She and her team went on to emphasize that few, if any, other community-based pediatric hospital programs existed in our area. All the same, they warned that the current and anticipated economics of healthcare would be more of a hurdle for pediatrics in comparison to adult medicine.

The voice from the screen concluded, "Despite your success to date, you need to be realistic. We recommend that, if you are to have any chance of success, you align with a tertiary-center partner as your next step to take advantage of new technologies such as telemedicine."

As we proceeded through the meeting, only the two pediatricians in the group, myself and the chairperson, had any relevant questions for the consultants. We spent the last hour in a relatively vacuous "group exercise" typical of such forums. As we finished, I felt like someone had tried to sell me snake oil for a cold that I did not yet have but was sure to catch in the near future. The whole "retreat" felt so sterile and staged. The administration instructed us that we should await the consultant team's formal report before we took any further steps. It could take up to three months before we received the consultant's final report. I felt powerless. The program was officially in limbo. I hated waiting.

As 2017 came to a close, one very significant change to the pediatric program took place. Seemingly out of the blue, the private mega-group relinquished complete control of the pediatric hospitalist program to the hospital. Five years before, in the 11th hour of negotiations, they had mysteriously become the only remaining candidate when the Westchester tertiary center bowed out of the process. Now we were essentially 360 degrees back to my initial advice to the administration—under the auspices of the hospital, the pediatric hospitalist service could remain neutral to all referral groups and more in control of the entire pediatric program's destiny.

Though I should have been inwardly thrilled by this turn of events and was admittedly feeling an "I told you so" moment, I was uneasy. It all seemed too staged. The timing just after the retreat was suspicious. It was so atypical for the large practice to release all contractual restraints on these hospitalist physicians. I again wished that I could have been a fly on the wall or tapped into the phone conversation that led to this "mutual" understanding. What was the price of this exchange? My spidey senses were tingling, so to speak. I worried that, somehow, this would be detrimental to our small pediatric program.

Through discussions with several of my physician colleagues, the truth emerged. Apparently, multiple players were involved in this deal.

Montefiore was courting a partnership with the mega-practice that just let go of the pediatric hospitalists. In one fell swoop, Montefiore would attain access to a significant share of the local hospital's patient population.

In one of our early morning meetings, Kathy expressed her concerns. "If Montefiore aligns with the local practice that now sends us the majority of our patients, this will not be good for our hospital. We could be in for a return to the past, with a huge outmigration of patients down to the city. I fear there is little we can do about it."

I chimed in, "Mr. Batson is not going to be happy."

Kathy nodded in agreement. Interestingly, my own very new alliance with my former competitors, under the Boston Children's banner, seemed inconsequential relative to this clash of titans. Once again, the main flow of local healthcare dollars relied on the control of adult medical services. As stressed in my past dealings at Columbia and Montefiore, and reinforced by the consultants at our recent pediatric retreat, pediatrics was just too small financially to matter.

The leadership of Boston Children's was also rightfully concerned about the regional impact of any alliance between the large physician group and Montefiore. After one of our weekly patient conferences, Dr. Gewitz confided in me, "Every child that goes to Montefiore is one less for us. If the pediatricians from the large group stop sending patients to our offices or our medical centers, this could be very bad for our fledgling combined practice under Boston. Keep me updated if you hear anything important."

As this complex web of deals on the regional medical Monopoly board expanded, a nagging question reemerged for me. "Is this really why I went into medicine? Is all this local politics and business strategizing worth it for me professionally?" More savvy and battle-tested than ever before, I decided to enter the ring in an attempt to pull our pediatric service out of any quagmire that could deter our goals for the local children. I was fully at peace with this decision because it was not based on my desire for personal gain or prestige. I truly had a strong vision of how I wanted to practice local pediatric medicine in the next few years, and pediatrics needed to be part of the local health-care equation. To give our children a voice at the bargaining table, I was ready to dig in and get muddy. My calling had grown larger and more all-encompassing than ever. I decided to step back, pull all my professional resources together, and plan my strategy, especially my initial move. First, I needed to get out of town, as far away as possible, for a clear perspective.

Our family of four welcomed 2018 on the other side of the world in my wife's native country of Thailand. The capital city of Bangkok knows how to celebrate. After dinner at a riverside restaurant in the middle of the city, Viyada and I boarded a water taxi on the Chao Phraya River, the main waterway that served as the city's lifeblood for centuries. Dozens of multicolored flashing fireworks could be seen and heard in all directions, amplified by the reflections off the river's waters. We shed the thoughts of cold snow back home as we wandered in our short sleeves with thousands of other happy people through the bright lantern-lit temples along the streets of the Yan Nawa district. Thanks to the magic of text messaging, we soon met up with our two sons along the Sukhumvit Road and walked back to our hotel in the bustling Khlong Toei district, exhausted but fully satisfied with our decision to bring in the New Year together in Viyada's homeland.

I ran through Bangkok's streets and parks almost every morning to start my day and clear my mind and soul. Everywhere I turned, I saw people setting up small street-side food carts already crowded by commuters on their way to work. I thought about this morning routine repeating itself across the world with millions of hardworking people all striving for the same basic dignity to be able to provide for themselves and their loved ones. In the tree-covered parks, I paused to marvel at the small groups of elderly people welcoming their day with their bodies flowing through the motions of yoga and tai chi under centuries-old pagodas. I hoped that I would be as flexible and healthy when I was their age.

On these runs, as the miles passed, I spent a lot of time thinking. I looked back at the United States from the vantage of Thailand's relatively new democracy and economic power. With the recent death of the beloved octogenarian king in October 2016, and a subsequent national year of mourning, the stability of the monarchy and democracy were simultaneously in question. The patience of the Thai people was stretched thin as the elections they had been promised were repeatedly delayed by the current military government. Though the new year brought hope and optimism for a better reality for the people, this was tempered by the wisdom of Buddhist philosophy that permeates Thai life. Though current conditions of our lives may appear to be all-consuming, Buddhism reminds us that life is a conscious journey toward a better state of being—the enlightenment. How we handle today will determine our chance of successfully achieving this nirvana. Amongst these people, my American sense of the importance of the individual was tempered by a view that we are merely a small part, a cog, in this larger wheel of life. I felt wonderfully small.

We spent hours in philosophical and political discussions over outdoor street-side meals, sharing mediocre but thirst-quenching beers in the heat of the day with my sons. As Daniel and Christopher fought over the last morsel of salted fish or grilled prawns alongside sticky rice and mango, they argued with me that Bernie Sanders's progressive views on healthcare and economics were essential for our own nation's future.

"He may seem radical to your generation, Mom and Dad," they explained as they swigged down another cold beer, "but we need an overhaul of our system if there is going to be any meaningful change."

In between bites of spicy papaya salad, Viyada replied, “Yes, but people aren’t ready for such a drastic overhaul.”

I chimed in, “Isn’t it better to meet everyone somewhere in the middle?”

We took a side trip to Cambodia to visit one of the world’s great wonders, the temple ruins of Angkor Wat. We again were humbled by the land and the wonderful people. As the morning sun broke the night, we stood across the pond in a hushed crowd to witness the mirage of the spires of this magnificent, sprawling twelfth-century palace—the seat of the once-dominant Khmer Empire and still the world’s largest religious monument—become the reality of a living architectural legend that rivaled the Taj Mahal, built 500 years later.

As we returned back to the States together, I felt rejuvenated with my renewed perspective. I was ready to move ahead on the next phase of the local pediatric program and my own medical practice. Our trip to Thailand and Cambodia reinforced many old lessons that I learned working in large and small community settings alike. It helped me remember that, when it came to many of my projects, I needed to balance my enthusiasm with patience. People may initially understand my ideas intellectually, but they will not take any initiative toward these visions until they are emotionally and philosophically ready.

Changing the existing paradigms of local pediatric care might very well prove to be a frustrating process that threatened to stifle my motivation and enthusiasm. All too often, the process manifested as the “hurry up and wait” effect. How many times had someone asked me urgently to provide details or information on a subject, only to stall and say they would get back to me later when everyone else was ready? My trip to Southeast Asia taught me that, if something is truly important, you sometimes just have to be patient. However, my American sensitivities reminded me to set a time limit on my patience so that I was not left stranded or frustrated. The combined summary of these different lessons is that the wisdom learned from having more grey hair and experience has the potential to move the process along.

The 21-hour journey back home across half the globe, across multiple time zones, gave me time to reflect on the complex dynamics of American healthcare that were now directly impacting the future course of our local pediatric program. The federal and state policies driving healthcare reform created a high-stakes, competitive environment in New York's Greater Hudson Valley. Much of this impact was intentional and meant to improve standards, but a significant component was purely motivated by the government's desire to reduce the runaway costs of healthcare.

Hospital and medical practice mergers were now par for the course and seen as the only way to survive. The small private medical practices were merging with each other to create a degree of improved tolerance to the stresses of private practice management. As operational systems and requirements became more bureaucratic, it was proving virtually impossible for small or solo practices to continue to focus on direct patient care without being overwhelmed by all of the new policies, protocols, and paperwork. Highly regulated electronic medical records, increased requirements to participate in the ever-changing third-party payor system, and perpetual continuing medical education requirements topped the long list of government mandates.

Many of the larger physician-driven practices still wanted to maintain their autonomy from the hospitals. An increasing number of doctors simply wanted to focus on patient care and go home at the end of the day. They did not want anything to do with running a practice in the current regulatory environment and readily signed up to become employees of hospital-run practices. Hospital partnerships and networks with each other and larger institutions were likewise driven by the need for economic and operational efficiencies.

The hospital's consultants would soon present their formal report on our pediatric program. I was chomping at the bit for the opportunity to get back on track from where we left off when everything had been put on hold several months earlier. While away, I had to admit to myself that I was deeply concerned about how the current regional healthcare dynamics would impact their conclusions and recommendations.

In late January 2018, three months after what was referred to as the pediatric strategic planning session, the official consultant's report came back. This report included 12 specific initiatives. The administration formally asked those who participated in the October 2017 session to rate these initiatives from highest to lowest priority. When all was said and done, the top two priorities were the development of a strategic partnership with a regional or nationally recognized children's hospital and the implementation of a pediatric telemedicine program. However, on the list was also the recommendation that the hospital create its own outpatient pediatric practice. This particular item took me back to my original concerns about excluding, literally disinviting, the other pediatricians from the October meeting.

Within three weeks of receiving the report, the new administrative project manager, Daniel Simms, came to the year's first monthly Pediatric Department meeting to give a full slide presentation summarizing the consultant's report and our subsequent priority rankings. For the first 30 minutes, he sounded very optimistic.

"I am proud to say that we in the administration and our consultant both agree that significant achievements have been made by the pediatric leadership over the first five years. This bodes well for the success of our program in the future." He continued in his positive tone with the full list of initiatives still projected on the screen behind him, despite the obvious agitation growing amongst the pediatricians. "We are now officially informing you, our community referral base, that the hospital is ready to move forward to the next phases of program development."

As soon as Mr. Simms opened the meeting for questions and feedback, one by one, the pediatricians leaped forward verbally and at times almost physically. A tall, lean, middle-aged, and balding gentleman stood up from his chair, looking Mr. Simms directly in the eyes, and sternly explained, "You are not fooling anyone here. You may indeed have a lot to be proud of on your list, but do not attempt to gloss over the particular item that most directly affects each of our livelihoods. You are now officially declaring your intent to compete directly with all of us by starting your own hospital-based outpatient pediatric program." Mr. Simms's response was weak at best as he made no attempt to deny this accusation.

One of the younger women physicians expressed her own fundamental conflict with supporting the program moving forward, "Why should we, the same doctors who blessed this program at its inception and have functioned as your supportive referral base, continue to send any of our patients to the hospital from now on?"

The "yeahs" muttered in the audience in reaction to her statement appeared to be unanimous. For the next half an hour after the presentation, nothing else besides this contentious topic was discussed. Mr. Simms did his best to deflect any animosity and hide his surprise at the level of resentment my colleagues felt.

I found myself atypically speechless and oppressed by a mixture of emotions and thoughts. I was awkwardly caught in the middle between my directorship role in the hospital and my status as one of the community physicians. As the physicians spoke, they repeatedly said that they did not blame me or the Pediatric Chairperson but held the hospital administration accountable for this aggressive stance. Despite this reassurance in my regard, I once again felt like my most valued principle—trust—was threatened. I was potentially at risk of losing the very trust that my colleagues bestowed upon me at the initiation of the program and as a reliable colleague to whom they could refer their patients. *Déjà vu* memories began to surface, harkening back to the collapse of Columbia's support of local pediatric services years before. I felt nauseous.

In an instant, the whole outpatient pediatrician contingent dropped their mutual rivalries and was united against the hospital's intentions. The large mega-group was now also an enemy of the common enemy—the untrustworthy local medical center that just openly declared a return to the pre-1980s pattern of direct competition with the local doctors. The most frustrating part of the whole scenario for me was that I had foreseen this as a significant flaw in the medical center's strategy when they decided to not include the pediatricians in the retreat. Had this been intentional all along? In retrospect, the administration's mindset was actually quite consistent. In the new year, they had completely abandoned any efforts on developing a pediatric surgical team with the doctors I recruited in favor of expanding their own outpatient surgical practice, to include a small, but expanded, component of pediatric services.

To deny that I was significantly angered and felt willfully abandoned by this process that unfolded before our eyes would be dishonest. However, I was still blinded by my desire to leave behind a better pediatric healthcare standard than the one I discovered when I first arrived in the area. Our pediatric program had come too far, and my internal drive still had a degree of forward momentum. I thus tried to remain constructive in my efforts with all of my clinical and administrative colleagues while addressing the pediatricians' concerns head-on. I frankly discussed these matters with the administration and argued for more transparency and creativity. I suggested that, if the hospital was planning to establish its own outpatient pediatric practice, then it should be for the purpose of serving unclaimed patients and to collaborate with smaller single or two-provider practices that were otherwise unable to compete with the larger mega-groups.

Underneath my slightly political veneer, I had to concede that the hospital demonstrated no intention of being anything but fully aggressive in their campaign to create their outpatient pediatric practice. To proceed with some sense of purpose still intact, I had to recognize that, similar to the case for the large private mega-group practices, the existing economic and government-stimulated factors were major incentives behind the hospital's decisions.

I even halfheartedly suggested to Dana, "Maybe we should come out with a constructive response to the medical community, stating that healthy competition could potentially raise the standard of outpatient care for children and should thus not distract us from further progress on the inpatient service."

She chuckled weakly in response.

On a more serious note in a formal meeting, I admonished, "This abrasive interaction with the pediatricians should serve as a learning experience, a reminder to the hospital—as an institution of the community—to recognize those whose shoulders we stand upon. I earnestly hope that this situation does not create an impasse that results in the end of our efforts. The community's children remain our common focus, and we should move ahead together with this in mind." Was anyone listening, or were they all too caught up in their own agendas?

Money often talks louder than politics. Politics often follows the money. I have always been convinced that healthcare should be as neutral as possible to both money and politics. I felt compelled to keep both money and politics from dissuading the hospital administration from keeping the pediatric program amongst their highest priorities. Initially, I had to pick myself up, despite a nagging despair that we were already too late. I then urged those around me to remain constructive by addressing two of the major items on the consultant's recommendation list—creating a telehealth service and choosing a tertiary partner. Even before the pediatric retreat meeting, I met with hospital leadership in several forums to discuss these two topics.

"We must await the consultant's report before we proceed," was the apparently rehearsed response I received each time I suggested that we should at least begin to lay the foundation for a telehealth service. Deep down, I sensed that we lost so much time, only to come back to where we left off several months before.

Telehealth is the use of a computer as a means of communication between a healthcare provider and their patient. By taking advantage of the visual, audio, and other media interfaces of newer computer technology, patients can now access their physicians or other healthcare professionals from work, home, or even remote areas. This concept of telehealth was slowly gaining momentum in the United States. Understandably, the regions with fewer physicians and medical facilities, as well as those with less dense populations who were often quite remote from comprehensive medical services, were the first to accept and promote telehealth.

At a physician leadership conference in 2015, I discussed the benefits of telehealth with colleagues of mine from Arizona who clearly "drank the Kool-Aid."

"It's the wave of the future," espoused one very energetic nurse practitioner.

"You'll see. It will eventually make it to New York, so you should get ahead of the curve," insisted a middle-aged pediatric radiologist.

Taking their advice to heart, right after the meeting, I actually made several proposals to my tertiary-center partners and the local hospital. No one seemed the least bit interested.

The problem with telehealth was not that it didn't make sense. The main impediment was actually that each state had a different approach to how they planned to "phase in" or "roll out" telehealth over the next few years. Some states were more aggressive than others in implementing telehealth. Most states had yet to agree to allow their Medicaid and Medicare programs to reimburse providers and medical facilities for medical services delivered through telehealth at a level comparable or equal to in-person services. Those that did could claim full "parity" of telehealth with traditional patient-physician encounters.

Each state adopted its own guidelines for acceptable high-quality telehealth services. Many states and older physicians were still struggling to implement comprehensive, computer-based medical record services and were in no position to even consider taking the next step toward telehealth. This created a patchwork of varying degrees of telehealth in each state that literally required a color-coded map to understand it all. It just so happened that, at the time of our consultant's report, New York was not fully on board with telehealth.

As anyone who recently received medical services knows, the COVID-19 pandemic jumpstarted telehealth across the country. Overnight, all the barriers to telehealth-based care—reimbursements to providers, limited hardware and software, and strict definitions for qualifying telehealth services—miraculously vanished. The proverbial question on everyone's mind is whether or not telehealth will remain intact once the pandemic subsides.

The second topic—electing a pediatric partner from a tertiary medical center for our local pediatric program—appeared, on the surface, to be less controversial. However, given the politics between the urban medical centers and the huge financial stakes implicit in any formal collaboration that involved large patient populations, this recommendation from the consultant was also more complicated than initially anticipated. The inclination for the local hospital administration to be as self-sufficient as possible was also a deterrent to making a quick decision about any such alliance.

With the consultant's "official" stamp of approval, I took the opportunity to readdress these categories of telehealth and designation of a tertiary partner with the local hospital administration. To my pleasant surprise, Kathy informed me that the hospital had in fact already begun exploring telehealth opportunities with the adult counterparts of my new tertiary partner. This dialogue was specifically focused on establishing a telehealth service for their highly utilized adult psychiatry service.

During my monthly meeting with Kathy, she advised, "You should join us at our next meeting so that you can get some ideas for fleshing out a pediatric offshoot modeled on our intended psychiatric telemedicine collaboration. Mr. Simms has taken on the task of developing our telehealth programs, and you should work with him to develop our pediatric telehealth services." With these words, I was once again reenergized to roll up my sleeves and get to work.

In the same administration boardroom where our pediatric retreat was held, I participated in several of the formal meetings discussing psychiatric telehealth. At its essence, telehealth appeared to be a very democratic force that leveled the way health services were accessed. I readily appreciated that the technology allowed people in need of psychiatric counseling and guidance to access these resources free of the barriers of distance or transportation. I could envision that, in times of individual or more global crisis, telehealth could save lives. Little did I know that the COVID-19 pandemic would engender a whole industry of online psychiatry services sponsored by celebrities like Michael Phelps.

After a couple of weeks focusing on psychiatric telehealth, my ideas started to flow, and I set about designing a pediatric telehealth program. Mr. Simms and I steadily fleshed out a full pediatric telehealth proposal for our hospital program. Our model combined the state-of-the art computer-based communication technology together with the existing and proven reliable clinical services.

Over the prior several years since we established the local pediatric program, the number and range of such specialized pediatric services available at the hospital bedside or in a local medical office had grown.

The initial expansion of these services had been rapid. Specialties with many clinicians, such as gastroenterology, neurology, endocrinology, and pulmonology, readily diverted their resources to our growing and ever more sophisticated program. After several months, the momentum slowed as we sought access to medical care from fields such as pediatric surgery, nephrology, and infectious disease, which had far fewer clinicians. Even before the consultant's report, I envisioned telehealth as the best solution to accessing these less available pediatric specialty services.

It is important to emphasize that my decision to concentrate on both telehealth and the designation of a tertiary ally was not arbitrary. The two go hand in hand. They are symbiotic and complementary. I was convinced that any effective telehealth platform should be built upon a strong and trusted clinical foundation. To do otherwise would be paramount to placing the cart before the horse. The existing local and tertiary-center alliance with the Westchester-based pediatric specialists had been supported by the local clinicians, hospitals, and patients for decades. It predated my arrival to the area by over a decade. After almost two decades during which I competed with this group, while developing the first drafts of the pediatric telehealth resource, I finally began to appreciate the longevity of their clinical presence. We did not need to start from scratch and choose another partner. The community had already chosen. We could invite others to join us later, but for now, all we had to do was build the telehealth service as an extension of their current presence. Mr. Simms agreed and suggested that we present our proposal along with representatives from the Boston Children's administration to the Chief Medical Officer, Dana Brodsky, and her team the following month, March 2018.

Everyone involved in the planning appeared supportive and excited about the potential of a telehealth approach to regional pediatric care. There was a constructive excitement in the air. I collaborated with Kathy, Mr. Simms, and the leadership of the pediatric inpatient service and emergency room, creating documents and diagrams to include in our slide presentation. I was encouraged by my local administrators to visit the command center of the adult psychiatry and intensive care telehealth operations at the Westchester Medical Center because they were the likely partner for our local hospital. Again, we would not have to recreate the wheel, just carve out a pediatric space from this existing operation.

As the final details of our presentation were underway, I met with Kathy and the hospital Medical Director, Dr. Oslo, in his office. Several years prior, Dr. Oslo had left his emergency room practice to succeed the now-retired Dr. Norm Samuels, one of my original mentors. He now wanted to clarify my decision to merge my private practice with my longstanding competitor.

"I think you should know that Mr. Batson and others are suspicious about your motives to join the former Westchester group, now under Boston Children's. I have no concerns about your commitments, but they are not assured of your true allegiances," Dr. Oslo quietly professed.

Somewhat defensively, I replied, "Please tell them I gave up everything, my 20 years of autonomy to run my own practice, for the benefit of this local hospital program. I have become convinced that the competition between us was detrimental to the program's future and was creating divided allegiances among the pediatricians that refer their patients to this young program. United we are stronger." I paused to see his response, but then added, "The icing on the cake that finally convinced me was that the best pediatric hospital in the nation, Boston Children's, was now involved. With their support and resources, our program could take huge leaps forward. It seemed like a no-brainer."

Kathy interjected, "That makes sense. I have worked with him since the beginning and never doubted his intentions."

Dr. Oslo leaned back in his chair. "I have never doubted Dr. Fethke. I just hope the others are convinced of his good intentions."

The night before our March 2018 meeting, at which I was to officially present the pediatric telehealth proposal, I was so excited that I had trouble falling asleep. I had the full computer-based slide presentation all cued up and backed up on extra drives in case of technical difficulties. Mr. Simms, Dr. Oslo, Kathy, and the Pediatric Chairman had all reviewed and approved the contents of this presentation in detail over the prior weeks. I had not altered it in any way. This meeting was simply a formality.

It was the final forum for the administrative leadership in attendance—specifically the same Chief Medical Officer, Dana Brodsky, who presided over the failed pediatric surgery proposal—to make any constructive suggestions and hopefully officially bless our moving forward to make the region's first pediatric telehealth program a reality. Dana sat toward the head of the long boardroom table directly across from me and removed by at least two chairs from anyone else in attendance, including the acting Pediatric Chairman. The Boston Children's Chief Operations Officer—a warm and burly middle-aged man named Mr. Sanders—and Mr. Simms sat on either side of me.

I was so nervous that, years later, I do not specifically recall who else among the 10 attendees was there. After my 20-minute presentation, I was commended by all present for my hard work and a very thorough and thoughtful proposal—all, that is, except Dana Brodsky.

She simply stood up, asked no questions, and officially ended the meeting by stating, "We will let you know our decision in a few days. Have a good day." With that, she left the room, rendering silent everyone remaining.

In hindsight, I do not recall if Dana actually made any comments at all before or during the presentation. She did not convey even the slightest hint of interest in the subject matter of my proposal. She imparted no guidance or blessing for us to proceed and make pediatric telehealth operational for our community. When a letter with Mr. Batson's "CEO" title on the envelope arrived at my office two days later, I thought for sure that it must contain the official green light for the telehealth project. It took me several reviews of the two paragraphs on this one page for the message to begin to sink in. I expected we would move forward together, which could not have been further from the truth.

CHAPTER 5

MY OWN BROKEN HEART

On the cold and damp Thanksgiving weekend of 1964, Gilbert was 22 years old, and Dr. Humphreys and Dr. Malm ultimately determined it necessary to perform his third and final heart surgery. They waited as long as possible, per Gilbert's father's wishes. It was now time to use the more established heart bypass machine that Dr. Malm helped develop to go around and empty Gilbert's heart while he entered the bottom heart chambers to close the large hole in the muscle dividing these two chambers. Dr. Malm notified the Tremain family that Gilbert was going to need a lot of blood for the surgery to fill the tubing in the bypass pump, so Gilbert called the college that he then attended and asked if they would be having one of their regular blood drives soon. Luckily, there was one coming up, and they were more than willing to donate and designate some of the blood to be used in Gilbert's surgery.

Years later, Gilbert fondly and gratefully boasted, "It only cost me a $35 lab fee for the blood transfusion used during my last operation." He proudly recalled, "A man who headed a store chain donated a lot of money to Columbia to build a top-of-the-line heart surgery recovery room. Following my last surgery, I spent some time recovering there. I got myself in trouble playing with the electronics, especially the heart monitor. I learned that if I put the probe in a specific place on my toe and wiggled my leg back and forth, then every line on the monitor would go crazy. The first time I did it, the nurses could not figure out what caused the temporary problem, and I stopped before they had time to call the surgeon. The second time, I was not as lucky, and the surgeon came running in. Fortunately, I stopped waving my foot by then and pretended to be asleep, but he realized what I was doing. The surgeon pulled the covers off of my feet and put the probe back in its proper place on my hand."

In the 1960s, there were three bays of six patient beds each on the 14th floor of Columbia Hospital and several individual rooms in between. Toward the end of the hall, there was a five-bed ward that was for cardiac patients. This was where Gilbert was transferred after being well enough to leave the recovery room.

There, he met a kid who had spent almost his entire life at Columbia. This boy was six years old and had only been home with his parents for one month in total. The doctors at Columbia managed to keep him alive, and he was doing fairly well, but he still had heart problems that needed to be fixed and kept him in the hospital. Gilbert recalled that his next heart surgery was imminent and tried to cheer him up. While sharing a room together, Gilbert let him in on the trick with the heart monitor probe, which by then the nurses had figured out.

One of the nurses became so mad when the two boys kept fiddling with the heart probe, she stormed into their room and sternly threatened Gilbert, "We're meant to save lives here, but if you tell one more person about this little game with the probe, I'll have to kill you with my bare hands."

Gilbert had fond memories of many of the nurses he met during his stay at Columbia-Presbyterian Hospital. The nurse caring for him after his first surgery noted that his tonsils were very swollen. She recommended to Gilbert's family that he should have a tonsillectomy before they caused any problems down the road. Because of Gilbert's heart condition, the local doctors refused to do it. Thus, he had to go back down to Columbia for a straightforward tonsillectomy.

To his surprise, after surgery, he was roomed on the fourth floor and assigned the same nurse from the previous visit who advised that he get his tonsils removed. They became good friends during his stay. Even more amusing to Gilbert was that she was also the head of nursing on the surgical floor following his second heart operation.

He laughed as he recalled, "She may have saved my butt a bit. The ward nurse, who was known as the Little Corporal, would snap at everyone, especially me. To my knowledge, no one really liked her. One afternoon, there was a nurse on special duty who had been assigned to remain in a particular patient's room unless his wife was able to be there. I was one for wandering around and getting to know people. This nurse could not leave the room, but she would stand in the doorway, and we would chat. When the Little Corporal saw me there, she got very mad. My friend, the head nurse, stepped in and vouched for me. I did not get in trouble."

Gilbert also recognized the important role of the candy stripers who were hospital volunteers that helped the patients and relieved the nurses of some tasks. One morning, an attractive candy striper asked Gilbert if he needed anything.

He cleverly responded, "Why yes, thank you. My doctors instructed me to walk around, but I am having trouble." As he hoped, she offered to help, and they regularly walked up and down the halls together. That is, until the Little Corporal took notice and figured out what he was up to. She told the candy striper that Gilbert was taking advantage of her company and had recovered enough that he could walk just as well as she could.

In another instance, Gilbert nonchalantly walked into the nurses' break room, not knowing that this was a restricted area for patients. He started chatting with the nurses who sat there, drinking orange juice and having a good time, when the Little Corporal arrived. She threw him out of the room and threatened to report him. Once again, his friend, the head nurse, came to his rescue, and he did not get into trouble.

A few days after entering the nurses' break room, he marched up to the front desk and told the Little Corporal, "I need to go to Dr. Humphreys's office and the blood bank to pay my bill." She told him not to leave the floor, but he replied, "You're not big enough to stop me. I'm going no matter what, but you could send a candy striper with me if this would be more by the rules."

The candy striper and Gilbert first went up to the blood bank and then down to Dr. Humphreys's office on the first floor. When they got there, Mrs. Humphreys was seated at the front desk. She had been Dr. Humphreys's nurse for as long as he could remember and knew Gilbert very well.

Gilbert greeted her warmly and triumphantly announced, "I promised Dr. Humphreys last spring, when I was able to get up and walk around after this last surgery, and not until then, I would come by and pay him what I owe him. I am here to make good and settle up." She smiled back fondly at him. As Gilbert and his candy striper guide hurried back up to the floor, they again ran into the Little Corporal just as they were coming out of the elevator.

"Did you really leave to pay your bills?" she scoffed disapprovingly.

Just then, Dr. Humphreys exited the adjacent elevator and jested loudly, "Just spoke to my nurse. Great to see that you are doing well enough to finally pay my bill." Gilbert and the candy striper couldn't help laughing out loud as the Little Corporal stormed off in defeat while Dr. Humphreys remained both puzzled and amused.

Years later, during a visit with me in my outpatient office, Gilbert explained to my medical student, "As a young doctor, you need to understand the importance of a good relationship between a patient and their medical team. When you can have the kind of rapport that I had with the caliber of people such as my two great surgeons, it means a lot for your well-being. The ease with which I could talk to them made my many stays in the hospital much more enjoyable, despite my fears and pain."

He recalls that Dr. Malm was quite easygoing. When he came to check on Gilbert the day after surgery, despite being in a lot of pain, out of a show of respect and determination, Gilbert tried to get up. At that moment, Dr. Malm extended his hand to Gilbert and helped him first to a sitting and then a standing position.

Dr. Malm then faced Gilbert and, with a twinkle in his eyes, admiringly asked, "Have you ever let anything get in your way, young man? Your will to get better is amazing. I have never cut through so much muscle in a man's chest, and I've been doing this for quite a few years."

Only after I read Mr. Batson's two-paragraph letter for the third time, the implications of his communication finally sank in. I was officially relieved from my directorship position due to a "conflict of interest" inherent in my work on his hospital's pediatric telehealth project. This letter—penned by the same person newly arrived five years prior who used my initial proposal on the neonatal program as a bargaining chip to gain regional control of the neonatal intensive care services for his hospital—now blamed me for favoring my new tertiary alliance with Boston Children's over the best interest of the very same community hospital's pediatric program that seven years before I brought to life with his blessing. He indicated that in four months, the young director of the new pediatric hospitalist service, who I fostered and promoted as an integral part of my initial proposal for the program, would take over my responsibilities under her recently acquired title of Pediatric Chairman. She would also soon be garnered with the position of director of the hospital's own private pediatric practice, which they planned to inaugurate in the next few months.

I was being fired.

I had been deliberately and unknowingly ambushed. At my next and last program meeting, I notified everyone that I was given a few months to wind my directorship down. No one, even the young pediatric director who I supported from the beginning, spoke up on my behalf.

In a state of disbelief, I also tried to review the letter with everyone who worked closely with me on the telehealth project. On the top of my list was the Chief Medical Officer, Dana Brodsky, who never returned my emails or calls. I have actually never met or spoken to her since the proposal meeting. None of them offered any valuable insight regarding the loss of my directorship position. To be fair, several of my colleagues who were recruited to participate in the pediatric program under my directorship apologized for not being able to alter the final decision of the CEO. They too felt helpless.

When I briefly communicated with Mr. Batson by telephone, he stood by his decision but added some parting comments as if to soften the blow. "We all still feel that you are a great doctor and an asset to our community. No one can take that away from you."

Though these words from his mouth sounded empty and completely condescending at first, I later concluded that they contained some subtle truth. The one consistent factor in my professional life was indeed my patient practice. The part of his argument that continued to strike viciously against my core was his attack on my value system. He was the first and only person to officially accuse me of being unethical in any way, especially as a medical professional. I was pissed off and resentful.

Many of my trusted colleagues tried to reassure me by explaining that Mr. Batson's intentions were politically and financially motivated, not personal. I was just once again one of his scapegoats, as was a growing cadre of other local practitioners. After one of the early morning monthly pediatric department hospital meetings, the pediatric director of one of the larger local private practices noted that I was unusually quiet.

He discreetly pulled me aside in the hallway and attempted to console me by explaining, "Don't let this Batson nonsense get you down. It is his loss, not yours. You are just an easy target that he needed to get out of the way to effectively pursue his own agenda. He plans to compete with all of us by establishing a large local hospital-based outpatient practice. He believes that your recent partnership with a large group threatens this goal. He can't see that you remain dedicated to the local program because he is clouded by his own aspirations and ways of seeing the business world of healthcare."

With similar feedback from other colleagues, I initially made some feigned attempts to fight back the accusations in Mr. Batson's letter. I met in person with the handful of remaining administrators who had been around since I arrived in the community and knew me well. After a couple of weeks, when it became clear that they too were helpless to provide any solutions on my behalf, I gave up trying.

In the end, I remained unwilling to change my value system and could see no benefit in even trying to work in any official way with the hospital. I put my head down at night without regret, knowing that all my intentions, including the merger with Boston, were dedicated to the children. The majority of the local hospital-based services that I started remain the operational backbone of their pediatric program to this day. The program is still intact, though not very resilient and less advanced than I had envisioned. The children's emergency room, Child Life, and pediatric hospitalist services are still moderately busy and remain the only such pediatric-dedicated resources in the region. Perhaps it was now someone else's turn to take the reins of the local pediatric program, though the handoff could have been more honorable.

I do not deny that I am a rosy-eyed fool. I had been in the position to start local pediatric clinical programs all too many times over the years, only to have the rug later pulled out underneath my feet. I should have learned by now. I experienced the negative repercussions on my practice of the NYPH network's removal of the pediatric neurology colleague under my leadership, followed by their exclusion of my involvement in the NICU service at the local St. Luke's Hospital. I struggled through two years of fruitless negotiations in the hopes of merging with Montefiore so that I could return my full attention to patient care and expand reliable pediatric subspecialty services to my community. I was coaxed back into official service several times by the CEO of the new community hospital, only to be accused of not knowing my true allegiances.

One of my dearest pediatric colleagues said during a weekend bike ride, "Dude, you have too many arrows in your back to even care anymore about what others say or do. The only thing that matters is that you've done great things along the way and that you're still here." My friend was right. What he may not have realized was that the cumulative effect of those arrows was that they had injured my heart.

When I took a step back, I could see that my alma mater and other institutions were not reliable because they were dealing with their own stresses in the current healthcare upheavals. The local hospitals had the right to their own agendas, but I knew now that I was done with this phase of my career. I would never again seek an administrative position with a hospital. My career path changed, and I needed to chart my own course for the next half of my professional life.

I was now at the point in my life and career that I was comfortably confident with who I had become. I could now be selective about where I expended my efforts and shared my skillsets. It took several weeks, but finally, I was at peace with what happened. I was no longer concerned about the pediatric program that I designed and envisioned on behalf of the local institution because they had become mired in a local battle for political and financial survival. I chose not to remain bitter because this negative energy was too distracting. Pediatrics was no longer on their high-priority list, but it was and always would be on mine. I remain satisfied that, along the way, I left my small mark by caring for the Brittanys of the world. I once again returned to my patient care as the bedrock of my local efforts to promote high-quality pediatric care and education.

One year after the pediatric retreat session, the local hospital put up a large billboard advertising their own pediatric outpatient practice, publicly announcing their intention to fully compete with the other preexisting practices. The community pediatric telehealth service still does not exist. Time will tell.

Here ended my second decade of hospital-based institutional leadership. It was at this point, 20 years after I first arrived green behind the ears in the Hudson Valley, that I began some deep soul-searching. I sensed that my time from now on would be best spent evaluating myself and not judging the merits of the actions or intentions of others. I no longer wished to spend my efforts and emotions on influencing others who had chosen a different path than mine or who did not share my values.

My retrospective self-review convinced me that even if I had been a fool, I was still proud and happy with my past. More importantly, I remained optimistic about the future. I had been for the most part protected from seeing the darker sides of business and politics within healthcare institutions that had become preoccupied with short-sighted competition over collaboration. Much of my ability to remain unscathed was due to my unwavering family support, my dedicated staff whom I remained so proud of, and the positive feedback from my patients. Without my wife's tolerance of the political and financial ups and downs I experienced, I knew that I would never have come this far. She literally kept our household financially solvent and covered our boys' college tuition while I was just trying to keep my doors open and staff employed during the toughest financial times of my practice.

I also remain stubbornly optimistic and determined to always see more of the good than the bad in every person or situation. As the hospital-based teams I worked with waxed and waned in their commitment to building strong local pediatric services, I was fortunate to fall back on my own practice. I owed it to my practice and patients to not be dragged away by the tidal waves of others' agendas.

During my training over 30 years ago, Dr. Gersony repeatedly reminded us, "You should always guide your professional careers like a large ship aimed at the highest-quality healthcare on behalf of your patients. No matter what others around you tell you or do, no matter how rough the waters or strong the rains and winds, stay steady on the course you know is right and true." His words had sounded reasonable back then but now resounded like a bullhorn in the deep fog guiding me forward. I would continue to steer my little ship, my practice, straight ahead. My place is with my practice, where I am dedicated to continued growth with my team while I attempt to keep them less affected by, but never completely free of, outside dynamics.

If I remain naive or ingenuous, so be it. I prefer to have my spirit motivated by the positive force of a physician's call to do the best I can on behalf of the children I serve. I realize that I have often been blinded to the ulterior motives of others in healthcare that do not share this same guiding principle. Their profit and power-oriented mindsets made me vulnerable to being deterred from achieving my own goals. I am not judging their decisions—even the flimsy ones proposed in letters—because I do not purport to know their full rationale. At this turning point, I am no longer part of their rat race. I am at peace. I have made a decisive pact with myself to not expend excessive efforts to please anyone else but me. Trust in myself has become my standard, my litmus test.

Moving forward, I worked only with people who shared my passion, optimism, and vision for a better healthcare system. I soon found myself joined by a strong core of people who reenergized me with their contributions to my patient care and a constant supply of stimulating questions about the need for healthcare reform. The past two decades taught me a lot about our healthcare system, much of which I now realized I was not very proud of and actually strongly disagreed with. I started to realize that students, laypeople, and colleagues saw me as a reputable source of information about the problems and solutions in our healthcare system.

Reluctantly, I had to admit this was partly because I had become older and worked through so many changes in this system. I was still standing, and there were lessons to be shared in this survival. I regularly found myself in deep conversations with friends and students about the "big picture" of medicine in the United States.

"Where are we heading?" asked my medical students.

"Why is the health insurance system so complex?" expressed an exasperated patient's parent.

"I have visited other countries that are poorer than us but where everyone has decent healthcare coverage. It just doesn't seem right that so many people in a nation as wealthy as ours do not have access to good medical care," shouted a neighbor over an evening bonfire.

I began writing essays about my experiences and ideas, initially as self-therapy and later for anyone who was interested. I soon found that many others—laypeople and medical professionals alike—agreed with me or found my ideas stimulating and provocative. My students and colleagues suggested that I turn my writings, which by then numbered over 1,000 pages, into at least one book. They urged me to overcome my apprehension about public scrutiny to tell my own career story as a synopsis of the misguided direction that healthcare in the United States has taken for the past several decades. Thus began the very venture that defines this work and comprises the bulk of the subject for the remaining chapters. My heart was whole again and beating strongly.

PART II

MY THOUGHTS

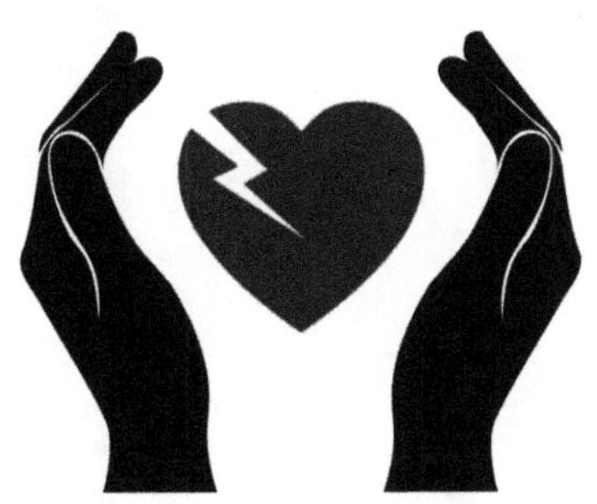

CHAPTER 6

OVERWHELMING BUREAUCRATIC BS

"Sorry to bother you so late at night, Doctor, but I am feeling lightheaded, and my heart is racing," explained Marianne breathlessly. She sounded exhausted. "My husband's away on business. I'm alone with the twins. I didn't know who else to call."

Marianne was born with the right half of her heart missing. As an infant, she began a series of three heart operations that progressively allowed her circulation to increase the oxygen content to her body. However, her heart muscle had become more tired, and the surgical scars in her heart chambers became a source of frequent, irregular, and rapid heartbeats. Marianne was on medications to control these abnormal heart rhythms, but they made her tired. She tried to time her naps to coincide with that of her one-year-old twins.

Miraculously, her heart had been strong enough that she was able to carry twins herself. During the pregnancy, her heart was closely monitored by a team of specialized high-risk obstetricians and congenital cardiologists at a Midwest tertiary medical center. After a successful C-section at 32-weeks' gestation, Marianne underwent a tubal ligation because her entire medical care team agreed that it would be too dangerous for her to have any more children. Originally hoping to be able to have even one baby, she and her husband considered themselves extremely fortunate to now have two healthy infants. She had made motherhood a priority, but there was a price to pay—the pregnancy aggravated her heart condition.

In the spring of 2009, just months after the twins were born, her young family relocated from the Midwest to New York because her husband was offered a promising new job. She had been referred to me by her original cardiologist when they notified him that they planned to move. After receiving her extensive medical records, I saved an hour-long appointment in my schedule for this wholesome-appearing young couple who now sat before me, a sleeping infant in each of their laps.

"We did our research, and, Dr. Fethke, your name kept coming up. We even chose our new house so that we would not be too far from your office," she explained excitedly during our first outpatient visit.

Right then and there, I did something I rarely do. I gave her my personal cell phone number in case of an emergency. It just felt like the right move.

"Thank you so much for being so available, Doc," sighed her husband in relief at the end of the visit. "I travel a lot, and it's reassuring to know that Marianne is in good hands—you know, especially being alone with the kids and all. We will only bother you with a direct call if there is a real emergency, I promise."

This transition to a new company required that they change their health insurance provider. The insurance company Marianne had been with throughout her life and pregnancy did not operate in New York and was not even an option in her husband's new company. Even more concerning, every health insurance option under the New York employer considered Marianne's congenital heart defect to be a "preexisting condition." Most would not cover the majority of costs related to medical care for her heart. Because of her heart condition, the family had to settle for one of the health insurance carriers that provided most of her ongoing medical needs, yet at a much higher annual premium than her old insurer, as well as an extremely high deductible and copay up front. They were stuck and had no other choice.

Given the professional opportunity for the family and the potential economic upsides, they crossed their fingers and moved to New York. They were hanging on the hope that Marianne, now 23 years old, would not need any major medical care until they were more financially secure.

However, six months after arriving in New York, her heart was screaming for attention. Now at 3:00 a.m., on a cold, winter morning in upstate New York, she explained to me between gasps of breath that, because her insurance did not cover the costs of her heart medications, she had been taking only half the dose to minimize her out-of-pocket expenses. She woke in her bed with immense pressure over her chest and shortness of breath.

Her mind raced as she weighed the balance between the huge out-of-pocket costs of going to the emergency room versus waiting it out to see what would happen. The doors of the ER were literally across the street from their home. She took an additional heart medication pill to hopefully slow down her racing heart, but after 30 minutes, she felt no better. She started panicking. She knew she needed immediate medical help, but on her way to her infants' room to take them with her to the emergency room, she passed out. She awoke to find herself on the landing that divided her stairway between the two floors of the new home. Marianne was so disoriented and confused that she didn't know why she had been on the stairs in the first place. It made no sense to be there because the children were on the same floor as her bedroom.

She sat on this landing talking to me on her cell phone. "What should I do, Doctor? I'm scared, my husband's away, and I can't drive in this condition. I can't leave the twins alone. I don't know anyone who can come and watch them. I could walk to the ER, but it's very cold. I'm not sure I can carry the twins."

I took her cell number and told her that I would call the local ER and ambulance myself. Despite my best-laid plans, I got stuck on the phone waiting for the ER nurse or doctor in charge to pick up. I dared not hang up, but I also wanted to notify the ambulance. Just as I was about ready to hang up with the ER, a doctor responded. I started to explain the situation.

He interrupted me politely. "What does your patient look like?" he asked. "A twenty-something blonde with twins?"

"Yes! Do you know her? " I asked, somewhat surprised.

"No, but I think she just walked in through our doors in her nightgown, snow in her hair, with a child in each arm!"

Marianne made the heroic decision to choose health over costs and crossed the several blocks in the dark to reach the ER on foot. While a nurse's aide kept an eye on one of the twins, the other nestled fast asleep under Marianne's right arm while she received IV fluids in her left hand and a dose of strong medication to calm her still-racing heartbeat.

After I made sure with the ER doctor that she was stable, we transferred her to the city hospital where colleagues could best take care of her as an adult with a birth-related heart condition. Fortunately, she not only survived this life-threatening event, she sought professional care early enough to stop the abnormal heart rhythms so that she suffered no additional injury to her already weakened heart muscles. She was lucky to be alive, and she knew it.

Marianne's husband rushed back from his business trip that same night. The very next day, from her ICU hospital bed, they made plans to move back to the Midwest. His original employer, happy to have a valued employee back, agreed to reinstate their original healthcare coverage. The following week, as I completed their last visit with me in my office, we exchanged hugs. I took one last look at her beautiful twins and wished them Godspeed.

MONEY GETS IN THE WAY

As many men do, my buddies and I like to solve the world's problems over a beer, on a bike ride, at a golf course, or while participating in weekend warrior sporting activities. Two of my closest friends are also physicians. As we approach our midlife years, the three of us often reflect upon the reason we wanted to be in healthcare in the first place and also how much has changed since we decided to enter college to pursue a premedical path.

We also sense that since about 2010, it feels like US healthcare has taken us hostage on a roller coaster ride with so many emotional, physical, and economic highs and lows. During this time, the control of physicians' decision-making and finances has become increasingly dictated by the health insurance companies. We are all too often encouraged by these third-party payors to ignore what we know through our training and experience is best for our patients and choose cheaper and less effective options. Reimbursements have decreased significantly, practice management costs have increased, and we are spending less time with our patients.

We worry that we are all increasingly at risk of losing track of our core values that are essential to being a good doctor. Doctors are also being forced to join large hospitals or other practices and give up their personal identity and relationships with their patients, which were at the heart of our choice to become doctors in the first place.

"Healthcare reform" has become the buzzword of the day, yet the course of this reformation seems often misguided and heading directly away from the patient-physician relationship. Most notably, American society—the average consumer, policymakers, and, yes, sometimes even physicians themselves—appear to be confused as to what type of healthcare we truly want our doctors and health institutions to provide.

Several components of society's priorities appear to be in direct conflict with each other. People demand the best and latest medical care, yet they want to spend only 15 to 20 minutes and as little money as possible to receive this care. In the past five to 10 years, this "fast food" version of healthcare has replaced the prior concern of patients that they were not receiving enough time and attention from their clinicians. Medical care joined the realm of a commodity like groceries and other items to purchase and find immediate satisfaction on the Internet.

Every day, I encounter at least one or two patients who have no hesitancy to look up from their smartphones, point to their watches, and express that they waited five to 10 minutes beyond their scheduled visit time. Plus, they have to be somewhere else in 10 minutes, so can I please move it along and quickly assess their child's possibly serious heart condition so they can go. It is as if people expect so little from their medical providers that they gave up trying to push for more.

"It is what it is, so we just have to accept and live with it," extolled one of my patient's parents, who also happened to be a doctor. If spending more and more on health insurance premiums and out-of-pocket costs like deductibles and copays bought better service or care, then this pattern of cheap-and-quick sadly makes some sense. Since the end product is often getting worse, not improving, I just can't help but think that this attitude is so defeatist and unacceptable. We should and can do better.

Since I began my medical training in 1987, I noted that each time our nation experiences economic hardships, American healthcare policymakers in government and industry fall back on the same formulaic pattern of trying to balance good access to healthcare against their primary goal of cost containment. There have been many complex financial models proposed and implemented over the past few decades. These include the managed care boom of the 1980s, capitation, fee-for-service, ACOs, government insurance, and the ACA.

The variety and complexity of these models continues to grow exponentially. It feels like a healthcare professional needs another education degree simply to understand all of the acronyms and suffocating bureaucracy. Ultimately, I sense that each variation falls short financially and operationally. Eventually, they all succumb to the path of least resistance and become money counters doing everything they can to save a dime while ignoring the desired end product of uniformly accessible, high-quality care. The holy grail of excellent population health remains a distant vision.

Until the ACA, many of these models restricted access to care for individuals with complex medical needs because they were deemed cost-prohibitive in the system. Therefore, patients with severe disabilities, mental illness, and complex chronic medical conditions often could not afford or even access health insurance coverage. As the COVID-19 pandemic revealed, we have not been very successful as a nation. There remain too many gaps in access to care for far too many people. We all end up paying more than we should in both economic and emotional costs because the formula is inherently flawed. Healthcare is not a simple commodity that follows the basic rules of economics. Anyone who has tried to tackle US healthcare reform quickly learned that it is far more complicated and intrinsically highly personal to Americans.

I am convinced that the current US healthcare system has become much too unwieldy and virtually self-serving. It has grown so many arms and legs, supporting a whole branch of the economically influential healthcare industry, that it is almost unrealistic to assume it can be dismantled without initially creating downstream significant negative economic consequences. The health insurance companies, pharmaceutical and medical technology industries, large hospitals, and mega-group medical practices justify their existence not on the basis of their excellent results but rather on the fact that they now employ a significant part of the workforce.

Employers responsible for the majority of individuals' health insurance coverage under the current paradigm are overburdened by the increasing costs of medical care. When politicians or healthcare leaders look around at other developed nations with universal or socialized healthcare systems, they realize that they can no longer point to their poor outcomes relative to the United States. The majority of them are doing much better for far less money. Anyone paying even slight attention to the political debates at all levels will now hear that economic justification has replaced the quest for quality as the main argument against dismantling the current system in favor of universal healthcare. Equity of access to care barely surfaced in the debates until the COVID-19 pandemic rubbed it in our faces.

If we are to finally achieve meaningful healthcare reform, we have to step back and take stock of our priorities. We must review our prior attempts and shortcomings through the prism of clearly defined national goals and values. This national soul-searching will not be easy or without significant pain, but it must now be seen as a prerequisite to moving forward on healthcare reform.

There are some very basic questions that we have left on the table for far too long. Who are we as a people when it comes to caring for each other and those who come to our shores? Can we truly achieve our enshrined national pursuit of life, liberty, and happiness for each individual if we cannot deliver the best medical care possible to everyone? Can we hope to remain a model of democracy to the world if we continue to rank so poorly in healthcare statistics relative to other developed nations? When we finally answer these fundamental issues, I believe that the solutions to our healthcare problems will be strikingly clear, far less complicated, and more meaningful.

OUR CURRENT HEALTHCARE MODELS IN LAYMEN'S TERMS

To determine where we should progress with healthcare reform, we must first take stock of where we currently are and from where we have come. Lately, I often find myself explaining the alphabet soup of healthcare terminology to students, laypeople, and colleagues to best orient them to the dauntingly elaborate and confusing models that inundated the health profession over the past few decades. I have become more knowledgeable in this area than many of my non-self-employed or academic colleagues simply to adapt and survive professionally.

If I were to have any chance of developing community-based pediatric services and maintaining a successful highly specialized pediatric subspecialty practice in a suburban community, far removed from any urban tertiary medical center, I needed to be adept and directly involved in the evolution of healthcare models. Like many of my nonacademic private medical leader colleagues, our education in these matters was through the school of hard knocks. We learned on our feet with daily real-life applications of the information we acquired. When we failed, we had no one else to turn to and just had to pick ourselves back up and forge ahead. Many of my colleagues with university degrees in healthcare policy or management still come to me as a resource for practical applications of their virtual knowledge. It is refreshing to see that, lately, universities such as Harvard and Dartmouth created degree programs in healthcare policy catering to on-the-ground, seasoned physicians such as myself. This is a testament to the value of experience combined with education.

In the following section of this chapter, I share some of my main insights regarding this all-too-complex system. This is not meant to be an exhaustive academic review, since many others, far more knowledgeable on the details and intricacies of the US healthcare machine than I, have previously accomplished this Herculean task. Rather, I aim to portray my sense of the system as someone who has been one of many end-users of a program designed by policymakers. I have spent almost three decades trying to navigate this increasingly tangled forest and lately begun asking whether there is merit in considering an alternate path to reach the sought-after valley on the other side. Sometimes I even wonder if the trek through the woods has become more important and all-consuming, while the original goal of achieving a healthy society has been kept too far out of sight.

COST-REDUCTION STRATEGIES

I first became aware of the financial aspects of healthcare in 1994. I just finished my three-year general pediatrics training at Columbia, and Viyada and I decided to take a step back from training to spend some quality time with our eldest son, Daniel. We both did some regular moonlighting work in Columbia's NYPH emergency rooms, and I joined a relatively new and growing pediatric practice in the Washington Heights community of Manhattan, just a few blocks south in the shadow of my training program at Columbia's Babies and Children's Hospital.

The founder and director of this practice, a handsome and energetic force with an exceedingly warm charisma in his early 30s, Dr. Juan Tapia, provided my first exposure to a physician entrepreneur. He combined business savvy with a commitment to providing top-notch medicine to the children of his historically healthcare-starved neighborhood. He worked hard to establish a strong financial foundation for his practice by availing himself of the Medicaid reimbursements and associated incentives for physicians choosing to work in such underserved communities. He clearly was driven by a higher vision of what healthcare should be, as made evident in the forward-thinking name he gave his practice—Pediatrics 2000. The community responded very positively to the presence of the local Dominican doctor from Pediatrics Dos Mil who had come to serve his own.

Though Columbia had a well-established, robust outpatient clinic program, Dr. Tapia's model seemed to be more familiar and approachable to many of the local residents. He worked at least 12-hour days and could be seen opening his office at off hours just to help a single child, even after over 100 kids had passed through his roughly 1,200-square-foot office. He maximized the flow of patients through this space and utilized the services of other Dominican and Latinx providers, as well as young doctors like me. He ran the financial books with just as much care, emphasizing that wasted money could make the difference of the practice's survival. He took nothing for granted in the operations and set an indelible lifelong impression on my sense of local healthcare.

Dr. Tapia's model soon proved to be so successful that he expanded with a second office site to the other Heights, the melting pot of the world known as Jackson Heights of Queens, New York. I split my time between the two offices and looked forward to exploring the streets of Jackson Heights, where I regularly sampled some of the most aromatic food I have ever eaten. Columbia University soon realized that they could no longer ignore his substantial clinical presence and welcomed him into the academic faculty. Here too he left many students and training residents with a different sense of healthcare than the traditional ivory-tower model. He placed boots on the ground in the middle of where people lived, instead of clinics housed deep in the often-scary facilities of large institutions.

Because he and I remained affiliated in good standing with Columbia and agreed to care for a significant portion of adolescents, we were both designated by New York Medicaid as preferred providers. This label was the first of many policy-driven terms that I became familiar with during my career. It symbolized a policy-driven concept by our state government to deliberately select and financially incentivize a subset of physicians to provide high-quality care to those most in need. They put their money to good use to improve the accessibility and quality of healthcare and, ultimately, to improve the overall health of communities most in need.

These Heights neighborhoods had become notoriously synonymous with crime, poverty, drug abuse, and some of the lowest healthcare conditions in the country. The hospitals in these neighborhoods struggled under the weight of providing complex healthcare to so many in need who could not pay anywhere near enough to cover the costs of this care. The preferred-provider policy aimed to end this cycle by investing upfront to establish a firm foundation of primary and preventative care so that the community would ultimately become healthier and less in need of treatments for emergencies and chronic illness. This approach turned on a lightbulb in my mind that remains illuminated to this day as an ideal that we have yet to achieve. Could healthcare policies such as this, driven by our own government, truly make a difference? Could I forever be a part of this?

As I began working with Pediatrics 2000, I unknowingly entered the world of managed care through my preferred provider designation. Managed care is a uniquely American construct that has significantly morphed since its origins in the late nineteenth century, accelerating as if on adrenaline in the 1980s and 1990s. The basic concept is simple. The managed care company acts like a general contractor in a building project. It contracts directly with the customer—the large company or union—to provide predetermined medical services instead of a house or building. It takes full responsibility for the end product of these health services and acts as a buffer between the patients and clinicians when it comes to any major financial negotiations. It gathers the subcontractors—in this case, doctors, nurses, and medical facilities instead of carpenters, roofers, and electricians—on behalf of the patient customer, who, like a homeowner providing residence to family members, then offers these benefits to their members.

In theory, everyone should be happy with the arrangement if the objective is to provide the best built facility or home for the inhabitants at the lowest cost possible. By assuming the role of general contractor, a good managed care company can control costs while providing high-quality, comprehensive health services through the large pool of participating health professionals under their banner. Through the intermediary of the managed care entity, physicians potentially benefit by collectively contracting out their medical services to larger organizations such as unions, companies, and even the government.

In the early twentieth century, this guaranteed patient base was the main driver of the first managed care arrangements. Individuals choosing to receive their health services through this arrangement pay a predetermined portion of the premium or membership fee in exchange for unlimited access to healthcare services by the assigned physicians. In theory, this is a win-win for all parties because the doctors are guaranteed to have an upfront income, the employers can better manage the soaring costs of their employees' health benefits, and the patient members obtain high-quality medical care at a lower cost than they could arrange if they negotiated on their own.

As these managed care arrangements proceeded through the Great Depression era of the 1930s, there were only a few private insurance options. The main alternative was the nonprofit Blue Cross and Blue Shield plans. Around World War II, early managed care companies, such as Kaiser and Health Insurance Plan of Greater New York, coordinated their clinical services through a network of prepaid group practices referred to as health maintenance organizations (HMOs). The doctors and hospitals in the HMO network agree to accept lower rates for plan members or policyholders. The policyholding members were required to select a primary care physician (PCP) from within the HMO's network of participating providers.

The rationale behind HMO requirements for each member to select a PCP is financially motivated and not based on the clinical grounds that having a PCP improves care. Since the 1970s, when healthcare costs began to rise significantly, there has thus been a concerted focus by private and public health insurance companies, employers, government, and policymakers to reduce costs by implementing processes that impact the ideal port of entry of the patient into the medical system—the visits with the primary general physician. Under these policies, PCPs were designated as "gatekeepers" appointed to the onerous task of literally "holding the fort" against the onslaught of the economic foes, known as waste and high-cost medical services. Therefore, in addition to the patient being restricted to using only providers in the network, one of HMOs' main cost-control features is that the gatekeeper PCP approves and coordinates only essential referrals to specialists and hospitals deemed "essential."

The only other private health insurance option was indemnity plans—aka fee-for-service plans—that function similarly to fire or homeowner's insurance. The policy owner pays an annual premium with the benefit that the insurance company will pay a predetermined percentage of the fee-for-service medical bill for any doctor or hospital the policy-owning patient chooses. These plans were generally more expensive than HMOs because of the level of the policy owner's freedom of health provider choice. In sharp contrast to HMOs, most indemnity plans did not even require that the policy owner designate a primary physician.

The HMOs were all initially nonprofit and viewed by organized medicine—such as the American Medical Association and, by extension, local and state medical societies—as a threat to their jurisdiction over US healthcare. In the 1950s, these medical societies originally tried to compete with the group practice HMOs by creating their own alliances with individual healthcare providers, known as independent practice associations (IPAs). Like private insurance indemnity plans, the IPA physicians were reimbursed on a predetermined fee-for-service basis. This meant that each service a provider rendered had a price tag, and there were essentially no limitations to how many items the healthcare provider could put on a patient's invoice or bill of services.

Eventually, many IPAs tried to keep costs down by implementing a capitation system, in which providers were paid a monthly amount per patient regardless of the services they provided.

Through the 1970s, the federal government under President Nixon stimulated employer-based health insurance through the 1973 Health Maintenance Organization Act. In this political environment, the group HMOs blossomed as employers were required to provide two federally approved HMOs in addition to indemnity plans to each employee. With this mandate, private industry and the government became allies, thus ending local and state medical societies' attempt to compete against the HMOs. After President Carter established federal regulations to approve HMOs, the HMOs never looked back as their numbers boomed until 2008. In the 1990s, the government joined the bandwagon by procuring HMO arrangements for Medicare and Medicaid, which increased the number of Medicare beneficiaries under HMO contracts from 1.3 to 6.3 million over the course of a decade.

In the late 1970s through the 1980s, the variation on the HMO model, known as a preferred provider organization (PPO), emerged. This is the very same designation that I first achieved at Pediatrics 2000 through New York State Medicaid. The managed care models contracted directly with designated individual providers or facilities to create their provider networks. Compared to HMOs, PPOs have larger provider networks with greater geographic presence, do not require PCPs to act as gatekeepers for referrals to specialists or hospitals, and cover out-of-network providers. An even stricter version of this PPO model is known as an exclusive provider organization (EPO), which does not cover any costs if the patient seeks care outside the managed care entity. The EPO also abandons the use of a gatekeeper or even the requirement to select a PCP.

The main restrictions of the HMOs having fallen to the wayside in these PPO models were not without a downside, as the costs to the policyholders were significantly higher. Despite being more expensive, by the 1990s, driven by their innate ability to contract with large companies with offices spread across the country, the PPOs' market share steadily surpassed that of the private HMOs.

After a one-year dive into private practice with Pediatrics 2000, I took a three-year hiatus from thinking about the financial administration of medical care during my fellowship training in pediatric cardiology at Columbia. My next tangible and career-long exposure to managed care through the HMO model abruptly reemerged when I accepted my position with the NYPH network and started my outpatient practice in New York's Hudson Valley.

As a full-time faculty member at Babies and Children's Hospital, and because my practice therefore belonged not to me but to the hospital, I was enrolled as one of over 1,000 academic physicians in the Columbia-Presbyterian Physician Network (CPPN). The CPPN served as a management agency that administered the day-to-day operations of the outpatient practices for all the physician members. This alleviated the burden on the doctors of having to think about staffing, supplies, and the day-to-day details of running a practice.

Though this practice-management feature was much appreciated, the most notable feature of CPPN was that it could collectively bargain for better reimbursements from the managed care HMOs on the behalf of the member physicians. Through the guidance of my administrative advisor at the local Horton Hospital, Mr. Jay Wilson, I was introduced to the practical applications of this feature within the first month of hanging up my shingle. During a weekly meeting in his office, he laid out some blank spreadsheets on a table as he looked up at me like a proud teacher with a new student.

"It is time that you formally set up the fees for your individual services that we will bill to the insurance companies."

I stared at him with my mouth hung open before uttering, "What? I was never taught how to do this. How do I know what to charge?"

"Well, that's where I come in handy," he boasted with an excited twinkle in his eye. "I have collected examples of what the local adult cardiologists charge for each item of service they provide. Each item is designated by a code, whether it is the actual visit or a test. Just choose the highest amount reimbursed from my survey and add at least 20 percent as your official fee."

"Why 20 percent? Where did you get that figure?" I asked, now full of curiosity.

He paused, as if holding back the big reveal. "Ah, you forget, I worked at Columbia with the dean, where I negotiated fees with the HMOs on behalf of the CPPN physicians. Because you are a CPPN member, you are entitled to higher reimbursements than our local doctors. I was actually recruited up here to try and do the same thing for the community physicians under our new four-hospital system."

OK, so these are the rules of the game, I thought to myself as I walked out of his office with the pile of spreadsheets rolled under my arm.

ECONOMIES OF SCALE

Over the next two years that I remained a full-time faculty member at Columbia, my enhanced fees under the CPPN remained the bedrock of my ability for my fledgling practice to survive and grow. When I officially received the blessing from Dr. Gersony to become a part-time faculty member and attempt to run my outpatient practice independent of Columbia, the rules changed. I was now required to meet with the local representatives from the health insurance companies to negotiate my fees as an individual private practice. I no longer had the clout of the CPPN directly behind me, but the CPPN had filled my sails with winds that had blown me out into the open ocean, where I would sink or swim.

For the next decade, I remained steady and afloat while the hospitals, medical practices, and health insurance companies began to merge with each other in an attempt to better compete in the patient marketplace for the healthcare dollar. By 2012, the pool of local health insurance representatives I met with annually to negotiate my fees dried up. Only a handful remained, and they only talked with the large practices and hospitals. The wind in my sails went still.

After a few months of getting nowhere by paddling alone, and concerned that I could be stuck in limbo for quite a while, I attempted to catch another good wind by hopping aboard a newly formed local IPA model. By 2010, several well-respected tertiary medical institutions, including Mount Sinai and Montefiore, were reaching out to suburban communities like mine to enroll private practice physicians and local hospitals into their IPA networks. As competition amongst the major urban institutions escalated, the Greater Hudson Valley was now on their radars as a potential untapped patient marketplace. Starting in 2010, abandoned by the HMOs' negotiating teams, several of my local physician colleagues had already signed up with at least one of these IPAs. They now encouraged me to do the same.

Since the original IPAs of the 1950s, the newer IPAs evolved to become more of a large medical practice management agency that offered single doctors or small practices the chance to compete more effectively with the onslaught of the larger mega-groups. The modern IPAs are varied in their legal and corporate structures, which allow them to fulfill several valuable functions. They act as an additional intermediary between the HMOs and physicians under their association to help contract the collective medical services of the participating clinicians to HMOs, while the doctors may still remain operationally private in their own offices.

Though clearly directed by legislation, such as the Federal Trade Commission Act, that prohibits the IPA from negotiating with the health insurance companies the providers participate in on behalf of all the IPA member physicians as one group, they are allowed to collectively negotiate when implementing a capitation financial model. Despite these limitations that essentially forbid the formation of physician unions, in the real world, the combined clout of many individual smaller doctors creates a significant degree of leverage when sitting down with the insurance company representatives that now ignore the small medical groups to discuss reimbursement fee-for-service schedules and capitation or flat fee rates.

The less-debated amenity of the IPA is that they can coordinate management service organization (MSO) resources. An MSO is essentially a cooperative entity that harnesses the buying power of many smaller medical practices under one large umbrella to provide economies of scale when financing supplies, technology, and personnel management services. I literally have seen the price of a box of blank printer paper sold by a supply company to an MSO for one-tenth the price I paid as a small practice. With the exponential growth of separate compliance requirements over the last few decades, the MSO can also hire staff dedicated to alleviating the oppressive burden of licensing and regulations for insurance and hospital privileges, physician billing, diagnostic testing, electronic medical records, patient privacy, marketing, and employment requirements. In theory, health providers should have much more freedom physically, intellectually, and emotionally to return their focus to patient care.

When I first met John McEwan in 2010, he was newly recruited by Montefiore with the main objective of establishing an IPA network from the Bronx out to the southern New York region, including the Hudson Valley. In recognition of both my experience with the CPPN and my success establishing high-quality pediatric subspecialty care in the local community, the administration at Montefiore requested that I meet with Mr. McEwan to share my experiences. In his well-tailored dark suit, this middle-aged, slightly graying, affable administrator sat with me in his city office or my office conference room in several two-hour sessions to pick my brain about the essential building blocks of an IPA in the community I served. As I provided him with insights procured through a decade of my experiences, he took copious notes.

After our final meeting, he indicated that it would be some time before he could create a fully functional IPA for Montefiore, but he specifically stressed his appreciation for my contributions. "When we are up and running, I will contact you right away so that you can be one of the first to join our IPA. I know that it has been tough for you to be on your own lately. The IPA will help ensure reasonable reimbursement levels and provide needed operational relief for your practice in this increasingly tumultuous healthcare marketplace." I was encouraged that I, in some small way, contributed to regional healthcare reform.

Four years later, my new manager, Kerry-Ann, brought to my attention a meeting to be held at one of the local hospitals for physicians interested in joining a new IPA to the Hudson Valley. The meeting was run by a Mr. John McEwan. She asked if I knew him. I was stunned. I had received no advanced notice nor any feedback for that matter since he and I last met. Honestly, I had completely forgotten our series of meetings. My curiosity piqued, I asked her to sign both of us up for the IPA introductory meeting. Actually, at that time, my interest was more than casual. We were still operating as a small private practice with almost no ability to successfully negotiate our own reimbursements from the health insurers. Initially, I hired some consultants to help, but to no avail.

On a late summer evening in 2014, Kerry-Ann and I sat quietly in the back row of the newly renovated, fresh-paint-scented, St. Luke's Cornwall Hospital's main meeting room. I recognized about two dozen other local doctors amidst the audience. They represented the last of a dying breed—the single practitioners or two-doctor to three-doctor practices. By the end of the Montefiore IPA meeting, Kerry-Ann and I were completely convinced that this IPA was sufficiently well established and that we should strongly consider joining. I stayed back until most of the attendees left and reintroduced myself to Mr. McEwan.

He had aged somewhat, but he clearly appeared more confident than when we first met.

"Hello, again. Do you remember me?" I asked politely.

"Dr. Fethke! I thought that I recognized you in the audience. How have you been?" he inquired somewhat awkwardly.

"We are fine, but more than ever, I definitely could benefit from participating in an IPA such as the one you just presented. Looks very similar to that which we discussed several years ago," I hinted.

He paused, as if regretful. "Yes, many of the elements you and I discussed have been incorporated. The problem is that you and your practice are likely not to benefit at all from this IPA model. This is why I have not contacted you."

"I don't understand," came my abrupt retort.

"The basis of our IPA design is that it encourages practitioners that are not yet meeting certain standards of care to join so that they can adopt our tertiary institution's best practices and thus improve their overall medical care, while lowering costs and becoming more efficient. Since you and I met, we have become a federally accredited ACO, which has to meet certain government-defined benchmarks. If our IPA members provide good care at a cost that is significantly lower than before they joined, they can share in some of these savings and increase their reimbursement levels through the HMOs. As an ACO, our IPA members must officially demonstrate such improvements to tap into these incentivized payment schedules," he explained with honest clarity but obvious disappointment. "Many of the doctors that came to the meeting today have room for significant improvements, according to our ACO-based IPA arrangements. This doesn't work for you. You're already the standard of care in your field in this region. You have no significant potential to improve your operations to attain such incentives through our IPA. Essentially, you've already done a great job. You should be proud."

I stood in place, somewhat shocked by this encounter. As we drove home, Kerry-Ann and I reflected that this whole process was extremely counterintuitive. It basically rewarded those practitioners who practiced well below the standard of care, instead of encouraging those who performed well to continue onward and lead as a local example to the others. It was analogous to exclusively rewarding only a D-level student who finally got a C on a test while ignoring the student who always worked hard to maintain an A or A-plus average. Why should the A student not become discouraged in such an environment? What could stimulate the struggling A student to continue to maintain A-level performance or even to remain at the school? Who thought of such an IPA in the first place?

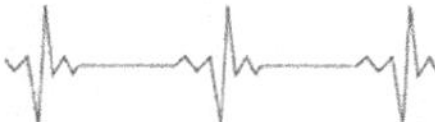

After my decades of experiences with HMOs and their byproducts, such as IPAs and PPOs, I have concluded that managed care has fallen far short of its objectives. It was originally proposed to Americans as the best way to run our healthcare system by balancing runaway costs with the need to still provide excellent healthcare. At times, I confess that I am even more cynical and wonder if the policymakers behind managed care have become lost and confused or really ever intended to place the quality of healthcare on par with their cost-containment strategies. From my vantage point on the ground level of community medical care, I am increasingly perplexed by the HMOs' cost-reduction strategies. They just don't make sense in the real world.

The most striking example of mixed-up priorities in creating a healthcare budget amongst the managed care entities is exemplified by their ubiquitous adoption of a "for-profit" business model starting in the 1970s. Once companies such as the Blue Cross Blue Shield plans caved into the pressure to compete with private insurance companies, the race to keep the shareholders happy officially began. When these companies all started sharing features of the HMO models, the for-profit component became the driving force behind their cost-containment efforts.

A simple mathematical analysis at an elementary school level could predict that, if a certain percentage of the money generated by medical services had to be skimmed off the top and committed to shareholders, then only two options were available. The providers either had to increase the volumes of their services or overhead costs had to be reduced. This led to reductions in the salaries and benefits of health providers through negotiated contracts on a reduced fee-for-service or capitation basis. Enter the administrative tool known as "denial of services" to significantly reduce or even eliminate many more expensive diagnostic tests and treatment options available to the providers. Push the limits one step further, and denial of care based on "preexisting conditions" was born. I am still waiting for someone to convincingly explain to me how these maneuvers actually improve medical care.

The HMOs along with other health insurers camouflaged their service restriction policies under the seemingly more palatable description of "oversight" responsibilities. The public has seen straight through this charade. Originally, this task was assigned to the PCPs, who soon found themselves trapped in a conflict of interest between what was best for their patients versus what saved the most money for the HMO that paid them. Medical education does not teach a physician how to factor cost into the equation of disease management or prevention. We are taught to provide the best care possible on behalf of our patients, who expect nothing less. This "gatekeeper" role that defined HMOs was thus a nonstarter before the policy even left the gate. When this situation eroded the patients' trust of their PCPs, ineffectively as it was saving the HMOs money, and policyholders returned to private indemnity plans with more patient choice, the HMOs readily abandoned this feature of their insurance policies.

The policyholders did not suddenly disappear from the scene, forcing the HMOs to persist in their cost-reduction attempts. They shifted their oversight responsibilities to nonclinical administrators of the HMO companies and focused a disproportionate amount of their energy on controlling the practice patterns of the health providers through financial incentives or punishments. The doctors who utilized below a certain threshold of predetermined tests such as CT scans, and thus tapped into less of the HMO coffers, were rewarded with a financial bonus. Those that overutilized such services were the target of punitive measures in the form of salary reductions. Again, the PCPs or other physicians were caught off-guard because their clinical education remained void of financial constraints. They all too often feel as if they have no choice but to work through an HMO because these companies now control the lion's share of the healthcare market.

"What do you think about the newer docs coming out of school with high student loan debts when they join the mega-groups or work for the HMOs?" I opened the conversation at a small physician gathering one weekend as we sat down to a socially distanced bonfire.

"I don't blame them. I could never have started a successful practice by myself in the current healthcare environment. The big guys hold all the cards nowadays. I don't even know how much longer I can hold out," professed an obviously tired local pediatrician as the pizzas and beers from a local brewery were served.

Many of my colleagues are so exasperated by the HMOs' denials of the tests or medications they order that they are increasingly discouraged. "I can't practice good medicine like this. If something doesn't change, I'm out of here. I may change my career altogether," screamed a middle-aged physician colleague of mine trying to get an ultrasound test for one of his patients.

As the HMOs adopted these finance-driven strategies, the public saw them as the enemy of good healthcare, rather than the savior. The original lack of physician choice and the need for a referral to a specialist was a hard pill to swallow, but these newer money-saving strategies seemed to cross the lines of decency, especially when so many others were siphoning huge profits off the system.

By the 1990s, the court of public opinion swayed the HMOs to blur the lines regarding patient choice of doctors and hospitals amongst their categories of pure HMO, PPOs, and EPOs. The miscalculation of the HMOs was their assumption that the now more-appeased policyholders would not mind the introduction of even harsher budgeting strategies. They soon realized that their for-profit HMOs, the corporations they serviced, and the healthcare providers and institutions that worked with them were all viewed as prioritizing profits over quality patient care. This sentiment was heightened and concentrated more than ever during the COVID-19 pandemic, when individuals suffered medically and economically while health insurers recorded record profits.[17]

As one of my patients who just lost a grandparent so eloquently expressed behind a wall of tears, "How many people like my grandfather might have survived or avoided COVID-19 if the managed care companies had allocated even a small portion of their profits to battling this public enemy?"

I am somewhat surprised that the policymakers could not see the basic weakness in the managed care model. When big money is to be made, it ultimately always comes down to greed. When I undertook my largest building projects, I learned that the integrity of the process always came down to having an honest and capable general contractor (GC). Good GCs are easy to identify because they are extremely transparent and organized before accepting and starting a project. Their proposals leave little, if any, doubt in the division of responsibilities for all parties involved. They use high-quality materials

---

17 Burns, Joseph, "The Pandemic One Year In: Despite Large Profits in 2020 Health Insurers See Volatility Ahead," Managed Healthcare Executive, Mar 11, 2021, Vol 31, Issue 3 (online), https://www.managedhealthcareexecutive.com/view/the-pandemic-one-year-in-despite-large-profits-in-2020-health-insurers-see-volatility-ahead.

and skilled labor. The finances are crystal clear, as are any contingency plans. There are no hidden or blanket clauses in the contracts, and they remain approachable throughout the project, including regularly scheduled communications. The end product is often completed ahead of schedule and becomes a wonderful home or medical facility in which all are proud to live or work.

A bad GC on the other hand tries to make more profit by "low-balling" the initial cost proposal and using the cheapest labor and materials along the way. The process is frustrating for all involved, and the communication and transparency are very poor. The completion of the end product is often delayed. The building is rarely even inhabitable without further alterations.

Many managed care organizations have taken the path of the less capable or less scrupulous GC whose goal is to make off with as much money as possible, regardless of the quality or structural integrity of the final building. To maximize profits, the HMOs have consistently promoted the cheapest alternatives in testing and medications. Because their arrangements with employers or other large groups allow them exclusive access to large pools of patients, they are able to squeeze as much work out of the care providers for the lowest reimbursement levels the market will allow. Even with this advantage, mergers between managed care companies and the exponential growth of their operations have stressed the system and led to many poor management decisions.

Michael Reese was a normal and active boy until about nine years old. After it was clear that he appeared to be clumsier and weaker, his parents took him to several different doctors who ultimately diagnosed him with a progressive form of nerve and muscle disease—a muscular dystrophy called Duchenne's. Over the years, his situation became progressively worse. Initially, he required a walker. Then, a couple of years later, he needed a regular wheelchair to get around. Eventually, he needed a special machine to help him breathe at night. Within the past few years, he needs this machine every moment of his life.

Around the time he first came to me to make sure his heart muscles were not affected by his disease, we noticed that he was developing a severe bend—essentially a collapsing—of his spine due to extreme weakness of his back and abdominal muscles. This scoliosis was so severe that when he sat in his wheelchair, his head was still below the back of the seat. It is not hard to imagine why this situation also compressed his ribcage and lungs, making it even harder to breathe.

Initially, no one wanted to offer him surgery to straighten his back because they thought that his lifespan would be too short to benefit from the procedure. More to the point, he was deemed "too high a risk" to even survive the procedure by most doctors and institutions. The insurance companies therefore felt that they had justification to deny paying for the procedure. The family and I could not accept this as a done deal.

I therefore called many of my colleagues from different institutions to see if they could help. Eventually, we created a team of specialists in scoliosis surgery, lung disease, nerve and muscle disease, intensive care, heart doctors, special anesthesiologists, and highly skilled breathing and rehabilitation therapists. It took months for all of us to put this team together. His mother also contacted local politicians to put pressure on the insurance company to cover the costs related to his surgery.

Michael not only survived the surgery—he thrived. With the support of metal rods to straighten his spine and excellent lung care, his head now rose higher than the back of his seat, and he could breathe much more freely and with less dependence on the respirator machine. More importantly, he was now smiling again.

That was over 10 years ago, and he is now in his late 20s. The quality of his life was much improved by the scoliosis surgery, but within the past two years, his disease has progressed. He has become weaker and is now fully dependent on the breathing machine. His heart has also now started to weaken. To make matters even worse, the insurance company has steadily withdrawn home nursing support, so his older brother stepped in to become his main caretaker.

Recently, he lost the ability to swallow even soft food by mouth. He lost so much weight that his heart and lungs became even more compromised. At one point, after he ended up choking and breathing in his food, he ended up in the hospital with life-threatening pneumonia. He once again beat this infection too. He admitted that he was afraid to eat and concerned about his nutrition, but he did not want to undergo another surgery to place in a tube through his abdomen to give him nutrition directly into his stomach. He was stuck between two difficult choices. We also again had to fight with the insurance companies for the same reasons they initially denied his back surgery a decade earlier.

Because of our long relationship with each other, including my attending most of his birthday parties since he turned 20, I was able to convince him to have the feeding tube placed. My wife, Viyada, a gifted and experienced gastroenterologist, now manages his nutrition, and I am glad to say that he has regained his weight and looks much healthier. In fact, he now complains in good humor that he looks too heavy. Even more miraculously, his heart has become much stronger. He is smiling again and refocused his energies on a podcast that he hosts as a champion for people with disabilities.

After surviving all of this, including the recent COVID-19 pandemic and jumping through hurdles, last month, his health insurance company terminated payments for his physical therapy. They declared his therapy to be unnecessary because they conclude that there is no hope for improvement—only maintenance of his current situation at best. Needless to say, we are all ready to challenge this opinion and persist.

I am not opposed to minimizing economically wasteful healthcare practices. My main contention with the managed care system is that it focuses on cost-reduction solutions that are extremely misguided. Their solutions directly and adversely impact the quality of care of many patients like Matthew. Instead of achieving effective cost control, their increasing bureaucracies added additional costs, lack of productivity, and more waste to the system. I am convinced that there are much better avenues to saving money that also allow for the maintenance or improvements in the quality of care. I wonder whether the HMOs just do not see these alternatives or simply choose not to venture into less lucrative, more controversial, or less politically advantageous solutions.

Several of the approaches that make the most sense to me as a physician and educator are briefly mentioned here. Later sections are devoted to fuller review of some of these options. They include the following: reducing the physicians' student loan burden; reforming the medicolegal liability process that fosters defensive medical care practices; incorporating medical economics and policy into the medical education curriculum; simplifying the mountain of regulatory requirements; fostering and promoting a more robust primary and preventative care physician workforce; expanding and facilitating the integration of ancillary healthcare professionals; reinvigorating and expanding our public health sector; and capping the exorbitant costs of medications and medical technology. I would limit the profit margin of shareholders in any industry that directly impacts healthcare, including health insurance, pharmaceutical, and medical device companies. The remaining profits should be mandatorily returned to the front lines of healthcare for education, primary care, and infrastructure updates. These and similar tactics are not punitive in nature. The health providers are not constantly attacked, and the patients are more able to access the services that represent the best care possible in our nation.

The other main flaw in the current design of managed care that I believe can no longer be ignored is the premise that health insurance should be so tightly connected to one's employer. Though the initial well-intentioned benefit policy was meant to place the onus of ensuring employees' healthcare coverage squarely on the back of the employer, all parties involved are no longer able to assure or tolerate this arrangement. Several large corporations including General Motors suffered financially under the burden of rising healthcare costs for their current and retired workforce. As the COVID-19 pandemic harshly demonstrated, when unemployment rises significantly, thousands of people suddenly lose their healthcare benefits at the time they most need medical attention. In the end, the whole system virtually crumbles under the additional weight of providing medical services without a mechanism for reimbursement. Even worse, the health of the entire population is severely reduced for years to come. We urgently need an alternative health coverage system that is not intrinsically linked to employment.

MANAGED CARE ON STEROIDS

By the 2000s, the federal government could no longer ignore the elephant in the room. The enormous national deficit was in large part fueled by rising healthcare costs of an increasingly older and disabled population. Their solution[18] was to reorganize and build upon the HMO model of managed care. Enter the ACO, the culmination of an initial concept proposed in 2006 by the government entity responsible for advising Congress on how to run the Medicare program—the Medicare Payment Advisory Committee. By 2009, the ACO philosophy came to the scene as a major component of the ACA, often referred to as Obamacare. Since consumer confidence in the 1990s opposed the HMOs' focus on cost reductions through limitations on patient members' choice of providers and restrictions of often necessary medical services, the ACO model needed to directly address these concerns.

18 Gold, Jenny, "Urgent Care," *KFF Health News*, September 14, 2015 (online), https://khn.org/news/aco-accountable-care-organization-faq/.

The ACO concept was therefore designed to both lift the restrictions on health service referrals and return to an emphasis on improving healthcare quality and outcomes that had been recklessly abandoned by the HMOs. Most notably, the ACO structure decisively returned to an emphasis on primary and preventative care as a bedrock of the healthcare system.

As with all service-oriented systems, the ACO needed a business model to support its operations. The Medicare policymakers, through the Department of Health and Human Services (DHHS), essentially chose to place the burden of both quality and cost of care directly on the back of the primary healthcare providers. The makeup of these providers was deliberately broad, ranging from groups of clinicians to extensive networks of health facilities and support services.

The DHHS program delegated the responsibility of creating guidelines to become an ACO to the Center for Medicare and Medicaid Services (CMS), who established the Medicare Shared Savings Program (MSSP) in 2011. This opened the door in 2012 for ACOs to contract directly with the Medicare system. This may all sound too complicated, but the rules of the game essentially boil down to two main components—the achievement of specific health-quality benchmarks and the reduction of expenditures from the Medicare trust funds.

The incentive or "carrot on the stick" for any entity to seek ACO status from the Secretary of DHHS is fairly basic. An officially recognized ACO can now share in a significant portion of any savings to the Medicare funds attributed to the ACO's efforts. The catch is that the ACO has to both exceed a predetermined amount of savings as defined by the MSSP and also meet enough of the CMS-defined quality benchmarks. CMS essentially retains the sole power to move the carrot closer or farther away by altering these savings thresholds and benchmark criteria. In the initial pilot trials of the ACO model, these criteria were so onerous that only nine out of 32 entities were successful in attaining savings and remaining functional. This led to significant reductions in the number of CMS-designated quality benchmarks for the subsequent ACOs. Needless to say, the ACO model remains a work in progress.

I believe that it is important to reiterate that literally in the federal government's attempts to pull the nation out of debt in 2009, the Economic Recovery Act focused a large part of their efforts on streamlining healthcare operations. The policymakers decided they had to publicly recognize that the inefficiencies of the US healthcare system were such chronic major contributors to our economy's problems that they had no choice but to finally address them through legislation. One of the first legislative steps they took to improve the healthcare situation through the Recovery Act was a push to establish a strong, consistent, and transparent electronic version of the paper medical chart. This gave rise to the Health Information Technology for Economic and Clinical Health (HITECH) Act. The main objectives were twofold—protect the privacy of patients' personal and medical information contained in these electronic charts and encourage the economically efficient use of this medical information to promote the health of individuals and the general population.

To jumpstart the adoption of electronic health records (EHRs), in 2011, CMS rolled out Medicare and Medicaid EHR incentive programs. These incentive programs were wrapped around a package of specific criteria that had to be met in three separate phases over several months—adoption of an approved EHR system, demonstration of appropriate use and data gathering with the EHR system, and promotion of quality healthcare. In the trenches, this whole program was referred to with some degree of disdain as the Meaningful Use (MU) criteria.

As each stage of the MU objectives were fulfilled, individual clinicians or medical facilities could obtain significant financial reimbursements—the incentives—to offset the software, hardware, and decreased productivity costs of implementing these EHR systems. Despite the often overwhelming bureaucracy required to adopt EHRs through these MU programs, within less than a decade, the prevalence of EHR systems increased[19] tenfold, and they were universally installed in the nation's clinical settings.

Currently, the ACOs could not operate or even exist if it were not for the EHR systems because they are so tied into their finances. I have no doubt that one of the main reasons my private practice was approached by several hospitals, large practices, and IPAs during this decade was the potential of thousands of dollars of incentive reimbursements that would now pass from our doctors to any new controlling entity. By 2018, this MU term left such a bad taste in the clinicians' mouths, CMS renamed it the Promoting Interoperability Program.

In the name of purported transparency, the CMS employed the ACOs' ubiquitous EHR systems to administer the essentially whole new language, including MU and Patient-Centered Medical Home (PCMH), they created to track all the components of the CMS requirements.[20] This expanded glossary of managed care terms was subsequently wrapped around the regionally defined standards of medical care and, when available, supported by the latest medical literature. These standards are classified as "evidence-based best practices."

These best practices are then introduced to the clinicians operating under a particular ACO-designated institution by creating algorithms for them to follow, like a recipe in a cookbook. These algorithms are codified in the ACO's EHR platform and reinforced administratively through routine orientation sessions, known as medical "in-services." The basic goal of this best-practices model is to establish uniformity

19 Tandon, Sanjeev, "Public Health and Electronic Health Records Meaningful Use," Course Hero, 2022, https://www.coursehero.com/file/p1tcm1br/CDC-the-meaningful-use-standard-is-made-up-of-five-pillars-Improving-quality/.

20 "Guide to Quality Performance Scoring Methods for Accountable Care Organizations," Centers for Medicare & Medicaid Services, 2012 (online), https://www.cms.gov/Medicare/Medicare-Fee-for-Service-Payment/sharedsavingsprogram/Downloads/2012-11-ACO-quality-scoring-supplement.pdf.

of the healthcare process in regards to common medical conditions treated by the participating clinicians. In fact, if a physician does not adhere consistently to these best practices, they run the risk of being called to task by their superiors.

This somewhat militaristic approach aims to improve consistency in healthcare delivery but potentially sacrifices flexibility and personal style—the art of medicine. The truth is, as all physicians were taught on the first day of their clinical education, there is never just one way to manage a particular medical condition. These best practices ironically may miss the point that medicine is not just a science with hard facts but is in fact a profession based on some inherent variations in practice, derived from one's cumulative experiences during training and practice.

Good leadership will realize this and view best practices as purely guidelines and not an ultimatum. However, when these large entities become too big, flexibility is often sacrificed in favor of consistency. Without good physician leaders, this consistency begins to look more and more like rigid dogma.

Because of the ACO model's preoccupation with saving or recouping monies, the historically supported standard of the medical note—now in electronic form as part of the EHR—has strayed far from its original intended purpose of clearly documenting and communicating the physician's encounter with a patient and the resulting treatment plan. It now mainly functions as a document that helps track the multiple highly bureaucratic MU, Medical Home, and Shared Incentive guidelines established for the ACOs by CMS. The actual clinical care of a particular patient is often buried so deep beneath these regulatory items that it is hard to decipher. The medical notes have essentially become useless. I often wonder if anyone knows how to write a good note anymore, and I know that my students are initially surprised when I put such emphasis on this skill.

When I first read this medical note from one of my colleagues, I couldn't believe my eyes. Why was so much nonsense so deliberately included in this EHR on our mutual patient? In the last part of their consult note, in the Assessment and Plan section, it read as follows:

- Reviewing chart (prior notes, new documentations, consult letters, labs performed in interim since last seen)
- Visit in the office including history review, physical exam, counseling for plans going forward based on history, physical, clinical status of patient
- Documentation in chart for maintenance of records
- Sending new prescriptions to pharmacy for patient care
- Creation and sending out of consult letters to outside physicians for communication including the pediatrician and other specialists who are co-managing the patient

For what it's worth, these items could simply have been summarized by writing, "See, everyone, I did do doctor stuff. I did my job." The more I read over these words, the more embarrassed, insulted, and angry I became. A very competent doctor had obviously been instructed by a medical records advisor to include these words in his note so that they could clearly document that MU criteria was met for adequate reimbursements.

All of these actions described are implicitly obvious to anyone who understands even a miniscule amount about what doctors do every day with each patient we meet. This documentation adds nothing at all to the value of the record, which is supposed to be done on behalf of the patient. The note is not meant to be a blatant inventory of work done for invoicing. In my opinion, it is disrespectful to the doctors and patients to intrude into this private document with such gibberish. I wondered if I was overreacting until I realized that no other profession stoops so low to justify the value of their work. Why not just come out fully and start this section by adding the following?

This is why I should be properly paid:

- I went to college and decided to pursue a premedical course
- After successfully completing my premedical requirements in college, I applied for medical school
- I got into medical school
- I completed medical school (thus becoming a legitimate doctor), internship, and residency (didn't sleep much)
- I then completed a specialty fellowship in pediatric cardiology (slept even less)
- I'm now a REAL DOCTOR because I care for patients in my office and the hospitals (I still don't get enough sleep)

One late fall evening in 2018, on our way home from work, Viyada—a private practice adult gastroenterologist—and I were talking to each other over our respective car phones.

"You sound tired. What kept you so late in the office today?" I asked.

She burst out a steady response. "It's because of these crazy MU requirements. When a patient comes to see me complaining of abdominal pain, I now have to stop my history-taking and physical exam to click multiple additional questions in a separate window or module in the EHR. On top of my standard evaluation and care for their abdominal pain, the MU requirements mandate that I now have to ask about and clearly document the patient's cigarette use, vaccination status, and other information that may not have anything to do with their chief complaint. I have to do all this each time they visit me, even if they already filled out this information on a recent visit or they have an established general primary physician whose main role is to handle such preventative issues. This slows everything down for me and the patients."

The EHRs of subspecialty physicians such as my wife and I are routinely scrutinized by insurance companies and the inspectors of CMS to determine whether or not any given doctor satisfactorily meets the MU standards. If they have not, the physician is now open to punitive measures, including denying or downgrading their reimbursements. Because the MU modules in the EHR inherently demand extra time on the part of the physician, well above and beyond that required to deal with the actual issue for which the patient is seeing the specialist—the abdominal pain in my wife's patient's case—you can see why this system is cumbersome at best and detracts from patient care at worst.

There is no reimbursement incentive provided to lengthen each patient visit to account for the added MU process. To the contrary, the whole matter is handled in exactly the opposite manner, in the punitive form of decreased reimbursements should even one item of the designated MU criteria be omitted or incomplete. My colleagues and I are damned if we do and damned if we don't with this ridiculous requirement. We lose money if we spend the added time to complete the EHR-based MU materials because we are forced to see fewer patients or perform fewer procedures per day than before the advent of MU. If we maintain our previous patient and procedure volumes, we spend late night and weekend hours filling in the MU data or risk the punitive reimbursement deductions. This whole pattern is not tenable for the long term without physician burnout.

Finally, in this type of ACO environment, these MU "report cards" are used to determine if the ACO as a whole has in fact achieved the quality standards and improved healthcare outcomes required to maintain the ACO designation. The specific outcomes chosen to represent improved healthcare in a population under a given ACO's jurisdiction essentially boil down to items on multiple progress reports.

I repeatedly concluded that these reports are not valid because many of these items are not even medically relevant to the quality objective considered. They are thus more a reflection on a doctor's or clinical group's ability to race through clicking off the MU boxes than they are representative of actual clinical practice patterns. This resistance to using the MU formats in current EHRs has corrupted the data. I can't count how many times I heard an EHR instructor in a practice or hospital advise the following: "When you see these MU-related questions in our EHRs, don't stop to think about it. Just always fill in the box for the first item in this History section, and the last box for the Review of Systems section. This will save time, and no one will notice the difference." In the research world, the saying is "Garbage in leads to garbage out." The report cards have become inherently flawed and useless.

My physician colleagues and I find this system absolutely frustrating. We feel we are needlessly distracted from our main focus—truly meaningful patient care. Essentially, we sense that an outsider who is not privy to what the physicians actually do has been self-appointed to be the judge of merit or worth. The outcome criteria of MU have been predetermined by bureaucrats from the 50th floor penthouse. Given how obvious it should be to ask the doctors and patients who work on the ground floors to contribute more of their opinions on truly relevant information, it's not surprising that many doctors have become cynical about the whole EHR, ACO, and MU setup. Clinicians feel like there remains the stain of an ulterior motive behind all of this busywork. The main purpose of the ACO appears to be less focused on actually improving healthcare outcomes and more on lowering costs by using the MU criteria to justify denying payments to doctors.

REPEATEDLY FIXING SOMETHING THAT WASN'T NECESSARILY BROKEN IN THE FIRST PLACE

The idea behind the ACO model is predicated on the delivery of community-based "patient-centered" care regardless of whether the community is urban, suburban, rural, remote, rich, or poor. By enabling clinicians to provide preventative, medical, and support care closer to where their patients live, health service providers are less likely to rely on hospitals or emergency facilities. Any large and well-run medical organization that can provide such comprehensive and integrated healthcare services to their community has the best potential for success through the ACO model.

I fully agree that it makes more sense for a particular patient to be able to visit their doctor's office regularly when well and have easy access during an illness. This is infinitely preferable to people showing up at expensive hospital or urgent care facilities where they are less familiar to the caretakers. Creative solutions to a patient's medical problems more naturally arise when viewing healthcare from the community- and patient-centered vantage point. Providers are even able to return to the old-fashioned "home visit" model. They can set up smaller fixed or mobile satellite clinics that outreach to more remote sites. Ancillary care services, such as physical and substance abuse rehabilitation therapy, psychology counseling, eldercare, home nursing, nutrition, and patient education, become vital parts of the care model. Clinicians can now appropriately incorporate technologies, such as feeding and respiratory equipment, telemedicine, electronic monitoring, and reporting devices, as adjuncts when reaching a more distant patient at their home or distant hospital.

It is not a huge intellectual leap to understand how, over the past two decades, this more local approach to care delivery has lately been packaged into the "newest" and trendiest term on the block, the Patient-Centered Medical Home, sometimes referred to as advanced primary care practices. I actually remain astonished and somewhat saddened that anyone believes that the PCMH is a new idea.

As a pediatrician, I am proud to know that this idea was first proposed by the American Academy of Pediatrics in their 1967 version of the Standards of Child Healthcare as an approach to dealing with children with chronic and complex medical conditions.[21] Conceptually, this model advocates for the coordination of care by a designated PCP for all the clinical services that a patient or community of similar patients may require during their lifetime. This clinician functions as the patient's first contact with the medical facility.

The PCMH returns both the responsibility and authority of directing and organizing a continuous and comprehensive healthcare team to the primary care clinician assigned to a particular patient. The team members may also work for the same facility as the clinician or at another practice in the community. The PCP or other primary care clinician must provide their patients with ready access to subspecialty care, hospitals, home health agencies, and nursing homes as well as family, public, and private community-based services. The theory is that more enhanced patient access to clinical resources—telehealth, expanded office hours, transportation, or in-home services—the better the quality of care and health of patients and the general population served by the PCMH.

The reimbursement models for organizations achieving PCMH status are as varied as the growing numbers of PCMH themselves. Each particular arrangement, whether it be under an ACO, IPA, or private group practice, or with an HMO, PPO, nonprofit, for-profit, or other type of payment contract, is unique. Some use capitation algorithms, while others still employ fee-for-service. Value-based models or a mixture of any or all of the above also exist. This is clearly still a work in progress as far as the policymakers are concerned. The one

21 Council on Pediatric Practice (US), Standards of Child Health Care, American Academy of Pediatrics (1967).

common denominator is that most authorities agree that the PCMH appears to run more efficiently and at a lower cost than non-PCMH operations. The added bonus is that patients and clinicians also appear to be happier in this model.[22]

The PCMH concept touted by the ACOs initially sounded both intriguing and familiar to me. The idea of each patient having a "medical home," one umbrella agency from which to base their healthcare in this complex system, seems rational. Unfortunately, as appealing as the idea sounds, I soon found out that even this clinically sound model was tainted and driven by strong financial motives, which placed profits over people.

"Each of our practice sites must achieve a Medical Home designation because we cannot afford to lose thousands of dollars in denied reimbursements," our outpatient practice administrator explained during a meeting with my whole team as we sat together in our conference room. The doctors, nurses, technicians, and clerical teams shuffled in their seats uneasily.

"We already do all this stuff that you have listed as requirements for the Medical Home," piped in our site manager.

Forcing a smile, the administrator looked across from her seat at the head of our long table. "Your practice may very well already be meeting the necessary standards of the Medical Home. If that's the case, improved quality is not as important as not being denied payments. We just have to check off all the appropriate boxes on the application."

"How long will that take, and how much time do we have to spend beyond our already long patient hours to complete this application?" inquired my astute head nurse.

The administrator turned to her young assistant, who responded, "Not that long. Since you have already implemented many of the indicated items, we should be successful in achieving this designation

22 O'Dell, Michael L., "What is a Patient-Centered Medical Home?", *Mo Med.* 113 (4): 301-304, https://www.ncbi.nlm.nih.gov/pmc/articles/PMC6139911/.

at your site within three to six months. We will only need a few hours each month to sit with each of you."

The administrator punctuated this last piece with, "Great. I am confident that you all have the potential of significant incentive reimbursements for our whole group. Meeting adjourned."

Meeting adjourned? Why was I once again surprised? The rest of the evening, I could not stop thinking to myself that, of course, the ultimate outcome for the administrators was economic. I tossed the whole idea over and over again in my head. I was now worried. *Can the large physician practices such as ours or ACOs legitimately achieve higher health outcome standards using this PCMH system while simultaneously significantly decreasing the costs required to deliver this care?* I was all too aware that there were many inappropriate and ineffective ways to reduce costs that could fall under a group or ACO's administrative jurisdiction. These included reducing the total billing claims submitted by urging global reductions in both diagnostic testing and therapeutic measures such as medication prescriptions. Punitive measures, including reduced reimbursements to any particular care provider or site not meeting the current meaningful use or EHR demands of the PCHM, were all too easy to enforce. If monies got really tight, other readily available options involved the elimination of certain key personnel—including physicians—in the patient care process. Doctors could readily be replaced with physician extenders, such as nurse practitioners and physician assistants.

Some of these measures may actually make sense, particularly if significant operational inefficiencies or overutilized clinical services exist. My main concern remained that non-clinicians with little sense of what it took to deliver quality care were now entering my practice environment. I was all in favor of the PCMH as long as the focus on finances did not change the culture of my team who had worked so hard to create a patient-centered approach years before it became the current vogue.

Upfront, the ACO and PCMH concepts all sound great. Keep the patient healthy at a lower cost by providing better-organized care close to home. However, I notice that the patients themselves appear to have been left out in the dark and are very confused on how to access these increasingly complex ACO networks within ever-larger practices. They are often unknowingly receiving their healthcare through an ACO but not accessing any or all of the benefits it was designed to provide for them. In a very large ACO, the patient often loses direct contact with their original PCP and is bounced around amongst the other primary care clinicians in the group. The ACO is often only required by CMS to provide primary care, not to assure consistent access to the same provider.

The paradigm of such large ACOs appears to be more designed to reach large numbers of people than to establish protocols that will improve each patient's interactions with the ACO entity. In other words, the ends of increasing the patient pool under the jurisdiction of a particular ACO appear to justify the means that ignore vital components such as continuity of care. I highly doubt that such ends as increased access to care are of value without ensuring the proper means of healthcare delivery.

If access to care takes precedence over the spirit of the care, the patient-physician interactions are merely mechanical in nature. Such relationships are not satisfying nor sustainable. Patient trust of these larger entities fades under this type of ACO as they realize that all too often individuals and families cannot have any significant relationship with their PCPs.

"Save time and money to keep the system alive" becomes the publicly perceived mantra of these ACOs, while improvements in healthcare delivery and outcomes once again become an afterthought.

Maria first came to me as a six-month old-infant accompanied by her solely Spanish-speaking mother from Guatemala and her oldest of nine siblings, a bilingual, 14-year-old, confident-appearing sister. Maria had evidence of a moderate blockage of the main valve that leads from the right side of her heart to the lungs. At this age, it was highly likely that, within two years, she would need a serious medical intervention in the form of catheterization or surgery to relieve this blockage.

Before I even examined her heart, I noted that she appeared to have the facial features of a child with a possible genetic pattern known as Noonan Syndrome. If this was indeed the case, she could have other serious medical and developmental conditions in her future, and the family would need significant resources to successfully address these. I noted in the chart that, four months prior, a colleague of mine suggested to the mother that Maria undergo genetic evaluation and testing.

When I asked the mother if she had been able to do this, she stared at me blankly and then abruptly and loudly asked me a completely unrelated question, "Maria was very congested with a cough two days ago. Is this OK for her heart?" Through my own broken Spanish and the help of the older sister, I reassured her that this should not hurt her heart and again asked about the genetic testing. The mother looked over at the older sister, confused, and they began a mumbled dialogue eight feet in front of me, as if my two medical students and I were not even in the room.

"Does your mother understand that I am asking about genetic testing?" I softly but deliberately asked the elder daughter.

"I don't think so," she replied in clear and very good English.

"So then why do you think she is having trouble understanding my question?" I asked patiently.

"Oh, she is completely deaf in one ear from an accident and lately losing hearing in the good ear. It has been pretty hard for her to communicate with anyone lately. I am missing school a lot because I have to come to all my siblings' and parents' medical visits to help translate and speak into her one good ear," she responded matter-of-factly.

After an additional 30 minutes, we finally wrapped up the visit, and I immediately contacted Maria's pediatrician indicated on her medical record. The doctor was an excellent clinician part of a large ACO.

"Oh yes, I am somewhat familiar with this patient and family. I have seen them a couple of times, but they also have seen several of our other practitioners. Looking at her chart closer now, it seems that others noted that the mother seems to be intellectually delayed and overwhelmed. I can have one of the other doctors who saw her a few more times than me call you later today," she finished while excusing herself to return to her other waiting patients.

Within 10 minutes, the other pediatrician contacted me. We had worked together many times, and I was relieved to learn that she was involved. She summarized the situation as my team listened on the speakerphone.

"Hello. Yes, this mother appears to have several children, and I have met the father only a couple of times. He appears to be more able-minded, but the mother and some of the other kids are clearly handicapped."

I elaborated the situation. "I believe that Maria has a genetic syndrome. We have advised genetic testing, but the mother doesn't understand. I am also not sure that she truly appreciates the nature of her heart condition. Should we get Social Services involved?"

She replied, "Regretfully, we have tried this through the school system, but the social worker states that the mother wouldn't let anyone into the house. She just shook her head and denied the offer of services. They had no choice but to leave."

Now even further stunned, I interjected my last kernel of hope. "Did they know that the mother is virtually completely deaf? She probably didn't understand a word they were saying."

"What?!" replied my colleague. "None of us knew this. That changes everything."

Within two days, Social Services returned to the home with a notepad to write questions in Spanish. This time, the door opened with a warm welcome.

On the surface, the idea of seeking cost reductions and improved efficiencies in healthcare delivery while simultaneously improving healthcare outcomes appears to be reasonable and noble. Who wouldn't want this to happen, whether through government Medicare or private funding schemes? I also agree conceptually that, to achieve the objectives of the ACO model, allowing clinicians to lead the organization of comprehensive healthcare services is inherently a sound approach. The issue at hand is not whether such an approach is logical but rather if it is even feasible without drastically changing other components of our healthcare system.

A car company may want to create the ultimate vehicle for consumers. They can allow a highly skilled and experienced driver to organize the team of their choice with mechanics, designers, engineers, and sponsors who are not only the best in their field but also economically and operationally efficient as a team. However, this team will not be able to effectively test-drive their creation if the roads they are obliged to drive on are unfinished, full of potholes or tollbooths, and not well managed. Because their chance of getting the car on the road and thus earning their living is too remote, they will soon become disgruntled, less motivated, and far less productive. The drivers are destined to fail or get hurt if the road remains in shambles. The best guarantee for building a high-quality vehicle for consumers is if the roads are as well-designed and smooth as the production team expects.

At this time, my experience leads me to conclude that the federal government has not yet provided adequate infrastructure for the clinician-driven ACO model to be effective. Too many resources beyond the control of the ACO remain inadequate. These include the lack of consistent and strong community-based services, such as public health departments, drug addiction facilities, social work and housing agencies, psychiatric care, and crisis management systems. As long as there remain such significant deficiencies on the roads of our healthcare system, the PCPs should not be held responsible for any failure to meet the CMS objectives for any ACO. Only when both parties, the ACO and the government, fulfill their duties will models such as the ACO be successful.

I cannot overemphasize that the recent infatuation with PCMH appears quite forced and ingenuine to me. Why is such an old and basic idea touted as special? Who would be against working with a strong, trusted primary physician who has one's best interests in mind at all times? I can't imagine a patient of mine coming up to me and saying, "Yeah, you know, Doc, this whole having a primary care physician who knows me well and takes consistently good care of me is overrated. Who needs them anyway?" If such a person exists, they must belong to the same group of people who hates chocolate or cute little puppies.

There has been an increasing trend over the last decade for physicians or other licensed clinicians to take over the care of all patients while admitted to a hospital. One of these young pediatric hospitalists called me about one of my patients who was admitted to a local hospital for a fever.

"Hey, Dr. Fethke, thanks for returning my call. I have one of your kids, Alex Wilson, with a syndrome and complex neurological problems here with a fever. The mother says her son has been having recurrent spiking fevers for weeks now. The child is apparently also allergic to several antibiotics. What do you want us to do?"

After a 10-second pause, I took a deep breath and responded politely, "I saw him around birth because of his syndrome. He had a completely normal heart, and I discharged him from my pediatric cardiology care. Do you expect something wrong with his heart? Does the primary physician know the patient is there? Have you also called them?"

The hospitalist replied nonchalantly, "Nope, we called you instead. The mother doesn't remember the pediatrician's name."

As we were talking, I looked up the pediatrician information in my chart. "Hold on. I found the primary doctor in my EHR. I will contact them and have him call you back in five minutes."

"Great. Thank you so much," he sighed with relief as he hung up.

"Hello, Dr. Jansen. I thought that you should know that your patient, Alex Wilson, is in the emergency room with a fever, and the pediatric hospitalist there needs to speak with you."

Dr. Jansen responded in a harried tone, "Oh, hold on, I am super busy now. Let's see. Oh, yes, I saw this patient just once last month for a low-grade fever. I really don't know anything much about them. Sorry, but I can't really help you guys. Got to go, really crazy here." He hung up before I could respond or give him the hospitalist's contact information.

I wish this scenario was rare and unique. It is not. In fact, it is all too commonplace. The most shocking aspect of this to me is that the supposed primary care clinicians in these situations don't seem to think that this type of response is absurd. Their role as the patient's main physician advocate has been abandoned by the system, so why should they act on or feel any commitment to a particular patient? Why would any other member of a patient's medical team, such as the hospitalists, even bother to search for or call a primary care physician from a large, impersonal medical group? They have concluded that it's a waste of time, especially if the parents don't even know the doctor's name. Each time I or my nurses collide into such an impasse, we become disillusioned as well. We wonder how the whole system became so broken.

Would we accept this attitude and approach from a teacher saying, "Hmm, I don't know what happened to Lisa. She only came once to my first-grade class. Not my problem, really. Someone else will check on her." Thankfully, there are still a handful of our community PCPs who are aggressive on behalf of their patients. They know their patients so well that they can almost sense when something is wrong before the patient becomes obviously ill. We hold onto their coattails tightly for reassurance that all is not lost.

As I have discussed, the policy writers of the past several decades consistently wrestle with the best way to incorporate the PCP back into the system. At the turn of the twentieth century, the general physician was the gold standard of healthcare providers, with little or no outside interference in their relationship with patients. No one knew you better than your general physician. As managed care evolved, the role of the PCP has been tossed around repeatedly. Initially, they were the gatekeeper through which all of a patient's care must be directed and authorized. As the HMOs took different approaches to improve their tarnished public image, the PCP was literally pushed aside as no more than an entry-level clinician. If they chose to go elsewhere or have direct access to specialists or medical tests, the HMOs now allowed patients to bypass their PCP. In the current iteration of the PCMH, they have come full circle, back to the "Home" concept where we started decades earlier. The PCP has returned as the bedrock of care in the ACO, but now, in the face of a much more complex healthcare system than existed over 100 years ago, they hold the full weight of "accountability" and responsibility for managing this system placed in their laps.

I often wondered how, all these years, we physicians wandered so far off course clinically and administratively as a profession that we allowed or even invited outsiders to drag us through the mud, barely recognizable to our patients or ourselves. It is ironic that today's best minds in healthcare policy reinforced the essential and invaluable role of the PCP in enabling both high-quality and economically efficient medical care. I am not the least bit impressed by their efforts because they essentially recreated the equivalent of the wheel in healthcare. What astonishes me is that they are bold enough to try and sell back to the public something that belonged to us in the first place.

It's as if a slick salesman knocks on your door and says, "Hello, nice family. We have this wonderful gadget that we know you could use and are prepared to sell it to you at a bargain price. Interested?"

As the family of four gathers closely around the outstretched hands of the salesman for a closer look at this new tool, the youngest child of eight years suddenly interrupts, "Hey, I know that thing. It's from our attic and belonged to my great-grandpa. How did you get that?"

The salesman responds nervously with just a hint of sweat on his brow, "Oh, dear. Young lady, you must be mistaken. My partners and I invented this ourselves in our workshop. There is nothing else like it in the world."

Perhaps it has just been so long since we enjoyed the presence of a genuine PCP that we have either totally forgotten what they were like or too many of us never met one. In hindsight, we the people should never have let a multitude of bureaucrats come between the PCP and their patients. Would a master head chef let hordes of people with no culinary skills into the sanctuary of their kitchen to tell them how to cook? Of course not. They would raise their knives to chase the intruders out of their workspace. We must now step up and focus on educating a larger proportion of our next generation of physicians to be the best PCPs possible. We can then proudly and justifiably chase the unnecessary intruders out of our clinical spaces where the patient-physician relationship is sacrosanct, shouting, "Go back to your own offices and find a way to pay our primary care clinicians more. They deserve it, and without them, we are nothing."

CHAPTER 7

THE HYPOCRISY OF THE CURRENT HEALTHCARE SYSTEM

In 2014, on a cold winter evening in New York's Hudson Valley, just as I was finishing up my evening patient hours and the windswept snow outside my window was pressuring me to wrap up my work before the roads became treacherous, I received an urgent text to call back a community physician colleague, Dr. Ifran Sharma. This was my cue to clean the snow off my car and head home. As my hands-free system connected me to the cell number which he provided in his text, I started our conversation while driving slowly home. After some initial pleasantries, he cut to the point.

One of his young nieces, Emaan Ali, lived with her family in Pakistan. She had been born with a complex congenital heart defect that was palliated through a collaboration of local and Western physicians. "The family was under the impression that she had been cured by the surgery," Sharma explained anxiously. "But they are now taken by surprise that, over the past few months, Emaan, who is now five years old, is becoming rapidly ill right before their eyes. They contacted me as an esteemed family member because I am an established physician in America. They are desperate, but I am an adult gastroenterologist. This is not my field. Can you help us?" came the worried voice of a loving uncle.

Dr. Sharma went on to explain that almost seven years after receiving the lifesaving heart surgery, the skin over Emaan's entire body, especially her face, hands, and feet, was becoming progressively more purplish. We both knew how serious this was. The purple hue, a sign known as cyanosis, indicated that the oxygen levels in her bloodstream were dangerously declining. Emaan had been an active toddler and preschooler, easily keeping up with her cousins and classmates. Now she was constantly tired, hard to awaken in the mornings, and taking frequent naps at school and home. She couldn't run anymore. She couldn't even keep up with her elderly grandmother. Emaan's teachers were alarmed by her appearance. Afraid she was too sick, they were hesitant to even have her attend school. I was so lost in the conversation that I barely noticed the snow pounding on the windshield, limiting my forward visibility to only a few feet in front of me. With my eyes on distant taillights up ahead, I drove in the right direction from sheer memory.

Throughout my 30-minute drive, even as I pulled my car into the warm garage, Dr. Sharma's voice repeatedly broke with thick emotion as he explained this all to me. He put Emaan's dire situation into context. No one in the Pakistani health system could fully explain what was now wrong with her heart or how to fix it. The closest pediatric cardiologist was in the northern capital of Islamabad, miles away over rough mountain roads from Emaan's home in the southwest suburbs along the Indus River. Since her first surgery, no one had provided the family with an informative update of her cardiac diagnosis or what to expect. The family was understandably petrified that she may not survive without immediate treatment. As Annie's worried uncle, not as an American physician, Dr. Sharma reached out to me for guidance.

Pakistan's healthcare system remains a complex mix of subsystems delivered through the federal and local provincial governments. These systems are mainly based in the larger cities and in direct competition with the formal and informal private sector healthcare providers who are typically more reliable and accessible. Though Emaan's family was middle class relative to their compatriots, they could not afford the expensive healthcare costs necessary to even begin an analysis of why she was getting sicker. If Emaan ultimately needed another heart operation, they would have to rely on the combined resources of her extended family.

Their dear American uncle was willing to house and feed them, as well as raise money for the operation, but this would all be for naught if we were unable to overcome the logistical barriers of figuring out the details of Emaan's cardiac problem in the first place. We needed to obtain clear current images of her heart to understand why she was developing more cyanosis. This required someone who could perform a proper echocardiogram study of a complex heart condition in a child and transmit the images to us right away. Because technology at the time did not allow for large digital images to be sent over the Internet, this study would have to be recorded and brought back to New York by hand.

Fortune was on our side. One of my private practice colleagues, Dr. Vipul Mirza, was originally from Pakistan. He did his medical training in the United States and Canada and had just started working with me. It so happened that he had a trip planned for the following month to visit his parents who still lived in Pakistan. He offered to rent a car and travel over seven hours from his family's southern home near Pakistan's largest city—the seaside metropolis of Karachi—to meet Emaan at her cardiologist's satellite office. This idea sounded perfect to both Dr. Sharma and me.

Over both large highways and small treacherous mountain roads, just six weeks after her uncle first texted me, Dr. Mirza finally met Emaan and her mother at the local provincial hospital. The local pediatric cardiologist guided my road-weary colleague through the clinic hallways and into one of the exam rooms. Her doctor made sure that one of the hospital's precious echocardiogram machines was set up in the hopes that Dr. Mirza could decipher her complex heart condition.

I was anxiously on standby at my home office. After an hour of concentrated ultrasound imaging of her heart with the local and somewhat outdated echocardiogram machine, Dr. Mirza retrieved the information we needed. Via several slow-to-arrive text messages, he relayed back to me across the continents and oceans that some of the details regarding her heart were still unclear. However, despite the limitations of the old diagnostic imaging equipment, we were both certain that Emaan would only survive with an urgent and complex heart operation. The operation she needed required closing a large hole in the wall separating the two bottom chambers of her heart and recreating the bloodstream from her heart to her lungs so that her blood could receive the much-needed oxygen. It had to be performed by a highly skilled pediatric heart surgeon with a full complement of human and technical support services that existed in relatively few places in the world, including New York City.

Time was of the essence. The next morning, I began canvassing my colleagues from over the years at several of the tertiary pediatric medical centers in New York City to determine if they would take on Emaan's case from both a medical and financial standpoint. Over the next two days, I worked feverishly, sending out a dozen emails and text messages and making phone calls in between patient hours. Montefiore Medical Center in the Bronx came to the forefront with an offer to help. If I could get Emaan and her mother to the States, reassess the details of her heart problem, and take full professional and financial responsibility for her local cardiac care in my private office, before and after the operation, they would consider performing the surgery.

There were several necessary hurdles to overcome. I would have to formally present her case to the full medical team at Montefiore, including the pediatric cardiologists, heart surgeons, anesthesiologists, and intensive care pediatricians. Only if they then all concluded that

Emaan had a good chance of both surviving the surgery and safely returning as a healthy child back to Pakistan would they offer her the operation. They graciously also offered to accept whatever the family could afford in terms of payment toward hospital costs. My physician colleagues, including the surgeon, and I would provide all her care while at the hospital as a charity free of charge.

That afternoon, Emaan and her mom booked a flight to New York.

I AM STARTING TO SMELL BS

I have come to accept the reality that patient health and safety are not the true motives for many entities to seek ACO status. Once again, like with the HMOs before them, economics and control of the market share loom strong as the main driving forces. Even a casual observer is aware that promotion of the ACO concept further stimulated the preexisting trend of consolidation amongst medical practices, hospitals, and many other entities that provide healthcare. In my own southern New York region, on more than one occasion, the state and federal government have had to step in to slow down the growth of such large mega-groups under the ACO model to ensure that antitrust laws are not violated and these groups are not granted unrestrained ability to monopolize local care. Such monopolies, especially large hospital systems that employ many clinicians and ancillary care providers, threaten the very fabric of the ACO model's cost-containment initiatives. If left unchallenged, these large entities have the potential to dominate the market when negotiating HMO or Medicare reimbursements and thus ultimately increase the costs of healthcare.

I repeatedly noted that one of the consequences of government's or any large bureaucracy's extensive involvement in healthcare reform is that they often view the task at hand disproportionately through the standpoint of bottom-line economics. I recommend instead that they focus more on ensuring that the fundamentals of good healthcare are solidly in place. Funding strategies are proposed before fully determining the nature and design of the healthcare product we seek to develop. The current state of the ACOs are a good example of this overemphasis on finances.

On the surface, the basic concept and structure of this organizational model appears to be logical. The standards of certain institutions or large medical entities—such as mega-group private practices and hospitals—are identified as prototypes for the desired model of healthcare within their geographic region. At a quick glance, their ranking may appear to be justified. More likely, in their application for ACO status, these entities proposed that they hold a greater potential to achieve economic and quality improvements than others in their geographic area. A very large private practice may argue that their possession of the lion's share of a region's patient population gives them a unique advantage to wield significant influence on regional healthcare. Even if their current clinical standards are clearly subpar or not better than that of a smaller group in the area, in theory they could improve if some uniform approach to quality was adopted. What matters more than their initial quality standards is their relatively large economic leverage.

This economic thrust was the very rationale Mr. McEwan used to explain why the newly formed Montefiore-Hudson Valley IPA was not applicable to my needs. It was the bias of this IPA that I did not need the fiscal "carrot on the stick" because I already met and exceeded the CMS-driven quality benchmarks their ACO adopted for accessing any funds from the Medicare Shared Savings program. They blatantly ignored the fact that I could not sustain my high clinical standards for much longer without participating in the improved reimbursements afforded to their new members. The potential for increased monies derived from the ACO-IPA arrangement drove the system more than the achievement or maintenance of high standards.

To make matters worse, it is obvious to me that the growth in the number of ACOs significantly contributed to the increased bureaucracy of the American system. The support of these ACOs is a high-maintenance endeavor which further aggravates the already huge operational inefficiencies of our complex healthcare system. For years, many of my physician colleagues and I have felt that everyone wants to be in the healthcare game and get a piece of the action. The human and material resources required to run an ACO, including staff salaries and benefits, information technology teams to install and maintain the computerized electronic health records, billing software, personnel, and so much more, are just other examples of the administrative overload. Close scrutiny of the status of ACO programs[23] actually reveals that these administrative costs have been the main culprit in the failure of many former ACOs since the 2011 pilot program[24] was launched. In the United States, administrative costs alone are four times higher than any other comparable developed nation, totaling $940 per individual. I sense a clear irony, verging on hypocrisy, that this administrative amount is far greater than what we spend on other programs, such as preventative or long-term care, that could save money and improve our nation's health.

I would argue that the process dictated by the ACO model may eventually achieve the goal of cost reduction, but the standard of care remains the same or even deteriorates. The advancement of the quality of the care is not the true priority. Incentivizing the reduced use of MRIs or CT scans increases risk that a patient's cancer may continue undiagnosed until it is too late to treat. The focus on electronic medical records, MU, and best practices can easily take priority over actual medical care. In other words, any particular individual patient cared

23 Merlis, Mark, "Health Policy Brief: Accountable Care Organizations," *Health Affairs*, July 27, 2010 (online), https://www.healthaffairs.org/do/10.1377/hpb20100727.412894/full/.

24 Liao, Joshua M.; Navathe, Amol S.; Werner, Rachel M. "The Impact of Medicare's Alternative Payment Models on the Value of Care," *Annual Review of Public Health*, Vol. 41:551-565, April 2020, https://www.annualreviews.org/doi/abs/10.1146/annurev-publhealth-040119-094327.

for in the system may actually become worse. Because the increase in documentation requirements in the ACO model demands a disproportionately high percentage of a physician's time, a patient may also go undiagnosed because the physician simply does not have ample time to listen to a patient and obtain a good basic health history. Given time constraints, preventative care itself is often forced to take a backstage in the ACO environment.

Non-physicians, such as nurse practitioners (NPs) and physician assistants (PAs), may become a greater portion of the health provider workforce because their average salaries are lower than a doctor's. I trained many PAs and NPs, and they are a wonderful complement to the medical team. However, it is my opinion that they benefit from regular and appropriate physician supervision and guidance. When, in any clinical setting, there are too few physicians available to oversee the NPs or PAs, they spend more unsupervised time with patients. It is therefore not surprising that in my legal medical expert work, there has been an increasing proportion of malpractice suits against practices relying heavily on non-physician providers. Their expertise is often not sufficient to properly diagnose and treat patients with particularly rare and complex problems.

So we are in a Catch-22. Personnel costs may be reduced by employing non-physician caretakers, but any particularly ill patient may be poorly managed and become sicker than necessary. If a particular community has enough ill patients, the health outcomes for the whole ACO may be adversely affected. In addition to not meeting the shared savings advantages, such an ACO, burdened with an unhealthy population, will see the costs of care rise as these patients become critically ill because of their inherent mismanagement. A balanced clinical team—doctors, nurse practitioners, physician assistants, nurses, technicians, and medical assistants—with experienced physician involvement remains the best resource for excellent patient care.

The guideline-driven criteria may make it seem as if the standard of care has improved for any given ACO-supervised patient population, but the reality is that these are often artificial endpoints that don't reflect the true quality of care. As an obvious example, if the majority of people in a given population or community started out already very healthy, then the arrival of the ACO on the scene may have little to do with the outcomes. However, because the health data was initially not recorded in the ACO's EHR system, the ACO can still claim the credit for this healthy group simply by clicking the right items on the EHR.

Another issue is that geographic areas, known as medical deserts, with underserved or unserved patients exist throughout our inner cities or remote rural communities. Though some ACOs have started to reach out to these areas, as shown by the COVID-19 pandemic, access to such organized quality healthcare is still an issue in many places of our country. Such medical deserts won't even register on the radar screen of EHR-based criteria and thus continue to fall through the cracks of the ACO system.

The bottom line is that nothing, even a well-run ACO, can truly replace good clinical judgment and practice. These skills should exist as a prerequisite in any well-trained arsenal of medical professionals, with or without an ACO or IPA. When ACO healthcare models overemphasize irrelevant and time-consuming information-gathering, ignoring the essentials of high standards derived from good medical training, the quality of care decreases. The bureaucracy, paperwork, and negativity detracts from the potential and ability of the physician to make sound medical decisions and provide quality care. As ACOs function on punitive measures, rather than positive incentives—when they tear clinicians down, rather than lift them up—physician morale suffers. Nothing can or should replace the tools physicians learn in a good medical education, and these should be reinforced by any credible practice administration. A thoughtful and well-conducted medical history, examination, and clinically relevant assessment and plan of care remain the time-honored and proven benchmarks that allow for high-quality healthcare. If any component of this patient encounter process is eliminated or underrepresented, regardless of the available technology and electronic documentation, problems arise.

Lately, I have been concerned that young physicians are trained more toward how to achieve the predetermined, clinically irrelevant outcome standards than how to provide direct patient care. In medical school and residency programs, the focus on documentation and seeing patients quickly has become overwhelming. My students and residents tell me that they are actually trained to keep their patient visits under 15 minutes, with 10 minutes as the proposed benchmark of success during practical testing. Because of this time-crunch requirement, the students are not spending enough time with their patients to learn from them, thus jeopardizing the primary foundation of their clinical education. My new students certainly can write a very long and, on the surface, complex electronic medical note. However, when I ask them to talk about the live patient they just saw, I regret that they are often severely unprepared to do so. During my brief teaching time with them, I do all in my power to correct this deficit.

The main roadblock to achieving successful fiscal accountability in our current US healthcare environment is that all of the different payment models still floating around inherently conflict with each other. To best understand the incompatibilities and frustrations with trying to simultaneously juggle the different reimbursement systems, we must take an honest and detailed look at the ubiquitous and too often all-consuming RVU model. RVUs are basically an attempt by CMS and private payors to create a standardized method of physician payments. This system started just five years before my administrative mentor, Jay Wilson, at Horton Hospital advised me to sit down and create my first professional fee schedule. The fee-for-service (FFS) methodology essentially spawned an inventory list of all the different services and tests that physicians and medical facilities provided. My first exposure to this FFS process remains an indelible memory that foreshadowed many physicians' distaste with the myriad of payment methods created over the past three to four decades.

As I walked into the bustling outpatient clinic at Brown University on an early Monday morning, my stomach was all tied up in knots. This was my first live interview for a potential student position at a medical school. I prepared for weeks. Locked up in the library at Princeton, I pored over articles about medical practice terminology in an attempt to come across as up-to-date on current trends in the medical field. I was certain that I could answer virtually any reasonable question that came my way during an interview.

The clinic secretary pointed me in the direction of a doctor sitting at a desk behind the counter. As I approached this obviously senior physician in a white coat with a full shock of equally white hair, hunched over in deep thought, he did not look up once from the messy pile of papers barely inches from his face. I cleared my throat politely so as not to seem rude, and he looked up at me while simultaneously removing his dark-rimmed bifocals.

"Yes, can I help you, young man?" he mumbled as if somewhat relieved to have a moment of reprieve from his paperwork.

"Hello. Yes, sir, Dr. Ebert. I'm Eric Fethke. I'm here for my 9:30 medical school interview with you," I replied respectfully.

He paused for an awkward moment and gestured for me to sit down next to him as he acknowledged the situation. "Well, I can see that, young man. I guess this means that I have to ask you some relevant questions, don't I?" I decided to remain silent and just nod my head. "Well, here's my question for you then. You see this ridiculous pile of papers on the desk? This is an example of the latest nonsense that our administrators dished out to us doctors. It is a laundry list of all the procedures, including visits and tests, that we are allowed to bill for after seeing each patient. The writing is so small, I can barely read it. Some misguided idiot obviously decided that medical care should now boil down to a shopping list." I remained attentive on the outside but was inwardly lost in this conversation. "So here's my one and only question for you today, son." He continued with his monologue. "Give me one good reason why, here and now, I should not just quit medicine altogether instead of dealing with this bullshit!"

To this day, I do not remember my response to Dr. Ebert or how I got out of this first interview without long-lasting psychological trauma. No one ever asked me this question again in my other interviews. I do know that I felt very badly for him. I was sure that a physician with all his years of experience would rather have been with his patients than bogged down with all this extra paperwork. I wished that I could somehow have helped him to not be so despondent.

For decades, the FFS system resulted in a significant lack of consistency in physician compensation. In an attempt to create some uniformity of fee schedules, Medicare established the Customary, Prevailing, and Reasonable (CPR) charge system—contained in the paperwork sprawled across Dr. Ebert's desk. This CPR scale, based on a comparison of fees charged by other doctors for similar services in a given geographic area, did not keep up with the costs of advancing technologies[25] and the spread of more advanced care to suburban and rural communities such as mine.

In response to rising costs and increasing reimbursement inequities for similar services in the physician-directed CPR system, in 1992 CMS collaborated with the American Medical Association (AMA) to create the Resource-Based Relative Value Scale (RBRVS). This more broadly standardized physician fee schedule was based on the RVU algorithm,

25 AAPC Thought Leadership Team, "What Are Relative Value Units (RVUs)?", AAPC, June 21, 2022 (online), https://www.aapc.com/practice-management/amp/rvus.aspx.

which at its core was still an FFS method. As such, the RVU approach still fostered a volume-driven, rather than quality-driven, motivation.

The RBRVS morphed the CPR into the Current Procedural Terminology (CPT) system that fills up the EHR software I use today. Each CPT service or procedure code is assigned a number of RVUs based upon a calculation of how much it costs to provide the service compared to other CPTs. As with the elderly Dr. Ebert's concerns, physicians and medical facilities were prompted and encouraged to check off as many CPT boxes as possible in a profit-driven mindset to capture the greatest number of RVUs. This in turn led to an explosion of the medical billing industry because it now takes a fully dedicated and informed team of people to even keep up with the submissions, denials, and constantly changing rules of the CPT-based process. As you can imagine, despite the best of intentions, this RVU method is at heart still an FFS methodology, which potentially raised costs even more than before. The RVUs are just an FFS horse of a different color.

At a quick glance, the RVU equation appears intimidating to anyone easily overwhelmed by complex mathematics. Like an algebra equation, it has several components. On closer scrutiny, when deconstructing this algorithm, I concluded that it actually epitomizes so much of the hypocrisy that belies the financing of our healthcare system. The basic equation for each CPT code payment is as follows:

[(Work RVU x Work GPCI x CF) + (PE RVU x PE GPCI x CF) + (MP RVU x MP GPCI x CF)]

The three main components of the equation—Work, Practice Expense, and Malpractice—are each weighted geographically using the Geographic Practice Cost Index (GPCI), which is intended to account for the wide range of costs across different areas of the United States. Work is supposed to take into account the many provider-specific elements, to include time, training, effort, and skill. The Practice

Expense component encompasses all operational costs of providing the CPT service, including personnel salaries, rent, equipment, and utilities. Finally, the Malpractice piece reflects the burden of malpractice insurance required to render a medical service or procedure.

Each of the three components is not represented equally in the total RVU value. The pieces break down roughly as Work 50 percent, Practice Expense 46 percent, and Malpractice 4 percent. The Conversion Factor (CF) is set by Medicare and is a nationwide currency amount that a current RVU is worth. It is used to translate the three components into a dollar amount. As of 2021, the CF is $34.89, which is actually lower than the previous year's amount of $36.09.

I was stunned when I first saw the RVU formula. I couldn't believe that so many inherent biases were blatantly and unabashedly incorporated into an actual equation. It is as if simply taking the form of an equation creates legitimacy to any egregious nonsense. Once my disdain cooled down, I started to analytically dissect the RVU components and their implications. As I did so, I started to realize that the whole premise of our productivity and value assessment was based upon a seriously flawed hypocrisy. It suddenly made more sense why so much of our healthcare system was dysfunctional. I now fully call out the BS.

The first component, the Work RVU, claims to appropriately designate a worth to the specific component of the service or procedure delivered by the healthcare providers. It does not take long to realize that CPT codes rendered more often by specialists or surgeons are weighted significantly higher than the group consultation codes that the generalist physicians tend to use. It is crystal clear that the time and experience factors of a primary care physician are less valued.

If we truly include experience in the Work RVU, then why wouldn't a senior physician like Dr. Ebert or a well-recognized leading general physician receive a higher RVU work score than a brand-new physician? The fact is they are assigned the same RVU Work value, regardless of experience or reputation. If a physician is truly remarkable, more often than not, they stop accepting insurance payments and operate under a cash or credit-only basis.

As one such colleague of mine stated at a college and medical school class reunion, "I stopped taking insurance payments 10 years ago and never looked back. Now I get to choose who I can give a cost break to and see more relatively poor patients than ever. It's a win-win."

Even more disconcerting is that the mathematics of the RVU Work component reveals that, as a general physician becomes more efficient, their total salaries do not increase proportionately to their increased Work RVUs. A new pediatrician may start at a salary of $120,000 per year and expect to see about 2,000 patients per year. Within a couple of years, their productivity is often contractually required, as per RVU-based forecasting, to increase twofold to threefold to approximately 5,000 patients per year, while their annual salary is capped at $200,000. This scenario means that the new doctor earns nearly $60 per patient visit while a more seasoned doctor in the same practice earns $40 per the same CPT-coded patient visit. Physicians are probably one of the few professions who work more as the years progress yet earn less per service rendered than when they started—all couched under the RVU productivity model.

The second RVU component, Practice Expense (PE), could provide enough material to critique for a whole thesis. I will restrain myself for this review to the two main problematic biases. The first is that, once again, surgical or high-tech diagnostic procedures are given a higher PE score than the less-technical procedures because the required equipment costs are much higher. But are these costs justified? It has become common knowledge that procedures such as a CT imaging scan cost much more in the United States than other countries. This is because the manufacturers of this type of equipment make a much greater profit in the United States than elsewhere. This directly results in a higher RVU PE component than necessary, with the profits essentially accounted for and buried deep into the formula.

Even if the technology becomes cheaper with time, the RVU PE somehow does not decrease proportionately. The high profit margin of the equipment becomes the expense of the facility performing the CT scan, which in turn seeks to cover these inflated costs and generate a profit. The general physician has to literally perform hundreds of earwax removals over dozens of hours to generate the same reimbursement as a single 30-minute CT scan because there simply is a limit to how much a cotton swab can cost.

The second issue with the RVU PE is essentially the same problem as with the third RVU component, Malpractice cost (MP). As the administrative bureaucracy and liability risks of providing healthcare soared astronomically, instead of addressing these factors as a source of cost reduction, they simply jumped into the RVU algorithm. It is as if the RVU formula was a bandwagon for everyone to join and receive a piece of the action so that they might stake their legitimate claim to the monies.

As the MU, billing, computer, and compliance requirements multiplied, my own experience confirms that they clearly increased the costs to deliver medical services. Instead of addressing this issue, the creators of the RVU system simply squeezed them into the formula. I get the sense that streamlining and reducing such overhead costs would cut too many people out of the pie who have grown accustomed to sharing. Too many industries, including the pharmaceutical manufacturers, the office and medical supply companies, medical billing agencies, and the computer technology industry, now depend on the healthcare economic machine to let go easily. Instead of once and for all addressing tort reform to decrease the burden of malpractice claims, it appears that it was easier to just tack this cost onto the end of the RVU concept as well. These non-physician costs have led total health expenditures to skyrocket[26] from $74.1 billion in 1970 to $3.8 trillion in 2019.

We have barely left enough room in this crowded RVU space for the patients who pay the premiums and the doctors who provide the care. Even worse, every time finances become an issue, the solution has been to reach into the pockets of the doctors and the patients. The physician salaries remain vulnerable to punitive reductions if volume quotes or MU criteria are not met. Patients have watched their copays and deductibles soar, even as their portion of the premiums increased. Why are cost-reduction efforts not dealing with the multiple 300-pound gorillas in the room?

Soaring medical education costs and student debts, malpractice reforms, aggressive bargaining to reduce pharmaceutical and medical technology costs, and a consistent universal physician reimbursement model are just some of the many areas that appear to me to be much lower-hanging fruit for lowering healthcare costs. For the past few decades, the proportion of the US healthcare expenditure[27] due to physicians and other clinicians has been between 15 and 20 percent and not grown anywhere near as quickly as pharmaceutical, hospital, health insurance, and administrative costs,[28] which make up the lion's share at over 50 to 60 percent of the national total health expenditure.

26 Ortaliz, Jared; McGough, Matthew; Salaga, Meghan; Amin, Krutika; and Cox, Cynthia, "How Much and Why 2024 Premiums Are Expected to Grow in Affordable Care Act Marketplaces," Peterson-KFF Health System Tracker, Aug 4, 2023 (online), https://www.healthsystemtracker.org/chart-collection/u-s-spending-healthcare-changed-time/#item-usspendingovertime_8.

27 Parks, Troy, "Analysis of Health Care Spending: Where Do the Dollars Go?", AMA, March 4, 2016 (online), https://www.ama-assn.org/delivering-care/patient-support-advocacy/analysis-health-care-spending-where-do-dollars-go.

28 Ortaliz, Jared; McGough, Matthew; Salaga, Meghan; Amin, Krutika; and Cox, Cynthia, "How Much and Why 2024 Premiums Are Expected to Grow in Affordable Care Act Marketplaces," Peterson-KFF Health System Tracker, Aug 4, 2023 (online), https://www.healthsystemtracker.org/chart-collection/u-s-spending-healthcare-changed-time/#item-usspendingovertime_8.

I sense that many of these non-clinician related costs have not been aggressively addressed because of the inherent conflict of interest for all the other cost contributors who substantially benefited over the past few decades. They tapped into a cash cow, so why would they willingly let go?

Ultimately, my biggest problem with the RVU thought process is that it looks at the delivery of healthcare in pieces, instead of a whole. Yes, it is bad enough that it still fosters the high-volume mentality of the FFS approach. However, the worst offense of the RVU model is that it ignores that the best patient care comes from a great collaboration of many human, infrastructure, and technical resources. One hand literally feeds the other. Without the consummate PCP managing the overall health issues of a patient, a surgical or other invasive procedure can actually become dangerous. No anesthesiologist of any repute puts a patient under general anesthesia for a procedure unless the patient was first cleared medically to receive the anesthesia and to undergo the procedure.

We can't legitimately claim publicly that we value the role of the PCP on the one hand and place such a relatively low value on their services behind the scenes in the RVU system. I am convinced that the only correct way to provide patient care is to function like a symphony orchestra, where all musicians make a contribution to the musical performance. The audience benefits from a conductor who knows how to harness all these separate players to produce beautiful music. The patient benefits most only when the policymakers take a global approach that values all health providers equally. The current RVU model applied to either reimbursement or productivity clearly favors some components of the system, especially the non-clinicians, over others and, as such, just creates a lot of noise.

Despite the inherent fiscal weaknesses of the RVU system and the obvious biases embedded in the RVU formula, it persists like old gum to the bottom of a shoe. In many areas of the country, it is still the operational model by which clinicians are reimbursed. Even if a medical group such as an ACO contracted their services under a capitation or shared savings quality model, the RVU system remains as the bedrock by which they assess provider productivity. Like taskmasters, administrators in medical groups or facilities regularly inform each provider of their RVU-based productivity compared to their professional peers.

My colleagues in large private and academic practices consistently told me that their administrative reviews include discussions such as, "We know you're a great doctor, and the patients love you. However, to justify your salary, we need you to increase your monthly RVU totals by 15 percent. Otherwise, you may see a reduction in your take-home income."

"I don't know what they want from me anymore," bemoaned a younger colleague of mine, echoing Dr. Ebert's sentiments from over 30 years ago. "On the one hand, we are being ordered to perform fewer unnecessary procedures to meet MU and best practices standards. So I changed my practices accordingly and ordered fewer CT scans and other tests than I used to. It makes sense because my patients are doing just fine without these unnecessary tests and procedures. I only requested them when I first joined because my administrators urged us all to capture as many RVUs as possible for the sake of the group's financial survival. Now they want to reduce my salary because I don't have enough RVUs each month to meet my contractual obligations. I can't see enough patients to make up for the reduced tests I used to order because the tests definitely count for significantly more RVUs than my patient visits. I'm confused, exhausted, and fed up."

This 180-degree turn away from a high-volume paradigm has been a particularly difficult transition for many of my local physician colleagues. Most of them initially worked under a larger medical entity with the clear encouragement by their own physician leaders to keep the diagnostic testing and physician referrals within the walls of the entity so that the partner physicians could reap the profits and junior doctors might receive a bonus. This philosophy may have indeed led to a significant level of over-testing, but this whiplash response arising from the ACO model, now focused on decreasing testing, appears to have gone to the other extreme. Medically and realistically, the practice pattern pendulum likely should rest somewhere in the middle between these two extremes and be dictated by physician training, experience, and the best interests of the patient. However, I have all too often noted that medical common sense easily gives way to economic priorities.

I NOW CALL COMPLETE BS

Now for a sobering reality—the huge corporations that entered the healthcare market and became very rich over the past few decades directly interfere with the struggle to improve healthcare in America. Medical device and pharmaceutical companies, large hospitals, corporate medical practices, and the medical insurance industry itself all stand squarely in the way of better health outcomes. These entities are by design profit-driven. They are obliged to answer to their shareholders more than to their employed clinicians or their patient beneficiaries. I often asked myself if any of these industries would ever give up their strong hold on the American healthcare system without an aggressive fight. They have become fat off the present system and will not readily let go of their jackpot. They and their shareholders have too much equity at stake to risk allowing population or universal health models to become the new financial norm in American healthcare.

Let's start by looking at the fundamentals of how health insurance companies make money. They collect payments called premiums from employers, individuals, or families. These premiums entitle individual beneficiaries to be "covered" to varying degrees, depending on the specific contract plan for which they signed up, to offset the costs for their medical care. The total of all these premiums creates a pool of money maintained by the health insurance company. The ACA requires that the company must designate 80 to 85 percent of the funds in this pool for only two purposes—to cover the costs of healthcare claims by their member beneficiaries and to make improvements in the quality of the healthcare of their members.

The insurance company uses the other 15 to 20 percent of the premiums to cover the costs of conducting business. Anything left over is viewed as pure income or profit, which they are allowed to invest in the stock market, bonds, or real estate to further increase their bottom line. The ACA sets limits on how much profit a health insurance company can make and requires revenue generated above this cap level to be returned to the consumers who pay the premiums.

During the COVID-19 pandemic, the large health insurers literally made billions of dollars more profit than in the past because so many patients stayed home without undergoing surgeries or attending doctor visits. As of early 2021, the health insurers have not rebated their customers[29] as required and are holding onto huge cash reserves.

Anyone who has looked closely at a statement from their health insurance company—known in the medical world as an Explanation of Benefits (EOB)—after receiving medical attention is familiar with the somewhat convoluted process by which the bill of their health services is paid. The EOB is broken into three main categories:

1. the total charge by the care providers,

2. the contracted amount the insurance company agrees to pay these providers, and

3. the portion that remains the responsibility of the patient in the form of copays or deductibles.

When all this adds up, it rarely covers the total bill. Within six months of starting my own practice in 1998, I learned about this whole process

29 Abelson, Reed, "Major U.S. Health Insurers Record Big Profits, Benefitting from the Pandemic," *New York Times*, August 5, 2020 (online), https://www.nytimes.com/2020/08/05/health/covid-insurance-profits.html.

and was amazed that my predecessors ever let this whole situation become the accepted norm.

As one of my best friends remarked in astonishment after receiving an EOB in the mail, "This looks ridiculous. My doctor billed $500 for my recent specialty visit with him, and the statement says that, even with my portion, he will only get $275. Something has to be wrong with the numbers. Why am I paying such large premiums? This can't be correct, can it?"

I answered flatly, "Yeah, it's crazy, but that's the way it works with health insurance."

For-profit health insurers became very adept at increasing the amount of money that remains after paying patient benefits and running their operations, otherwise known as their net revenue. Before the ACA, they blatantly denied or delayed paying insurance claims. This behavior, which included the now political football of "denials for preexisting conditions," soon led to the aforementioned public distrust of insurance companies and managed care.

I clearly remember when one of my first patients who worked in the benefits department of a large health insurance company advised me, "Doc, you know you should send your bills for any of your services twice, one to two weeks apart. Though there will never be a written policy in any health insurance company like mine, it is understood by everyone who works there that we are to shred a significant portion of medical bills without even opening them. This keeps the premium pool from going down so the executives can pay their shareholders and themselves the big money." Sure enough, when I followed her advice, my cash flow improved tremendously.

With the arrival of the ACA, the insurance companies devised other tricks to hold onto their funds as long as possible. These included straightforward tactics such as raising their premium prices and reducing their staffing salaries through electronic automation. They also use less of their premium pool by creating a multitude of additional consumer costs they tack onto the already high baseline annual premiums. Like the airline industry, they have become rich on "hidden fees."

Through these insidious accounting schemes in their FFS model, they gave rise to several now-infamous terms—exceptions of benefits, denials for out-of-network doctors' services, and rising patient copays and deductible costs. More subtle maneuvers include holding on as long as possible to any excess funds from the claims-designated pool that are supposed to be rebated to the beneficiaries to invest them. Just over a year into the COVID-19 pandemic, these funds total billions of dollars.

The main issue with most of the health insurers is their for-profit model. Like other profit-motivated corporations, a for-profit health insurance company must keep their investors happy. This requires that they disburse a significant portion of the profits amongst the shareholders as dividends to keep them interested in the continued financial support of their company by owning and buying more stocks. It also cannot be ignored that many of the shareholders are actually the owners of the company and that the biggest shareholders are non-physicians who often sit on the company board where they can further influence how the monies are spent.

As a physician, I cannot help but worry that the focus on my patients' well-being is compromised much more than it would if this whole process was not so focused on making money for the executives, owners, and shareholders. This approach makes sense to me for a company that creates nonessential commodities but has always raised deep ethical issues in my gut when applied to any industry that significantly impacts the world of healthcare.

What about the pharmaceutical industry? Why do Americans pay far more for medications than any other nation? Because even more than the health insurance companies, the drug companies are profit-driven and beholden to their shareholders. The only limitations on their exorbitant drug pricing remains what the free market will bear.

Even worse, the drug companies' destinies are closely tied to both the government[30] through the Food and Drug Administration (FDA) and to the frontline giant medication distributors—corporate and hospital pharmacies.

The members of this triumvirate of bedfellows—the drug manufacturers, the FDA, and the pharmacies—have become legally interdependent in the United States, and this operational structure significantly contributes to keeping prescription drug prices so high. As soon as the FDA gives a patented and successfully tested medication approval to be prescribed by physicians, the manufacturer's marketing and distribution campaign is launched with a full-court press. The drug company has an average of 12 years of government-protected exclusivity to reap as much money as possible from their new medication before another competitor may release a generic or similarly effective new drug.

Though the ACA protects patients by preventing health insurers from increasing their premiums or denying access to people based upon preexisting health conditions, this component of the ACA threatens to significantly increase the insurers' operational costs and the total premiums they must pay. Basic math dictates that their profit margins would significantly reduce. In response to this threat, many insurers use their strong relationship with the pharmaceutical industry to create loopholes around this component of the ACA. US drug companies are free to set their own prices, but it is the insurers and pharmacies that decide how much the patients actually pay out of pocket.

To reduce the ACA-imposed financial burden associated with clients with chronic or serious preexisting medical conditions, the health insurers created a strong disincentive for such patients to enroll for benefits under their company. They simply increase the portion of medication costs that the patient must pay for long-term or very

---

30 Sachs, Rachel E., "Delinking Reimbursement," *Minnesota Law Review*, 102:2307 (2018), https://www.minnesotalawreview.org/wp-content/uploads/2018/07/Sachs_MLR.pdf.

expensive medications. Ultimately, this high copay cost that, say, a patient with diabetes must cover for insulin or a patient with HIV pays for their antiviral medication is determined through behind-the-scenes negotiations between the insurance company itself and the drug companies. The final negotiated price is driven by the financial motivations of the health insurers or the large employers, not by what is necessarily the best option for the patient-employee.

What the patient ends up paying at the pharmacy level is the difference between the price at which the insurance company's benefit manager agrees to buy the medication from the manufacturer and the portion of this the insurer decides to pay. If an insurance company ultimately makes the medication—or, in other cases, the equipment or physical therapy costs—high enough, this creates a disincentive for the patient to enroll for coverage through this particular company. These prohibitively high costs to the patient thus minimize the insurer's financial risk without having to violate the "preexisting conditions" requirements of the ACA. The patient is forced to pay high prices for critical medications or look elsewhere for insurance coverage. The insurers playing this game therefore can legally lower their portion of covered customers with high-risk expensive healthcare needs and thereby maximize their profits. Their pharmacy and drug manufacturer coconspirators also maximize their profits because these high-risk patients are a captive audience who eventually still have to buy these medications through some form of insurance coverage. It's evil, clever, and all currently legal.

It has now become kitchen-table conversation that the cost of medications in America are so high that people have to ration their medications or forgo fundamentals such as food and utilities to afford life-sustaining medications. During the COVID-19 pandemic, the gall of pharmaceutical companies that literally took advantage of a frightened and desperate public through price gouging with the antiviral drug Remdesivir—ultimately found to be mildly effective[31] in hospitalized patients with severe lower respiratory tract infection due to the SARS-CoV-2—once again raised the bipartisan cry for centralized regulation of drug prices. Because of such heinous practices, in 2019, the pharmaceutical industry made political headlines as the presidential candidates vowed to take on these corporate drug Goliaths in a battle to reduce medication costs to a level equivalent to that spent in other developed countries.

Even politicians as diverse from each other as Donald Trump and Bernie Sanders both campaigned on the same promise to establish federal legislation to regulate and reduce drug prices. However, many of these same political candidates' campaigns received enormous financial support from the economic giants of the pharmaceutical industry that they publicly declared to be the "enemies" of the average citizen. Where does this hypocrisy leave the public? We the people are now still holding our breaths to see if the words of this generation of politicians are as empty as they have been in the past, or if there is a chance that their promises will finally come to fruition.

Sadly, the type of scenario experienced by my patient Marianne, in which the health insurance company completely or partially denies coverage for medical care, is all too common. Many of my friends and colleagues are surprised when I tell them that such gaps in coverage based on preexisting conditions and many other factors still continue.

They all ask the same question, "Wasn't Obamacare supposed to stop all this nonsense once and for all?"

The simple answer is, "No, it did not."

31 Beigel, John H., et al., "Remdesivir for the Treatment of Covid-19-Final Report," *NEJM* 2020; 383:1813-1826, https://www.nejm.org/doi/full/10.1056/nejmoa2007764.

There are still many gaping loopholes in the system that allow patients like Marianne to suffer. Amongst these include the regulatory variations between different states. Not all states availed themselves of the opportunity to improve their state-based healthcare coverage for the poor or unemployed by adopting the "Medicaid expansion" portion of the ACA. Thus, many people in these states who are poor or do not have access to health insurance coverage through a job remain ineligible for the financial assistance that would allow them to access health insurance. As of 2019, almost 74 percent of uninsured adults openly admit that the high cost of insurance is the main reason they lack coverage.[32]

Another deficit in assuring nationwide comprehensive and affordable access to healthcare is that many preexisting health insurance policies—those purchased on or before March 23, 2010—are not required to follow the regulations of the ACA. This is because such policies were obtained by the agents and brokers of private insurance companies outside of the sphere of the federally operated ACA-established marketplace. They maintain the right to deny care coverage for any reason agreed upon in the original contract with their beneficiary and are not subject to any of the ACA-based consumer protections. Some of these plans were the so-called short-term or "junk insurance" options that many younger people bought in case of emergencies. The policy owner was well aware that these plans were never intended to provide for ongoing preventative care or preexisting conditions. However, when an emergency actually happened, these plans still placed an extremely high financial burden on the patients. These "junk insurance" scenarios

32 "Nearly 30 Million Americans Have No Health Insurance," Peter G. Peterson Foundation, November 17, 2021 (online), https://www.pgpf.org/blog/2022/11/nearly-30-million-americans-have-no-health-insurance.

only worsened when the Trump administration reversed many of the ACA regulations.[33]

People without health insurance or who find themselves trapped in those policies that fall outside the regulatory control of the ACA have to make life-altering choices every day. Do they seek emergency care and continue buying life-sustaining medications knowing the huge costs they will be forced to pay? How will they buy food, pay the rent and utilities, or provide childcare, clothing, and school supplies for their children?

My patient Marianne could not afford the ACA marketplace health insurance policies when she moved to New York and thus had to give up the private insurance provided by her husband's prior employer. As a temporary measure, she bought cheaper emergency coverage insurance when she moved to New York, but because this did not cover medications and routine outpatient visits with her doctors like me, this left her family strapped with a several-thousand-dollar medical bill to pay over the next few years.

Ironically, because of the emergency caused by her heart beating too fast without medications, her most recent short-term insurance company in New York was also on the hook for several more thousands of dollars to cover a large portion of the bill. All of this could have been avoidable if she had adequate insurance to afford the medications that would have kept her out of the hospital in the first place. In the end, everyone—the state, the insurance company, the local hospital ER, and the family—paid more than they would have if there had not been such gaps in her coverage.

To make the situation even worse, because of her uncontrolled abnormal heartbeats, her heart muscle weakened more rapidly than it would have if she stayed on her medications. This accelerated

33 Deam, Jenny, "He Bought Health Insurance for Emergencies. Then He Fell Into a $33,601 Trap," *ProPublica*, May 8, 2021 (online), https://www.propublica.org/article/junk-insurance.

deterioration in her heart condition ultimately increased the likelihood that she would require more expensive care earlier in life than necessary if the whole emergency situation never occurred in the first place.

Other patients of mine had to be taken by ambulance to the emergency room because their health insurance denied coverage for effective medications that they were on for years. Jack, 12 years old, successfully underwent curative heart surgery as an infant. Unfortunately, he also had severe asthma, which was well controlled as long as he took several long-acting medications. However, his insurance removed one of these potent medications, Advair, from their inventory list of covered medications. They gave him no alternative but to use another asthma medicine that he had already tried and which failed to work years ago. What happened next should have been expected. Jack almost died from the asthma attack that ensued a week after he started the approved medication. He survived a heart condition only to be rendered near death because of a forced medication change. Here's the kicker—the cost of the ambulance ride, the emergency room visit, and the three-day intensive care hospital stay could have paid for 10 years of Jack's original asthma medication.

Our healthy young adults face similar challenges to my heart patients. It is now a universal policy that young people "age out" of health insurance coverage under their parents' policies at 26 years old. Not everyone is fully employed or able to afford their own health insurance at that time in their lives. The ACA established the open marketplace at reduced costs for people making below a certain annual income to address this. However, many young people make too much money to qualify for access to the marketplace. A large portion of young people remain underinsured because, even if they qualify, they still find the cost of the marketplace insurance policies to be prohibitive.

In both of these economic scenarios, many choose short-term or Medicaid insurance instead. Even worse, millions remain completely uninsured. This age-based policy resulted in a huge increase in our nation's uninsured adults, from 19 million in the 19-to-25 age group to 39 million aged 26 to 34. With the ACA under political attack along party lines, improvements in the ACA marketplace that could render the policies more affordable remain vulnerable. The new Biden administration addressed this early on by providing subsidies to make the marketplace policies more affordable. Without such resources, young people do not receive preventative care and are more likely to seek medical attention in an emergency or when a health condition progresses too far. Again, the related costs to our society at this point are exorbitant, including the burden of huge healthcare debt to these young people if they survive their illness. Even if they recover sufficiently, they begin this early part of their lives financially behind the eight ball.

Extrapolating shortsighted scenarios such as those portrayed by Marianne, Jack, and our young adults to the many millions of patients across the country, I can just imagine the magnitude of the total costs to our nation. No one wins with such non-comprehensive and cost-prohibitive insurance policies. If we are to be truly successful in our healthcare reform platforms, Americans need to start seeing health insurance as covering peoples' lives, not their medical diagnoses. Marianne is not just a heart condition—she is a mother, wife, and survivor of congenital heart disease. She is an American citizen whose husband fought for years as a soldier in Iraq, and when she needed us most, she was cruelly forced to take extraordinary measures to save her own life and care for her children. Moving forward, we must do better.

Perhaps I sound cynical. I doubt that anyone truly is in love with their private health insurance company. In speaking with my patients and in my role as the main negotiator for my staff's health insurance coverage, I learned that people refer to their particular policy or coverage package, not the name of the actual company. Unlike a decade ago, none of us had any kind of personal relationship with these companies or their representatives. When we need to contact them, we find ourselves on hold for hours, passed from one faceless bureaucrat to another, asked to fill out redundant and meaningless paperwork, and too often left in the dark about how their decision to deny us the coverage we need for professionally directed healthcare was made.

People may not realize that most health insurance companies actually contract a third-party representative—a broker—to sell their insurance to clients ranging from individuals to large corporate employers. These brokers work on commissions or a flat-fee basis. Our broker for many years was a warmhearted, affable, and gentle giant of a man in his mid-40s, named Charlie Goodman. Every year, for almost two decades, my practice manager and I put on our benefits-coordinator hats in a several-hour-long meeting with Charlie to tailor the myriad of increasingly complex health coverage options to the needs of our employees.

In the end, these meetings always boiled down to a handful of health benefits "packages" in which my employees could choose to enroll. Each year, the cost of these benefits increased for both me as the employer and my employees, while the actual benefits became increasingly restrictive and less comprehensive. Because of this broker-coordinated process, the employees were never able to review all the possible options on the market. They had to trust that my manager and I had their best interests at heart. In the presence of the broker, we updated the employees about the latest medical insurances available to them at one of our regular staff meetings.

"Are these the only insurances we can choose from?" sighed a hardworking, young, single mother of two who, for the past decade, warmly greeted my patients as they entered the building.

"What's the point of pretending we have a choice? Looks like we are all getting the short end of the stick once again. Our premiums, copays, and deductibles are higher, while our medication coverage and choice of physicians are worse than ever," interjected my brutally honest senior nurse.

"Yes, I'm sorry to report that, despite strong-arming our kind broker next to me, we are told that this is the best we can do this year," I stated calmly.

Seeing that I could use an ally in the ring, Charlie softly but firmly added, "Dr. Fethke has thrown in a lot of his own money to provide this level of medical insurance to you all. No other physician group that I work with has been as generous given the currently difficult financial times in healthcare. The fact that you all enroll as a group is also still to your advantage. There definitely is no way that any one person could afford plans as good as these in today's market if they applied as an individual."

In the end, the staff was resigned to accept this process because they knew we had given it our best shot and trusted that Charlie told the truth.

My patients and neighbors consistently confess to me that they would readily switch to any other company or third-party payor as long as the most valued elements of their health insurance coverage—their wish-list items—are maintained. These common-sense priorities are not sophisticated or difficult to appreciate. They have also become major topics of the 2020 political candidates' healthcare-related debates and campaign promises. The seven top ranked items regarding the fundamental expectations of decent health benefits that I repeatedly hear from my patients, family, and friends include the following:

1. The ability to freely choose one's primary or specialty physician or medical facility

2. No limitations or restrictions on coverage for any prescribed medical services based on preexisting medical conditions

3. No restrictions on any prescribed testing, medications, or other therapies

4. Full coverage outside a person's home state or the country when traveling

5. Full coverage for emergency-related or disaster-related medical care

6. Truly affordable family coverage, including children up to 26 years old

7. Truly affordable deductibles, copays, and maximum annual expenditures

If anyone today actually has a health insurance policy that fulfills all of these criteria, they or their employer footing the premium bills must be extremely rich. To receive this kind of comprehensive coverage in our for-profit medical system, an individual or a small business must pay premiums of approximately $10,000 per year per insured patient.[34] This level rises to $20,000-$25,000 per year for a family. The costs also vary wildly between states, by age, and considering health status of the beneficiary. The 50 to 60 percent of small- to medium-sized companies nationwide that presently cover an average of 70 percent of these premiums for their employees cannot afford such comprehensive packages and therefore typically choose a more midrange plan that covers some of these items on the wish list. As with my employees, people are forced to pick and choose amongst these items from a preset menu, often with metallic names such as the bronze, silver, gold, or platinum plans. If you have the bronze plan, you might as well stay home in a bubble to avoid accident or

34 Porretta, Anna, "How Much Does Individual Health Insurance Cost?", eHealth, October 01, 2022 (online), https://www.ehealthinsurance.com/resources/individual-and-family/how-much-does-individual-health-insurance-cost.

limit your exposure to infections. Though the average premium cost of this lowest tier plan is about 40 percent of a premium or platinum plan, the costs for which the patients are contractually responsible, such as the deductibles, copays, and annual maximum out-of-pocket expenditures, can total as much as $25,000 per year for a family.

I often wondered why the various components of these different-level plans cost so much and are so complex in the first place. Designing any particular insurance plan is so complicated that even I, after two decades of experience, could never imagine doing this without a broker. This remains true even though many insurance companies provide online calculators similar to personal tax filing software to help with the process. Compiling an individual annual tax report form is much simpler than choosing the right combination of levels of deductibles, copays, and maximum out-of-pocket thresholds for any one person or family. The stakes are also much higher with medical insurance. Making an error in filing taxes is subject only to a defined and limited financial risk. Choosing the wrong insurance coverage can not only hurt one's wallet; it can leave them vulnerable to inappropriate or insufficient healthcare with life-changing implications. I certainly felt the pressure to make the right choices when working with Mr. Goodman to provide health benefits for my staff.

I also remain skeptical that the insurance companies actually use the different bronze to platinum packages as a smoke screen to minimize their own financial vulnerabilities. They use this system to create an advertising-driven impression that the consumer somehow gets a better deal for their money with the gold or platinum options than the bronze package. In the end, like a gambling casino, they are simply steering the healthcare consumer to pick the card from the deck that creates the least exposure to the dealer. The insurers raise the premiums so high for the platinum plans that, even if they make sense for a person's health needs, very few people throw all their chips into the bet upfront, despite a sometimes virtually guaranteed huge payoff.

After one of our annual health benefits staff meetings, a physician colleague sat down to pick my brains.

"My wife has been recently diagnosed with a chronic autoimmune illness and will be needing many doctors' visits with specialists and lifelong expensive medications," he informed me with obvious concern.

"I'm so sorry to hear that. How can I help?" I replied as I instinctively but consciously moved my chair closer to him.

He looked up, deep in thought. "I know the platinum plan will minimize my final costs because the deductibles, copays, and maximum amount I personally pay each year are much lower than the bronze or silver plans. I just can't see taking that much money from each paycheck before I even know what we will need. I wish I had a crystal ball to see the future and make the right financial decision. Why is health insurance so complicated?"

When I buy a car—an item that costs as much as the annual outlay for the average family's health insurance—I do not hesitate to research the value of the bundled components included in the highest-level EX Honda Accord compared to the midrange LX. My objective is to choose the best value in the short term while minimizing the losses in the long run. When we buy healthcare in America, we are forced to make similar calculated risks and value judgments. This lowers healthcare to the level of a simple commodity, rather than a right and a basic necessity we all need as much as food and shelter.

I also propose that by restricting or eliminating any of the seven priority items that people seek in their medical care coverage, the insurers are fooling themselves that they save money. If the high copays or deductibles of a lower-premium plan discourage a person from seeking preventative or semi-urgent medical attention, the chance that the beneficiary will end up with a more serious illness increases significantly.

The COVID-19 pandemic demonstrated this phenomena when people were afraid to venture outside their homes. Initially, this resulted in far fewer payouts from the insurance pool and associated record profits. Within months, many people finally reached the threshold of seeking medical attention for their recurring chest pain, only to find that they suffered permanent heart damage from untreated hypertension or mini-heart attacks. People with unexplained weight loss eventually went for the medical evaluation that diagnosed a now large and likely deadly malignant tumor that would have been much smaller and treatable when symptoms first appeared months before. Given these situations, the health insurers are sure to spend much more money for treatments and hospitalization with a now much lower chance of successful outcome. Any such disincentives or obstacles to regular or urgent healthcare, such as health plans with higher patient costs, run the same risk for worsening illness and higher costs for all involved. Thus, when I take a step back to scrutinize each of these seven components individually, I conclude that these are not just part of an ideal wish list. They are inherently crucial to any viable health insurance policy and successful healthcare system.

Though we in the United States claim to be a freely and openly capitalist system, my experience and travels lead me to conclude that we are actually much more of a socialist or government-controlled society than we like to admit. When Gilbert Tremain developed potentially life-threatening abnormal electrical signals from the bottom of his heart, known as ventricular tachycardia, I knew it was time we considered using a special pacemaker, known as an automated internal cardiac defibrillator (AICD). The use of this device was founded and promoted by a pioneer in medicine, Dr. Arthur J. Moss, and colleagues in the 1970s. When inserted in the chest of the patient, it saved countless lives by delivering a shock to the heart to quickly stop these tachycardias before they could result in a lethal, sudden cardiac arrest.

After months of discussion with Gilbert about the need to obtain an AICD, during one of his late-evening outpatient visits with me, I became concerned and spoke up. "Have you made a decision about the AICD I advised for you a few months ago? I am worried that your heart may suddenly speed up, and you are still without the protection that you deserve."

Gilbert looked me straight in the eye and with a tremor to his voice replied, "I know you have my best interest in mind, Doc. Believe me, I appreciate it and all that you have done for me. The problem is that my Medicare health insurance does not fully pay for most of the costs—the necessary tests, hospitalization, and the procedures involved. I'm not a rich man, and my ailing wife needs the money for her care more than I do. I'll just have to take my chances."

I knew he was sincere in his wishes to spend any of their life savings on helping his wife, rather than laying out thousands of dollars to pay for the AICD costs that his government-based insurance did not cover. I began calling and writing to my physician colleagues at several prestigious institutions to see if anyone could reduce the costs for the AICD. "This man is part of our medical legacy. Surely he deserves all that we can give him without worrying about going broke," I pleaded over and over. Before I received an answer, Gilbert passed away quietly at home, and I will never know if he suffered a preventable ventricular tachycardia-induced arrest.

Gilbert's final days and the stories of many of my patients force me to confront the proverbial elephant in the room that causes these problems. The insurers continue to call the shots and dictate the rules that limit or completely exclude necessary healthcare resources. All too often, physicians are unable to efficiently and equitably promote the utilization of indicated diagnostic testing, procedures, and therapies they know are best for their patients.

A landmark example of this was when public pressures and medical evidence finally led the ACA to fully cover seniors through Medicare for a colonoscopy as a screening tool for early detection of colorectal cancers. Though this could potentially save thousands of American lives, Medicare and the private insurers who followed suit first significantly reduced the reimbursements to the physicians and medical facilities for these tests. They also left a gaping loophole in the law that required patients to cover the costs of the removal of any intestinal masses, known as polyps, if they were later found to not contain any cancer. Many patients therefore continued to avoid this screening test, and it has taken almost a decade for Congress to pass the Removing Barriers to Colorectal Screening Act that will phase out this loophole by 2030.

Echocardiography, a very common, painless test used in adult cardiology to noninvasively image and evaluate the heart, was also subject to government cost-control measures. Beginning in the late 1990s and through the next two decades, CMS policies suddenly decreased reimbursements by over 50 percent for any echocardiograms performed in the non-hospital outpatient setting. CMS did not reduce their payments for any echocardiograms performed on hospital property. The tragic economic irony is that the US medical profession responded to these draconian reductions by simply performing double the echocardiograms in the hospital setting. In the end, this shortsighted intervention did not save[35] any money. It actually cost CMS, the taxpayers, and the patients hundreds of millions of dollars more.

If the free-market processes of the United States had truly been allowed to function, then perhaps other breakthrough technologies, such as modern genetic testing, would also have been pursued more equitably from the start. As my practice evolved in the first decade of the twenty-first century, I began recommending genetic evaluations for my patients with certain heart conditions. These tests identify patients carrying a potentially lethal gene that may be shared with other family

35 McKeown, L.A., "CMS Cuts to Office-Based Noninvasive Cardiac Tests Are Driving Costs Higher," *tctMD*, Oct. 17, 2019, https://www.tctmd.com/news/cms-cuts-office-based-noninvasive-cardiac-tests-are-driving-costs-higher.

members and also passed onto future generations. The ability to find such genetic patterns allows for life-saving, targeted treatments and preventative strategies that have revolutionized the medical field. People living with once universally deadly illnesses that resulted in premature deaths can now live long productive lives.

At the time, only a few select diagnostic laboratories were providers of high-quality medical genetic testing. They therefore had an essential monopoly in the market and were able to charge extremely high costs for these tests. Many of the insurance companies completely denied coverage for such expensive testing. Eventually, a minority of insurance companies approved this coverage, but this highly accepted and evidence-based medical tool was denied and thus out of reach to most of my patients. Recently, though, new startup private companies began to provide very high-quality genetic testing for a fraction of the cost that the original companies charged. Free-market competition without government involvement has just now opened access to these tests for everyone at an affordable level. Though I am happy that these tests are more equitably available, I cannot help but be conflicted and wonder how many lives were lost and at what cost to society. So many people were not aware that they carried these invisible, dangerous genetic patterns. Why didn't the government step in then to lower costs and reveal these silent killers?

These and many more examples reveal that the US government essentially stepped in as the most influential regulator of diagnostic testing and many therapeutic modalities. How are Medicare's policies regarding the standardization and reimbursements for colonoscopy and echocardiography any different than the Canadian government's role in paying for and regulating the costs of such tests in their country? The often-touted political rhetoric purports that, unlike foreign governments with socialized healthcare systems, the US government does not interfere in the free-market-based healthcare system. The reality is that they clearly do and quite often.

The problem is that, without appropriate medical and scientific guidance, these financially driven government decisions often waste money and cost lives. I am certain that government-based policies, such as those championed by CMS, focused solely on cost reduction should not be used as the template or the green light for the private payors to follow suit. If we are to achieve any significant level of quality and performance outcomes in the US healthcare system, evidence-based medical care must guide our policy and economic decisions.

A MATTER OF TRUST

It's so easy to just give up. It's so hard to give in. This is the internal, emotional turmoil that I and many of my physician colleagues have found ourselves dealing with over the past decade, one only amplified during the COVID-19 pandemic. As we go about our days caring for patients in our offices and hospitals, we return home each day with a heavier heart. Somewhere along the way, I sense that we have let go of the ideals that originally called us to join this once-noble field of medicine. What was once a source of immense pride—the privilege of caring for others—feels more and more like a burden weighing down on our souls. I have finished many of my long days wondering what underlies this heavy heart I try to conceal from my patients and from myself.

What could have so tarnished my pride in being an American physician that I was now beginning to think about early retirement? At first, I thought it was simply the accumulation of the escalating bureaucracy in my day-to-day routine. Had one more recent straw finally broken the camel's back? No, this was a necessary evil that, though not welcome, still did not rise to the level of outweighing my pleasure in being a physician. In the end, I kept coming back to the same conclusion. It was a matter of trust—specifically, the lack thereof at multiple levels, including between patients and their physicians and amongst physicians and the institutions we serve.

I often wonder where this mistrust originated. Perhaps it started in the past when, in other healthcare reform cycles, physicians all too readily gave up their leadership roles. They stepped away from making any meaningful contributions to the evolution of healthcare delivery systems. As an unforeseen consequence, they gradually lost their claim as the defender and protector of the physician-patient relationship. In abandoning this role, they lost their professional and cultural authority to lead the healthcare system. In other words, because the doctors themselves appeared to not want to be bothered with the policymaking that determined how patients accessed and received healthcare, patients felt abandoned, suspicious, and mistrustful of physicians' motives.

As a young mother so eloquently summarized, "It seems like for most of the physicians I have brought my daughter to with her complex medical problems over the years, money is actually more precious than getting to know and caring for my child."

I know that for most physicians, this label of being solely "money-driven" is far from the truth, but the misinterpretation by those outside of this relationship is perhaps understandable when viewed from the patients' vantage point. Doctors began to lose patient trust in the modern era when they appeared to represent the managed care industry more than their patients. This disillusionment with the lack of patient advocacy by physicians became more solidified as the HMOs and their progeny, including the government's healthcare agencies, relegated the primary physician to a more remote and less prominent position than the corporate profiteers.

My patients distrust anyone who treats them as a number, rather than a person, when they seek medical attention. As a young, confused, and disgruntled mother recently told me, "I literally had to take a number at the clinic where I have been taking my kids for years. They were recently taken over by a big corporation, and no one there even knows who we are anymore. I just want my doctor back."

During the 2016 presidential debates and the 2018 midterm elections, this lack of access to one's own doctor was a consistent part of the heated political debates regarding healthcare reform. As the 2020 presidential elections were underway, a policeman father of one of my handicapped patients summarized his concerns about the political process.

"Many of my colleagues on the force and the people in the communities we serve do not have access to the same privileged healthcare that the wealthy and powerful still have and are clearly keeping for themselves. These fat cats have made sure that they can always see their own doctors, but they are designing a system in which the rest of us have to fend for ourselves. Except for the occasional specialist like you, my kid never sees the same pediatrician anymore." In my experience, Americans highly value the ability to have a medical visit with their own regular physician. Without such access, they feel stranded and never form the patient-physician relationship that is essential to establishing trust in the system.

Reimbursement strategies and delivery mechanisms are constantly revised and implemented by those outside the medical field. A pediatrician colleague of mine hit the mark when, after a stressful and busy week with patients during the COVID-19 pandemic, he complained, "Did you see the crazy political debates last night? In the middle of the worst health crisis in a century, these policymakers don't even mention what us doctors and our patients are going through together. The bond I have with my patients is the only thing that is getting us through this. Nowhere in their proposals do they show me that they understand how important this patient-physician relationship is, not only to our healthcare reform but, right now, to our very survival. If they stop us from being able to know our patients, we're done."

As with this physician, I sense that the sanctity and security of the patient-physician relationship are highly vulnerable and too often the first elements sacrificed in many of the policy proposals. Over the years, I have interviewed hundreds of families about medical care, and they almost all say essentially the same thing. They want access to their doctors, time with their doctors, and affordably delivered individualized care. They desperately wish that those making important decisions of healthcare—the larger business-oriented models they work under, the private insurers, or the public clinics—would stop making changes without asking the patients or the physicians themselves to guide the process.

"Don't they trust us—you know, us people and you doctors—to know best what we need? Do they think we're just all about spending or making money? We want and need good care," prompted a perplexed, single grandmother raising her granddaughter in need of heart surgery as she left my clinic.

This woman's sentiment hits the nail on the head for me. She is acutely in tune with the prejudiced mixed messaging of policymakers, which translates as follows—physicians cannot be trusted because they all have an inherent conflict of interest that prevents them from establishing a resource-efficient healthcare delivery model. Doctors want to be the main economic benefactor in any such system, so don't rely on the doctors to organize medical practices or systems because they just get richer without benefitting society or the patients in any meaningful way.

The recent political battle between the two main parties over the nature of US healthcare reform further exacerbated the people's confusion and mistrust at a very fundamental level—access to medical services. For the past decade, the pieces of the ACA pertaining to the cost and criteria to enter the insurance marketplace have been tossed back and forth with every four-year cycle, depending on the party in the White House. This resulted in an understandable whiplash to the American psyche, a health coverage insecurity that left many doubtful that they can reliably make any long-lasting plans about how to receive routine and emergency medical care. This state of instability handicaps all parties involved in our healthcare system—policymakers, patients, medical care providers, and the healthcare industry at large—preventing them from confidently moving forward.

In the midst of the increasingly bureaucratic and cost-savings-motivated policies, physicians repeatedly demonstrated they still care to have their voices heard regarding the way the US provides medical care. Since its founding in 1847, the AMA remains determined to represent physicians' and patients' best interests. Across the nation, this spawned state- and community-wide medical associations that work tirelessly to keep the physician at the forefront of healthcare decision-making. However, the AMA's activities have not been free of controversy, repeatedly stirring up cries by the public and the medical profession regarding serious conflicts of interest.

Since the 1960s, for many of my physician colleagues, the AMA has also lost credibility as an agent of patient and physician advocacy. Too many medical societies seem to have succumbed to focusing more on economics and protecting the rights of the medical profession, rather than prioritizing the well-being of the physician-patient relationship. They may say otherwise when questioned directly, but the frequent communications by email and other literature I receive from the dozens of medical societies clearly demonstrate that they function mainly as a physician advocacy group. They primarily support doctors by countering the outside trends from third-party payors and government reform that threaten the financial interests of the physicians.

Though this physician advocacy may in fact be an important endeavor in the latest political environment, it appears it has become all-consuming, and little is said about the patients themselves and the quality of care. This sense that medical societies function like an exclusive medical guild resulted in a deep-seated mistrust of such institutions by medical professionals and policymakers determined not to lose sight of the patients' best interests. When finances become the main focus of medical societies, physicians instinctively begin to mistrust that their leadership is truly watching out for their individual professional interests and are more likely indebted to a small group seated at the top of these entities watching out for their own economic interests.

In other words, like patients and the public, physicians begin to mistrust their own leadership. "I keep getting letters requesting that I join the medical society. The dues are not cheap, and I'm not convinced that it's worth it," complained one of my physician friends. "I don't see anything changing for the better at work. Our supposed medical society representatives sit rubbing elbows with the politicians while we get buried deeper in BS. What have they really done for us and our ability to care for patients with all these dues?" A house divided has begun to fall.

One of the hardest lessons for me from the COVID-19 pandemic experience is the realization that the cost of such profound loss of trust amongst physicians, patients, and our medical institutions has been deadly. The possibility that even one COVID-19 death may have resulted from a mistrustful person not accepting the advice of the medical profession is bad enough. The fact that hundreds of thousands of our people may have died because they no longer had faith in the advice of the medical profession is emotionally and morally devastating to me as a physician. I fear that, if we are unable to reestablish this trust in our medical professionals, in addition to the already experienced economic downfall, US society at large is in peril of moral, political, and social collapse.

Rebuilding trust is now priority number one. As David Brooks writes in *The Atlantic*, "Unless we can find a way to rebuild trust, the nation does not function."[36] Do doctors and the healthcare system have an important role, a responsibility, to step in now during this moral crisis of mistrust, which Mr. Brooks conveys so well? As hard as it is,

36 Brooks, David, "America Is Having A Moral Convulsion," *The Atlantic*, October 5, 2020 (online), https://www.theatlantic.com/ideas/archive/2020/10/collapsing-levels-trust-are-devastating-america/616581/.

I think so, yes—and a critical role at that. We must both regain and protect this trust. If not medical professionals, then who? When society is as sick as I can remember in my lifetime, divided and mistrustful of institutions, government, other races, genders, and anything that appears to pose a personal threat, the need for trustworthy healthcare remains our common denominator.

Physicians must step up to build back medical institutions that learned from the past mistakes that led us to the edge of the culturally moral abyss. Once and for all, physicians must prove to society that we will care for all people. This is no longer material for philosophical banter. The pandemic has shown us the horrible price we pay for not providing healthcare equitably. I no longer wish to feel the shame, guilt, and disgust which this pandemic has left us with in the face of losing so many people we are sworn to protect. Untimely and unnecessary death is a physician's archenemy, and we can no longer be anywhere but on the frontlines of this battle, wherever it may take us.

My experience teaches me that the best way to gain trust of a community is to start with individuals and their families. Contrary to the image of a doctor as an erudite and high-powered professional, I teach my students that their best chance at achieving true authority amongst their patients is to practice humility. We don't have to always pretend that we know everything, only that we will use all our resources to know our patients well and provide them the best care possible. We earn trust when we finally realize we are privileged to be entrusted by others to enter into such personal aspects of their lives at such vulnerable times as an illness. This humble approach shows without a doubt that we care and can open the doors to healing at all levels of our lives. I know this not because I wear a white coat or hang Ivy League diplomas on my wall but because I have practiced this way all my professional life and experience the resulting faith in my abilities every day.

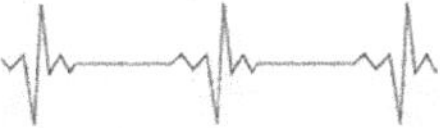

The young Haitian mother sat stoically in the exam room chair, eyes directed downward and avoiding my gaze. Her six-foot-three-inch tall husband shuffled quietly in the corner of the room opposite from the entrance door, staring at me without a word. I sensed I was being sized up before I even spoke. I soon learned that they had only just arrived from Haiti one month ago. Their home was devastated six months prior by the earthquake of January 2010. They just made it to the United States in time to give birth in New York.

They spoke very little English, but I am fluent in French because of my Parisian-born mother. "Give the baby to me," the father said sternly to the young mother as he reached out to take this wide-eyed, strikingly beautiful infant and lay her gently on the exam table. "Doc, the pediatrician says something is wrong with my baby's heart. What's going on?" he asked with a slightly angry tone when he realized I understood French. I read the hospital records and learned that an irregular heartbeat was noted in the newborn nursery. "No one told us anything," he went on. "They just sent us here, and we had to wait 10 days to see you."

I now sensed that, though he appeared brave and strong on the outside, he was internally petrified that his daughter was in danger of being very sick. In my southern New York offices and on the border of Haiti during medical charity work in the Dominican Republic, I had worked with many patients from their politically and environmentally ravaged country. You had to be tough and wear thick skin to survive there. Everyone had to fend for themselves. Trust was not readily granted because the people had been deceived and deprived too many times to count over the years. The journey to New York could not have been easy.

Before I proceeded to mechanically examine the baby, I picked her up in my arms and played with her a little while asking them about their family. I let them know that I had been to the Dominican Republic just after the earthquake and attended to several Haitian refugees. We talked about the tasty food there, and when I saw the parents shoulders begin to relax with an accompanying slight smile, I laid the infant down and completed my exam. Using pictures on a small whiteboard to help explain everything, I reassured them that the tests were normal, and the irregular heartbeats had resolved. I finished the visit by putting the baby back in the mother's arms.

As they stood up to leave, I reached out with one arm on each of their shoulders, saying, "You have a beautiful family. Your daughter is safe, and I wish you well here or wherever you may go." The mother began to tear up slightly as she now looked directly at me.

The father bent over to give me a bear hug, the barrier between us now melted away. "You're a good man, Doctor. Hopefully, we do not have to come back for our children, but we are glad we met you."

It's high time that the reflex response from a PCP, "I can't help because I only met the patient once," becomes unacceptable. We must educate our medical students to not accept this mindset early in their clinical rotations. Beginning from the moment they first encounter a patient, we must create a managed care culture that reinforces the PCP's role as the patient's rightful main advocate when it comes to their medical needs. When we assign legitimate trust to our PCPs, we empower them with the authority to deliver the best care available. This approach engenders a culture of trust amongst all parties involved in patient care.

My hardworking and dedicated staff have come to me several times on the verge of tears during the COVID-19 pandemic. "A mother just yelled at me on the phone that I did not care about her child's health," my medical assistant informed me as I sat down at my desk. "She accused me of refusing to provide needed medical care to her child and warned she was calling her lawyer to sue us."

The mother of this six-year-old girl became angered because, to prevent the spread of the virus, we advised postponing her visit until her daughter's cold symptoms of coughs and sneezing resolved. This was the practice's policy which came from our administration. My assistant was just doing her job. At this time in early 2020, testing for the SARS-CoV-2 virus was not readily available in outpatient offices like ours. Before speaking with the family about rescheduling the visit, we talked with the child's referring regular pediatrician to make sure he thought she could wait a bit longer to see us. This PCP had followed her since birth and noted what appeared to be a fairly benign heart murmur in a recent healthy child visit. He agreed that the pediatric cardiology visit with us was not urgent and could wait until the resolution of her cough and congestion.

There was still no convincing the mother. She vehemently blamed us for neglecting her daughter's health problems. Several nurses called to try and console her. I did too. She just did not understand why we were not allowing her coughing daughter to enter the building. She did not seem to care that others would be placed at risk by this action. For some intangible reason, at that time, she just did not seem to get it. Her actions, and the emotional impact on my staff, stood in stark contrast to the way we were treated by other patients' parents.

Many did "get it," acknowledging and respecting that we took extra precautions for the good of all. Some families even complimented the staff for this conscientiousness, despite all the extra steps required. "We truly appreciate that you guys are still here for us even in the face of the increased risk to yourselves," said one of the parents of a small infant who had just undergone heart surgery.

The pandemic taught me that immense stress makes it all too easy to judge others. We jump to place them into basic categories that are easier to process in the midst of this chaos: "Those who get it and those who don't." However, if we employ our emotional IQs better, the spotlight allows us to look deeper and be more compassionate. It is not so simple.

One week later, I again reached out to the mother who was so accusatory of my staff. Through sobs and tears, she apologized for her prior interaction with our team. She revealed that she is an emergency room nurse and was exhausted physically and emotionally at work because of the pandemic. She added that her husband just lost his job, and her mother had been hospitalized with COVID-19. In the midst of all of this, she became panicked that her daughter might now have a life-threatening heart condition that the pediatrician just picked up.

"I spoke with her pediatrician last week," she explained. "He told me that you all contacted him directly about everything, and he reassured me that I could trust your judgement about her safety. We trust him implicitly, and his words mean a lot to us. He apparently also thinks very highly of you all and said that he would send us to only the best."

I thanked her for her kind words and reassured her that we were here to help. Trust was established because we placed their beloved pediatrician at the forefront of the communications centered around her daughter's well-being. When I saw them for a consultation the following week, now cough- and congestion-free, I found that her heart was indeed normal. The mother cried tears of relief and apologized for not being able to hug each and every one of us. She has since referred several patients to our practice from her emergency room. The chocolates she left behind were an added bonus.

I cannot help but wonder if the advice to wear masks and the distribution and delivery of the miraculous COVID-19 vaccines would have been much more widely accepted if we maintained trust in our frontline healthcare workers and primary physicians in the first place. During the pandemic, the media and American public were in the justifiable habit of calling these healthcare professionals heroes. I believe this is because we recognize their honorable insistence on carrying out their professional roles despite the high risk to themselves. These nurses, doctors, technicians, and staff are not world leaders in healthcare, yet we are most proud of their efforts. They have earned our undying trust, and I believe they best represent the solution to regaining trust in the US healthcare system.

One of the most striking examples of this medical professionalism and earned trust is embodied in a news story I watched one evening with my wife. In the height of the pandemic in a California emergency room, a Jewish physician, Dr. Taylor Nichols, and his multiracial team found themselves caring for one of many deathly ill patients with respiratory failure. As they removed his shirt to attend to him, they were stunned by his many swastika Nazi tattoos. Despite the understandable personal fear and disgust they experienced when seeing these emblems of hate, they remained professional behind the layers of personal protective equipment that hid their religious identities. They treated this man with the same dignity and standard of care as any other patient. Their story spread across social media like a ray of hope. The doctor and his team were praised for their professionalism and humanity. They earned the nation's trust and respect.[37]

Given the intensely polarized political landscape of the American people, the only hope that we can come together again to heal our people during the multiple simultaneous pandemics, including

37 Palmer, Ewan, "Jewish Doctor Admits He 'Hesitated' Over Treating Man With Nazi Tattoos Amid COVID Stress," *Newsweek* 90, Dec. 1, 2020 (online), https://www.newsweek.com/jewish-doctor-hesitated-treating-man-nazi-tattoos-covid-stress-1551382.

COVID-19, gun violence, racism, domestic terrorism, housing and food insecurities, and the opiate crisis, is through the single acts of pure kindness such as those delivered by Dr. Nichols. Trust is reborn amongst people who fear and even despise each other when, ignoring such differences, we reach out to deliver care during our perceived enemy's most vulnerable times. This act of selflessness has the potential to leave a kernel of doubt about their prejudices in the mind of people like Dr. Nichols's patient. Today, this doubt spreads on social media like the seeds of hope in the wind. Here is where we begin to rebuild trust in the medical profession. Here is where healthcare breeds the heroes that heal our society.

THE BATTERED PHYSICIAN

Many physicians I know confide that, over the past two decades, they often feel like helpless bystanders watching policymakers, big businesses, and politicians making important decisions that directly and significantly impact their professional lives. As the winds of healthcare reform become stronger, the individual physician feels obligated to take the path of least resistance. It is definitely easier to be pushed by the wind than to march against it, but they question whether this is the right course of action. They are resigned to follow instead of lead, even when they don't necessarily agree with the direction healthcare in their community, state, or nation may be heading. Any effort to buck these gale-force winds—the "system"—seems futile.

"You know, there are all these extra steps—the credentialing nightmare, the malpractice costs, the crazy complicated electronic medical charting, MU and best-practices requirements to become a Medical Home, and more—just to see a patient. This has gotten beyond ridiculous and not why I became a doctor, " ranted an anesthesia colleague in the hallway after a hospital staff meeting. Suddenly more resigned, he continued, "Ah, well, what are ya gonna do? If you can't beat 'em,

I guess we just have to put our heads down, join 'em, and get out of healthcare before the shit hits the fan."

At times, I too feel like I am holding an umbrella against a hurricane. Perhaps this is why writing about what physicians are dealing with has become so therapeutic for me. It is like sending a message in a bottle during a storm from a small boat tossed by waves in the hopes that someone will read it and help us reach shore safely. My deep concern is that, because it appears like we physicians are all heading in the same direction, everyone around us, including our colleagues, may assume we are all complicit in the path we take—that our current course of US healthcare represents the medical profession's "common sense," rather than our mutual futility. If an individual doctor was to look over and ask one of their colleagues being pushed forward in the collective wind tunnel how they truly feel about their situation, they may be shocked to learn that this is not necessarily an exercise of free will. Sensing few reasonable alternatives, they too feel obliged to follow. If the physicians themselves feel helpless, I shudder to reflect how even more harmful of an impact this forced march may be for our patients.

In a November 2018 article in the journal *Medical Economics*, Dr. David Nash posed the alternative argument. He is the founding dean at the Jefferson College of Population Health and a leading physician voice with an emphasis on improving US healthcare. He has been a chief editor of several major peer-reviewed medical journals and a major advisor in academic and leadership forums about issues related to promoting population health since at least 2008. In the article, he expresses, "For folks on the frontlines, population health is an explicit recognition that the delivery of care is only 20 percent of the story." He explains that physicians essentially have no choice but to allow the policymakers to link physician income to performance measures through the implementation of population health guidelines. He concludes that, to survive, today's physicians must accept being part of the big business of medicine. "You can run, but you can't hide from it [population health]," he says at the end of the interview. "We are heading toward the total accountability for the outcome of care, and with no outcomes, there will be no income for doctors, and that is a sea change."[38]

Doctors have always written notes in a standardized way that document the visit with each patient. These notes include the patient's health story, our medical opinions about their health status or problem, and any plans to conduct other tests, refer for procedures, or treat with medications or other therapies. When we compile each patient's records in a binder, we call this a chart. Until the past two to three decades, our "charting" work was always handwritten or typed on paper. Today, it is entered into a computer version of the chart, the EMR, and explains why all too often, patients see their doctors' backs more than their faces as they remain hunched over computers.

What Dr. Nash fails to acknowledge is that, though his goals of improved population health are laudable, the way these goals are incorporated into the physicians' work has been at best ineffective. The data we are forced to enter into the EMRs at each patient visit is relatively meaningless and does not actually promote population health. At worst, the exponentially increased busywork of filling in the patients' medical charts misses the true mark and distracts doctors away from spending valuable time with their patients.

In my day-to-day work, the "population health outcomes" that Dr. Nash touts have been reduced to little more than superficial jargon. Like empty calories, they have so far manifested in our EMRs as abundant, but relatively meaningless (and time-wasting), boxes that the doctors or their medical staff reluctantly click through to complete the patient visit notes. Doctors view them as the annoying, tasteless, and nutrition-lacking fruits of our electronic charts. Doctors view

38 Todd Shryock (ed.), "Succeed at Population Health Management: How Practices Can Benefit from Data-driven Patient Care," *Medical Economics* 95 no. 22 (November 25, 2018), p. 22, 25.

this data entry as a nuisance of little relevance to clinical care on a personal or larger community level. In the name of very limited time available to spend on each patient visit, they simply jump mindlessly and as quickly as possible through these "hoops" to reach the end of the patient notes. There is rarely any real thought put into the choices they click.

If we think of the patient-physician relationship as analogous to the best fruit in the whole orchard, should we all start buying a tasteless and less nutritious fruit (clicking our way through all the MU criteria boxes in the EMR) simply because it is the more abundant and low-lying choice? How long can we, in good faith, keep ignoring the general consensus that more bad fruit is actually far less satisfying than less good fruit? Many of my colleagues already lament the loss of quality in favor of the quantity of this fruit.

Just because the wind is blowing everyone on the cliff toward the edge, this does not mean that everyone is obliged to plummet to their deaths on the rocks below. I would advocate that we need to grab hold of our colleagues who want to brave the winds and not be blown along en masse, unwittingly using someone else's road to population health. We need to call out the current notions of how to implement population health for what they truly are—a bureaucratic process added to the physician's already overwhelming daily responsibilities. The premise for population health may indeed be a good one. However, the specific roadway we must travel to successfully achieve better population health is not the one that Dr. Nash and others now propose. Their electronic path is errant at best and uninformed at the worst. Collectively, we physicians need to begin to place some stakes in the ground and hold tight to the core values of high-quality healthcare founded in a strong, compassionate, and patient-oriented manner.

We do not need to check boxes on a computer chart that only indicate virtual instructions to our patients. Instead, we should be given sufficient time to best guide our patients toward tangible ancillary services and resources that complement and promote our office-based care. The patients will trust us more if we actually sit with them, instead of making a computer entry that implies we did, when the truth is we actually did not have the time to do so. With this earned trust based upon true communication and mutual decision-making, stable economic efficiencies and improved outcomes will soon follow.

This result may not occur right away, and for a while, physicians who elect to buck the notion that they have no choice may find themselves few in number, standing firmly on the windy bluff. My experience indicates that when the wind subsides, these brave physician leaders will not have been tragically blown off the cliff into the "sea change" of which Dr. Nash warns us. They will not be seen as having run away or remaining on the sidelines in obscurity. On the contrary, they will have held this bluff in the name of their patients and thus earned the right to be true advocates of population health.

My patients like Marianne with complex congenital heart defects and Michael with muscular dystrophy are the patient population I serve and strive to keep healthy. They don't get access to needed health services outside of my offices because I check off the correct boxes in their electronic chart. On the contrary, I need to pull myself away from my computer and consistently speak to the vast team of people and agencies providing these services. I create a true medical home within the community when I pick up the phone and speak with the nurses, social workers, respiratory technicians, and other physician colleagues comanaging my patients. I reach out to wheelchair and breathing machine companies, politicians, and health insurance representatives.

This is how the work is accomplished that best benefits our patients, and no box in the computer can ever exist that will magically motivate a doctor to do this or fully represent the value of these efforts. A doctor either cares enough to do all this, or they don't. Physicians can only do this when the environment they work in grants them the full authority to represent patients outside the boundaries of their offices. For Dr. Nash's population health objectives to be reached, barriers placed by insurers and bureaucrats must be removed so that Marianne can afford her medications and Michael can receive home nursing care and physical therapy.

My main criticism with the present paradigm of managed care, including entities such as the ACOs, is that instead of designating the physician as the leader or clinical manager of the healthcare team, these models place the entire burden of population health outcome measurements on the backs of physicians. There are many elements, such as social work resources, rehabilitation and home care services, medical supplies, and psychological interventions that must come together to promote successful patient and community health outcomes. In the current setup, physicians have little or no direct control over most of these.

Physicians like me are forced by the current status quo to work with more expensive, inadequate, and less-efficient resources and should not be held liable for the associated inflated costs. As a primary example, for over two decades, my patients remained hospitalized in the large urban tertiary medical centers many days longer than necessary simply because, in my community, I have extremely limited child-appropriate home nursing and nutritional services available. At the current daily cost of inpatient care in these large hospitals, I am certain we could redirect these expenses toward establishing such services closer to my patients' homes. Within a couple of years, this would save the insurance providers—or, in the case of Medicaid, the taxpayers—thousands of dollars per year.

There are also many deep-rooted socioeconomic and political constructs that are uniquely American and significantly impact the medical profession's ability to successfully deliver quality healthcare.

The medical profession should not be treated as a scapegoat for America's inherent prejudices, including racism and gender inequalities, or the widening economic gaps between the extremely wealthy, middle class, and poor.

In my region of the Mid-Hudson Valley of New York, this socioeconomic issue is well illustrated by the microcosm of some of our poorest counties. Sullivan and Ulster counties lie within a two-hour drive north of Manhattan and halfway to New York's capital, Albany. Orange and Rockland counties, where I live and work, are halfway between Manhattan and Sullivan and Ulster counties. For comparison, as of the 2018 national census, the populations and geographic size of Orange and Rockland counties are 382,000 people in 839 square miles and 326,000 people in 199 square miles, respectively. Similar data for Albany and Saratoga counties around the state capital are 227,000 people in 22 square miles and 307,000 people in 844 square miles, respectively. There are far fewer residents in much larger spaces in Ulster and Sullivan counties, with 179,000 people in 1,161 square miles and 75,000 people in 997 square miles. The following 2018 US census data also illustrate the much lower annual household incomes in Ulster and Sullivan counties, compared to their immediately surrounding neighbors. Ranked from highest to lowest, these incomes are the following: Westchester, $95,000; Rockland, $90,000; Saratoga, $81,000; Orange, $76,000; Albany, $64,000; Ulster, $63,000; and Sullivan, $56,000. The bottom line is that, relative to nearby counties, Sullivan and Ulster counties have far fewer people living much farther apart and with much less income.

Given these demographics, these two poorest counties lie in stark contrast to their neighbors and serve as a microcosm of communities with scarce vital resources, including medical care and education. In fact, both counties were designated as "medical deserts" by the federal government in 2019 and in the 2021 HealtheConnections Regional Community Health Assessment of New York's Mid-Hudson Valley.

This designation means that these counties' inhabitants are amongst the 80 percent of rural Americans or 30 million Americans in rural and urban communities with sorely inadequate access to medical services, including acute-care hospitals. The HealtheConnections report highlights Ulster and Sullivan counties' many barriers to healthcare access compared to the other five counties in the region. In both places, the ratio of physicians to inhabitants is below a critical threshold that would allow for the delivery of even basic medical care. The COVID-19 pandemic placed such underserved areas front and center in the public's eye.[39]

The medical desert designation is supposed to identify these regions to open doorways to needed resources, including increasing the number of available physicians. The medical desert designation was used in my area of New York to bolster the creation of a brand-new medical school run by Touro University with the goal of placing graduates into these underserved regions. This school in fact opened its doors in July 2014 in Orange County, New York and literally set up residence with teachers, dormitories, and facilities in the same Horton Hospital where I began my medical career in 1998. The bulk of my current medical students come from this school.

While the creation of a new medical school to eventually send out graduates to serve in Ulster and Sullivan counties sounds like a good idea in theory, it's problematic for several reasons. Suggesting we can fix the medical deserts by building a medical school and then hoping some graduates will choose to practice in economically depressed areas again places the main emphasis on individual physicians. If these brand-new physician warriors fail to actually improve the population health grades, as determined by the state and federal governments'

---

39 Mathew, Jamie, *et al.*, "Mid-Hudson Region Community Health Assessment 2019-2021," (online), https://www.orangecountygov.com/DocumentCenter/View/14538/-Orange-County-Regional-Community-Health-Assessment-2019-2021-PDF.

criteria, these government policymakers reserve the right to implement financial penalties by reducing physicians' salaries.

An average medical-school education at Touro now costs near a staggering $250,000. My medical students repeatedly told me that this brand-new school enticed them to come to this university through several means. These included the promise of tuition forgiveness and the prospect of bonuses tied to potential improvements in the health of their patients if these students agreed to set up shop in areas such as Ulster and Sullivan counties. The reality that these young doctors quickly face is that physicians who work in underserved populations do not have direct control over the many factors that keep their patients unwell and prevent the doctors from achieving successful care outcomes. Patients in these communities have no access to transportation, poor education regarding how and when to use the health system, inability to pay their electric and heat bills, and decisions regarding buying food and paying a copay on medication.

During one of my morning group teaching sessions in late February, I noticed that one of the six medical students looked particularly tired.

"Is everything OK?" I asked.

"Not really," she quietly replied. "I just returned from spending a month training in one of the rural community medical practices in Sullivan. I was so excited because I planned to work there when I'm done with school. What I learned instead was that we don't make a dent in these patients' well-being because they can't even get to us. They have no transportation, and they are stuck in their homes wrapped up in blankets over a furnace fire just to stay warm in the winter," she explained in exasperation.

As she so succinctly encapsulated the issue, holding the physician solely responsible for these patients' morbidity or mortality makes little sense. I have been teaching cardiology and pediatrics to medical school, nursing, and physician assistant students for 30 years. Many of the students from this new Touro medical school start out enthusiastically, with altruistic visions of serving the region's medically underserved inhabitants. All too soon, they become disheartened by how little control they have over so many important factors that influence their ability to improve this region's population health. By the time they complete their fourth and final year, the majority of them choose to pursue further education or start their careers elsewhere.

"I hate to give up, but I really can't see how we young doctors can achieve what they are asking of us. The odds of success are stacked against us and our patients right from the beginning," emphatically added one of the other students.

How do we fix this unrealistic expectation that the medical professionals can solve these problems by themselves? All entities with a stake in achieving a successful population health model must share the risks and benefits of success and failure equally. It takes a village to educate and heal a community, not just a doctor. Patient lifestyle practices, physician services, and population resources, like access to nutritious food, must work together symbiotically.

The local government must provide social work services and effective public transportation. If they don't, they are partly to blame for poor patient health outcomes. If there is no quality home nursing or medical equipment services covered by a particular third-party payor, the payor is culpable of restricting a critical resource. If a patient can barely read the printed instructions on medications because of racial or language inequities and inadequate schooling, local public educators are also culpable for low population-health scores.

Like a police force trying to reduce crime without any outside help when people are unemployed, cold, hungry, and addicted, the medical force cannot single-handedly improve population health when major socioeconomic inequities make people sick. There must be a partnership where government, policymakers, academics, payors, allied healthcare professionals, and doctors are all held equally accountable. Doctors did not create or perpetuate the "holes" in the dam that prevent them from filling up the reservoir, and they certainly should not be expected to plug these holes by themselves. We all must desist from simultaneously idolizing and victimizing doctors in the name of "population health." The actual culprits at the heart of America's diseased soul include poverty, unchecked greed, racism, sexism, and power hunger. Only by calling out these pathogens together can we heal America.

It remains an honor and a privilege to be a doctor. As I gain more experience, I enjoy referrals for second and third opinions to solve complex medical problems. I am consistent in my approach to such cases, taking a step back to gain the big picture and then diving into the details during an often hour-long visit. When I conclude that one of my patients needs an invasive procedure, such as catheterization or heart surgery, my goal is to choose the optimum time for them to go under deep anesthesia and the knife. This sense of timing took years for me to develop.

Given the risks of such procedures, I do not take anything for granted. I am honest with the family about my choices of only the best surgeons for any particular cardiac situation. We are fortunate to be near New York City, where such medical resources are strong. In pediatrics, this decision must also include family logistics such as work schedule, childcare, and emotional readiness. The healthier the patient at the outset, the better the results afterward. Nothing can replace the feeling of warmth I feel when seeing a heart patient and family return home after a successful surgery, relief on the family's faces and the child much healthier than before.

Sometimes, though, it's inordinately frustrating to be a doctor. My main frustration with my own profession is that, all too often, doctors become caught up in a repetitive two- to three-decade cycle. Initially, most of us support altruism and complete devotion to their patients, followed by a sense of helpless futility with the "system." Then we relapse defiantly and passionately back to our fundamental mission of patient-centered care. Many doctors start off their education and careers believing strongly in the paramount importance of our relationship with our patients but are quick to give this up or be distracted from it when we become overwhelmed and times get rough. An honest look in the mirror that questions why, during these cycles, our profession all too easily abandons our patient focus may sadly reveal and lead us to admit that economics is indeed often at the core of this tendency.

I still have students admit to me that the main reason they want to be an American doctor is because they want to be wealthy and recognized by others as belonging to the prestigious echelons of American society. "My son, the rich doctor," remains a calling card for rubbing elbows with high society. For many non-physicians, the inclination of many doctors to seek wealth and fame creates resentment and a view of doctors as elitist and therefore incapable of understanding the people they serve. Yet I also found that this resentment is counterbalanced by patients' desires to have their doctors held in high esteem—that is, until they receive the medical bills from these same well-recognized doctors.

Americans are mainly torn by this dilemma to praise or criticize doctors because all too often it appears that only the wealthy can afford the best doctors. This situation is analogous to our nation's mixed-up priorities regarding the value of teachers in our education system. It should not be a revelation to anyone that the quality of an education in schools parallels the wealth of the community in which a school is situated. Higher taxes usually mean better schools. Better schools require higher taxes. Those with less income can only afford to live in communities with lower-quality schools. Private schools are clearly out of reach for most people.

However, like a great education, great healthcare affords individuals the advantages of success that those less fortunate may not have.

During the COVID-19 pandemic, these advantages literally spelled the difference between life and death. So why are opportunities such as education and healthcare still held out by the American mythos as equally available to anyone who works hard? Lately, I asked my students and colleagues if such inequities should be allowed in a United States that purports to be truly democratic.

America also does not seem to prioritize the value of healthcare relative to other things on which we spend money. Why are baseball players or other professional athletes paid so much more than teachers or physicians? In New York, the cost of even the cheapest major league baseball tickets is much higher than a copayment for a doctor's visit, yet it is highly unlikely that a sports fan will be heard publicly screaming and complaining at the ballpark about ticket prices. Throughout every week, my reception staff is worn down by several patients shouting at them across the desk—the waiting room filled with other young families in earshot of the commotion—about the costs of copays and deductibles. Only when a manager or head nurse intervenes and reminds the patient that doctors' offices do not set the fees of their particular medical insurance company do the voices begin to lower. An apology to the reception staff is a rare event.

At first glance, applying such a warped economic value system to physicians' services compared to less vital or recreational endeavors appears inconsistent and contradictory to the common assumption that medical care in the United States is worth the cost. You get what you pay for, right? Actually, no. For decades, policymakers have recognized that our healthcare delivery system and quality lag behind many countries. Instead of being among the most successful in the world, as of 2000, the World Health Organization ranks[40] the United States at 37th out of 191 nations in healthcare quality. According to

40 "World Health Organization Assesses the World's Health Systems," World Health Organization, Feb. 7, 2000 (online), https://www.who.int/news/item/07-02-2000-world-health-organization-assesses-the-world's-health-systems.

a 2014 Commonwealth Fund Report, when compared to 11 other comparable industrialized nations, despite spending far more than any other nation, the United States is ranked last "on measures of health system quality, efficiency, access to care, equity, and healthy lives."[41]

Even studies conducted within the United States[42] concluded that our healthcare system suffers from many major problems, including inequities in primary care access and inefficiencies in delivering health services, that pull it down compared to other, less-developed countries. I consistently tell my students that such self-assessments are not meant to be disparaging nor lead us to conclude that our healthcare system is so dysfunctional that it is beyond repair. To the contrary, these formal analyses and reflections are indicative of the esteem we have for our profession and essential if it is to meet its full potential.

Since the 1960s, this constructive self-criticism has led policymakers to wrestle with the inconsistency between our comparatively low-quality healthcare ranking in the world and the fact that the United States spends almost three times more on healthcare than the number-one-ranked nation—France. One proposed solution was to take a purely economic approach. This resulted in the cost-containment strategies reviewed previously in this chapter, including reductions in physician reimbursements through third-party payors. To try to bring the United States healthcare ranking back up within the top 11 by focusing solely on finances is both a meaningless and fruitless endeavor. As a physician, it also always makes me feel like I am professionally under attack and

41 "US Health System Ranks Last Among Eleven Countries on Measures of Access, Equity, Quality, Efficiency, and Healthy Lives," The Commonwealth Fund, June 16, 2014 (online), https://www.commonwealthfund.org/press-release/2014/us-health-system-ranks-last-among-eleven-countries-measures-access-equity.

42 Davis, Karen, *et al.*, "How the US System Compares Internationally," The Commonwealth Fund, June 16, 2014 (online), https://www.commonwealthfund.org/publications/fund-reports/2014/jun/mirror-mirror-wall-2014-update-how-us-health-care-system.

held as one of the guilty parties responsible for the majority of the runaway costs of healthcare.

I don't mean to ignore finances all together. Americans need to find a balance between always wanting the latest and greatest and the economically sound ways of keeping our people healthy. The proverbial pendulum cannot keep swinging to one extreme or the other but should be allowed to come closer to its natural resting place in the middle. As a doctor myself, I believe that we cannot ignore the tendencies of US physicians to heavily factor finances into their career choices and decisions. It is wrong for young people to want to be doctors solely because they want to get rich.

On the other hand, policymakers, thought leaders, and educators should determine a reasonable monetary value for good patient-centered healthcare. This value must factor in the myriad of costs, the often excessive financial burdens, involved in becoming and remaining a good and productive clinician. If a physician comes out of medical school hundreds of thousands of dollars in debt and has to pay exorbitant malpractice and management costs just to deliver care at the outset, they already feel the impetus to focus on economics just to keep up.

Medical school tuition was about $30,000 to $40,000 a year in my day during the 1990s. Today, my medical students[43] look at nearly $80,000 a year and come out of medical school with a median debt of $200,000. My wife and I finished medical school with over $100,000 in college and medical school debt. Though we were able to postpone some of the college debt through medical school and residency, as soon as we finished training, we were on the hook to begin paying these loans back. The monthly amounts of these loan payments were higher than the mortgage on our first little home.

43 "Tuition at Every Medical School in the United States (Updated 2022)," Shemmassian Academic Consulting (online), https://www.shemmassianconsulting.com/blog/medical-school-tuition.

As a comparison, the medical school tuition in some of the world's best medical schools in Canada[44] and Europe[45] is significantly lower. The tuition in these publicly funded schools is about $12,000 a year for citizens. Even for international students, the cost is about 50 percent of the American medical schools. This difference is even more striking because, after high school, it takes six years to become a doctor in Canada and Europe, compared to eight to 10 years in the United States. This time difference further increases the total cost to become a doctor in the United States, which is between $400,000 and $800,000, compared to $60,000 and $150,000 in these other countries. This would only make sense if American physicians' salaries were much higher than those in Canada and Europe, but a comparison as of 2020[46] reveals salaries are fairly comparable. In the end, I always stress that what someone keeps after expenses is much more important than what they make. When considering education debts and administrative costs, American physicians fall far behind other equally developed countries.

As a physician specialist, my annual malpractice insurance premiums were over $20,000 and today are closer to $30,000. This cost was initially factored into my contract with Columbia but fell completely into my lap when I started my private practice. As the years passed, even after I finally paid off my student loans, the exponentially increasing operational and management requirements for my practice became a major factor in my decision to give up control to the larger multi-physician group entity of Boston Children's Health Physicians.

44 "10 Best Medical Schools in Canada," Global Scholarships, (online), https://globalscholarships.com/best-medical-schools-canada/.

45 Chilaka, Mbagwu Amarachi, "10 Best Medical Schools in Europe for Americans in 2023," Kiiky, February 28, 2023, https://kiiky.com/medical-schools-in-europe-for-american-students/.

46 Sabin, Sara; Abbas, Ola, "10 Highest-Paying Countries for Doctors," Medic Footprints, Nov. 2022, (online), https://medicfootprints.org/10-highest-paying-countries-for-doctors/.

Most physicians I know made similar, albeit difficult, career decisions based on such financial stresses.

Ultimately, it has been the economics, the almighty dollar, that continue to drive the choices healthcare professionals and policymakers make regarding the course that the American healthcare system pursues. I remain convinced that money is clearly a misguided beacon to follow that has led us away from the equitable administration and delivery of healthcare, placed the financial benefits in shareholder or corporate pockets, and promoted the public's lack of trust and cynicism about the medical profession. If we continue to follow the money blindly, I fear we will all find ourselves falling over a cliff to our collective tragic demise. We must return to true patient-centered and population-centered care now before it is too late.

CHAPTER 8

BACK TO BASICS TO CLEAN UP THE MESS

"They said that her fast breathing, low oxygen levels, and poor appetite were due to her having a sick heart for so many years," explained the mom of one of my patients over the phone. There was desperation in her voice. "At the local urgent care center, they didn't even do any other tests and told us that we should just call our cardiologist in the morning. She's still breathing fast and does not look right. You know her better than anyone, Doctor. This isn't like Evelyn. She's usually nonstop talking and friendly with everyone. But now she's withdrawn and quiet. Dr. Fethke, I'm scared."

Evelyn had been my patient for over a decade. She was now 45 years old and had Down syndrome. People with Down syndrome, caused by an imbalance in the number of chromosomes before birth, often have malformed hearts and several other organs affected. In Evelyn's case, she had a complex birth defect of her heart that had not been surgically repaired as an infant. The entire center or core of her heart was missing because it never developed before she was born. This large hole between the two sides of her heart chambers allowed the right-sided, less-oxygenated blue blood to completely mix with the left-sided, oxygenated red blood. Over the first few years of her life, this led to many other problems, including abnormally elevated blood pressures in her lungs, known as pulmonary hypertension. While she grew, this in turn led to several traveling blood clots that cut off circulation to her brain—strokes—and her shortened left leg. I never learned why she was not considered a candidate for heart surgery as an infant. I didn't know her then, but if I had, I would have likely recommended surgery in the first year of life.

When I first met Evelyn in her 30s, her skin and lips were a grayish blue all over because the resting oxygen levels in her body decreased from a normal 95 percent or more to 75 percent. When she did the slightest exercise or became upset, these oxygen levels dropped to as low as 40 percent, risking sudden and life-threatening heart and brain damage. It was clear to me that heart surgery was no longer an option for her.

In the early 1960s, many great medical pioneers learned the hard way—with too many patients dying—that children like Evelyn with her heart condition and Down syndrome had a very short window of opportunity within the first couple years of life to undergo successful heart surgery. Because she never had the surgery in time, her heart and blood vessels had become too permanently damaged to tolerate the procedure without making her sicker or perhaps killing her. The lungs' blood vessels and the right side of her heart that pumped to them were under such severe strain that, left unchecked, within a couple of years, there would not be enough blood sent to her lungs to keep her alive. She was already using a wheelchair due to severe exercise intolerance and vulnerable to further problems with blood clots and infections. During her first visit with me, I recommended that we pursue life-sustaining medications that could mildly reverse and at least slow down the progression of her pulmonary hypertension. It worked, and her breathing, alertness, and exercise tolerance improved so much that it gave her a longer and better quality of life.

That was over 12 years ago, and together, we beat all the odds by over a decade. This was in large part because her mother was on top of everything and knew to call me with any concerns. It also helped that I was fortunate to learn from some of the original pioneers at Columbia University who studied and developed the medical treatments for pulmonary hypertension. After decades of caring for such patients under the watchful eye of these pioneers, I learned to recognize patients with pulmonary hypertension—a disease which most pediatricians will never see in their entire careers—from the moment I encountered them trying to walk down my office hallway.

Together, with an expanding group of pediatric cardiologists at several academic medical centers in the northeast, I continued to manage several such patients in my community practice. This limited the number of medical trips these patients had to make to the big cities. More importantly, it allowed me to recognize early warning signs that indicated their conditions might be worsening. For decades, I intervened in time to prevent what I knew could be a sudden loss of life in my patients with pulmonary hypertension. They had been living longer and happier lives.

My close connection to and frequent interactions with Evelyn's remarkably devoted mother also allowed me to recognize when her condition just did not make sense. The situation that her mother now described on the telephone was one of those circumstances. Her mom, 67 years old and always attentive to her daughter's health, had taken Evelyn to the nearest urgent care center covered by her health insurance that afternoon. There, her concerns about her daughter's health were dismissed, and they were sent home with no testing. So I advised her to take Evelyn to the local hospital emergency room, where I had some influence as one of the medical directors on staff. I called ahead to the doctors in the ER and in the intensive care unit and verbally updated them on Evelyn's full medical background. I explained that her heart situation was relatively stable and her current medical signs and symptoms were unlikely to be directly due to her heart problem. I stressed that I was suspicious that something else was making her sicker and could aggravate her heart condition.

Through our collaborative discussion, the hospital-based doctors and I developed a plan to test her for infections, including pneumonia, none of which was done earlier that day at the urgent care center. Within two hours, Evelyn was diagnosed with both pneumonia and a urinary tract infection. The emergency room physician informed me that the infection was so severe that, untreated, it would have likely overwhelmed her body and become a condition known as life-threatening sepsis. The medical director of the intensive care unit thanked me for being so involved and communicative.

"If you hadn't taken control of the situation, she'd be dead by tomorrow," she literally shouted when I went to see Evelyn that night. "What are they training these people in the urgent care sites today? They should have at least called you as her doctor before sending her home," she emphasized with a rewarding pat on my back. At the hospital, Evelyn was started on intravenous antibiotics. Forty-eight hours later, she was discharged home, already back to her usual talkative and affable self.

GETTING BACK TO THE FIELD

When I grew up, my parents and neighbors used to set up their folding chairs around a Little League baseball field to watch me and my friends practice and play baseball at least two nights a week. The spectators were always as much a part of the game as the players. Today, many who love baseball will tell you that a school or minor league game can be even more enjoyable than a professional major league game. As the sport becomes more and more of a business, the majority of the major league fans are left behind.

For many, they simply cannot afford the tickets and food, the tab running well over $200. The ballparks themselves are increasingly elaborate. There is only so much that can be done with the field itself. The stadiums, however, stand as monuments to the ancient coliseums of Rome and are extremely expensive to operate and maintain. The fancier the stadium, the higher the ticket prices and the more removed the general public becomes from the field of play. The connection between the players and the fans—once the main driving force of America's favorite sport—barely remains intact, like a strained fraying string. The economic future of the game at the major league level remains tenuous and vulnerable.

For such a beloved sport with roots in neighborhoods and community-based Little Leagues throughout the country, the current professional dynamic portrays a sense of abandonment of its foundation as a universally American pastime. The socioeconomics of American society are now reflected in the layout of the stadium seats. The more prestigious the team, the farther away from the field the spectators' seats are. Like the passengers on a cruise line from the turn of the twentieth century, the commoners are relegated farthest away from the action, while the richest are literally perched in fancy, elevated, enclosed boxes, barely even paying attention to the supposed main event. The game and the players now take a backseat to the food, drink, and hobnobbing that occur in the luxury boxes. The details of any particular team's rivalry—the hits, the runs batted in, and the errors—are lost in the highlights, which are just as easily broadcast on a smartphone. Why go to the ballpark at all?

In many ways, the evolution of the American healthcare system over the past century reminds me of the fate of major league baseball. As people struggled through the Great Depression of the 1930s, the United States created an environment that promoted affordable and equal access to medical care for its citizens. Health insurance was seen as a vital component of our struggling democracy, a ticket to promote our economic recovery that was actually offered door to door by the Boy Scouts. Everyone was to have equal seating around the healthcare field.

Beginning in the 1970s, the dynamics and priorities of the healthcare system gradually changed, and it became more and more of a business. Like baseball, big money was to be made by wealthy investors. Within

50 years of President Roosevelt's New Deal, the costs of healthcare became prohibitively high for many average citizens. Only the well-to-do could afford the best medical attention—the box seats of American medicine. The disparities in access to the current US healthcare system, like the attendance of a major league baseball game, now threatened the entire operation.

For the past four decades, reform of the US healthcare system has emerged front and center in the daily discourse of all who live here. I sense that the solutions our policymakers adopted so far have wandered far off the one and only true course we should take. Like major league baseball, we must return our attention back to the general audience. Though perhaps sounding drastic, the stadiums must be torn down so that the financial and intellectual resources they drained away from the game can be redirected back to the ground level—the field, where all the truly meaningful action takes place.

The patients sorely need to be invited back to their own healthcare at a level they can access as equals to all others seeking medical attention. As the COVID-19 pandemic so blatantly taught us when we ignored the essential workers, like the relationship between baseball's players and their fans, a well-functioning healthcare field rightfully belongs to the doctors and their patients. They should never have been pushed out and felt uninvited. It is now well past the time that we welcome them back home.

CONTINUITY OF CARE AND REESTABLISHING PATIENT TRUST

"Continuity of care" has become a buzz phrase among the US health insurance providers and government. I do not think either entity really understands how much being able to build a relationship with one's doctor means to people, how to best achieve it, and, most concerningly, how very critical it is to the success of our uniquely American healthcare system. To refer back to the earlier baseball analogy, continuity of care is achieved when the audience—the patients—truly sit close enough to know the players on the field—their physicians and the other clinicians that care for them. It is actually not a difficult concept to grasp when we step back to analyze the implications of this continuity.

As in any fruitful relationship, the more time that all parties invest in knowing each other, the stronger the bonds become. It is also fully consistent with this notion of continuity of care that people have the freedom to choose their own general or specialty physician. After working for over two decades as a physician, I am convinced that a personal and professional familiarity between the doctor and the patient is the sound bedrock from which the highest quality of medical care is possible. Patients have better health outcomes when they have providers who know them well over time, function as reliable healthcare advocates on their behalf, and remain in constant communication with others in the patient's healthcare team.

In the healing arts, this strong patient-physician relationship is clinically critical to promoting both physical and emotional health. When doctors know their patients well, they can often pick up subtle health or psychological issues that doctors less familiar with a patient may completely miss. The early recognition of a situation that doesn't "look right"—as my patient Evelyn's mother brought to my attention—is often the key to good medical care.

This awareness leads to early detection and timely diagnosis of medical conditions or emotional stressors that may negatively impact the patient's well-being or the effectiveness of prescribed treatments. How many times have we heard someone say, "They caught it too late?" When health conditions—including cancer, heart disease, and even autoimmune disorders—go untreated, the consequences can be dire. The cost of treating a very sick person for days and weeks in an intensive care unit is also many times higher than when we catch an illness early in its course and are able to keep the patient home or in a non-urgent hospital setting for only a couple of days. When health problems are caught early, we spend less money and save more lives.

Continuity of care also strengthens the component of trust between a doctor and a patient introduced earlier in this chapter. The more consistent the pattern of care between a person and their doctor, the stronger the trust grows. The stronger this trust becomes, the more that patient relies on a particular physician to guide them. The patient chooses to remain with the same doctor, rather than bounce between other clinicians or medical care facilities. Doctors can and should be the leading agents to encourage good preventative and maintenance health behaviors from our patients.

In my experience, my patients value my opinion. The single mother of a very overweight five-year-old, Alex, with a disease that started thickening his heart muscle even before he started kindergarten, latched onto my nutritional and exercise advice beyond my highest hopes. After joining a local gym together, where they spent the next decade following a disciplined regimen of moderate aerobic exercise four days every week, Alex grew up to be a tall, lean, and fit young man. Most notably, now well into his 20s, his heart muscle thickening actually never progressed to the point that any medical interventions were necessary.

When a doctor makes a concerted effort to create a relationship based upon open communication and trust, patients listen. However, to listen, patients need to feel that their doctors—and even the profession at large—genuinely care about their well-being. My adult patient Dana was born with an extremely complex heart condition at a time when over half the babies born with the same problem died in the first couple years of life. After undergoing multiple heart surgeries and invasive catheterizations before I even met her, at the end of her first visit with me, at 50 years old, her initially very quiet elderly mother stated, "You know, this is the first time that we have come to a doctor and actually clearly understand what happened to us. We have been through so much, and now it actually makes sense. Thank you."

Dana added, "Why don't the other doctors take the time to explain too? It didn't take that long for you to do it, and it was so very helpful."

Just one year later, with this foundation to our therapeutic relationship, both Dana and her mother followed my recommendation to receive the COVID-19 vaccine, despite being extremely confused and downright afraid amidst all the conflicting opinions in the media. During a visit for a sonographic study of her heart—an echocardiogram—Dana and her mom literally ran up to greet me in the hallway.

"We both did it, Doctor! Because of all you taught us, the time you took to treat us like we were special and capable of understanding the details of my health, and our trust in your advice, Mom and I went together and got both doses of the COVID-19 vaccine. We had no problems after and feel fine. Even better, a friend of ours came over to visit, and later, we found out she had the early symptoms of COVID-19 at the time. She got so sick, but we never even had a sniffle. Thank you, thank you." That was a good day for me too.

When my patients seek medical attention at a site other than their regular physician's office, such as an urgent care center, they often undergo an inappropriate number of diagnostic tests. If the provider is overly cautious by nature, they order too many unnecessary or irrelevant tests. If they operate more on the fast food model or are overworked, they typically do not do enough or do not pursue the correctly indicated tests. Much of this extreme variation could be rectified if they took a moment to obtain the necessary information by carrying out a thorough medical history or contacting the regular physician.

As I find myself saying repeatedly, we have more ways to communicate with each other than ever, yet we actually communicate more poorly than ever. When a doctor treats a stranger and has no context about their life or health history, besides perhaps a cursorily completed patient questionnaire, they can blatantly miss the mark in regards to the true etiology of the patient's health problems.

If the health insurance companies not only allowed, but insisted upon, the patient choosing and staying with their own physicians, I remain confident that both costs and quality would benefit. In the end, what anyone buying an important commodity, including medical care, seeks is the best value for the cost. Who wouldn't pay a little bit more for an appliance that works better and lasts two to three times as long as the cheaper model? Everyone with a basic business sense knows that this ultimately saves money.

The problem as I see it is that the funding scheme currently in place is too shortsighted to legitimately support the intrinsically long-term nature of the continuity-of-care model. By underpaying the primary care physicians who are supposedly the entry point and backbone of the healthcare system, the economic realities forces these physicians or their practice administrators to implement schedules that promote high volumes and short-duration visits with any physician with an open appointment spot. In every way, this approach is by definition the very antithesis of continuity of care. Despite this inherent conflict with the continuity model, the number of urgent care facilities actually exploded because they can significantly supplement the revenue of primary care providers. As one of my family practice colleagues recently explained, "If we hadn't opened our urgent care center when we did, I'm sure that we would be out of business by now."

I can't help but view this trend of finding ways for each PCP to maximize the number of patients they can see as an exercise similar to placing one's fingers in the cracks of a dam. If we do not fortify the wall of the dam properly, it is destined to give way and drown anyone downstream. If we are truly committed to supporting a continuity-of-care paradigm, then we should dedicate more funds toward primary care. The health insurers, including Medicare and Medicaid, should increase the reimbursements for primary care services. This would enable the medical facilities to increase the salaries of their general physicians, and more training physicians would then choose to work in primary care. Ultimately, this increased pool of primary care providers would lessen the burden of underserved geographic areas with too few providers in either densely populated or remote communities. With better income, primary care providers could spend more time with each patient and readily serve as any given patient's main physician. Though this model would cost more upfront, the continuity of care it promotes would save money in many ways. To begin with, patients would have more meaningful and productive visits with their regular doctors. They would thus decrease their inclination to use emergency room or urgent care services in the place of their primary care visits.

"Why should I go to my supposed primary physician group? We're just a number there," replied the mother of one of my patients when I asked why she had taken her 12-year-old son to an urgent care facility to be evaluated for two weeks of frequent mild dizziness and chest pain after eating. She continued in an aggravated tone, "We never get to see the first doctor who is supposed to be Johnny's regular pediatrician unless we book at least three months in advance. The nurse practitioner or other pediatrician they schedule us with doesn't know Johnny any better than the urgent care doctors anyway."

Her logic was hard to argue against because there was no continuity-of-care advantage with her pediatrician's large practice. It didn't make any difference to her. The insurance company paid the expensive bill to cover the dozen blood and imaging tests that the urgent care doctor ordered, which I thought were excessive and unnecessary.

Because the urgent care referred Johnny to me for a cardiac evaluation, during this visit, I called his pediatrician myself to discuss the medical situation. "I didn't know that he had gone to urgent care," said the pediatrician, Dr. Neilssen, in an apologetic tone. "Sorry to have wasted your time. I will call the family and try to squeeze him in to do more teaching about his stomach acid condition and possibly adjust his antacid medication."

Johnny and his family spent all this extra time with costly visits to an urgent care and a cardiac specialist before coming full circle to his primary doctor. If the urgent care provider had simply asked a few basic questions about Johnny's medical history, they could have learned that he suffered from a long-standing increased stomach acid condition, known as gastroesophageal reflux disease (GERD). If the mother had more confidence that they could see his primary doctor more consistently, she would have never gone to the urgent care facility in the first place. This regular pediatrician discovered Johnny's GERD problem years ago and would readily recognize this condition as the source of his pain. He would treat Johnny accordingly, relieving his pain days earlier and without any testing.

I know of one particular medical practice that stands out because it has fully and successfully embraced the continuity of care model. For the two years before COVID-19 hit the United States in 2020, one of my regular clinics was set up in an urgent care facility belonging to one of the largest multidisciplinary private medical practices in New York State. My desk at this very busy urgent care facility was within earshot of the reception desk. As I sat down at my computer between my own patient visits, with only a makeshift partition separating me from the view of the incoming patients, it was difficult not to overhear the pleasant but penetrating voice of the regular employee greeting the new arrivals.

Within the first six months of 2020, I noted that the receptionist made a significant change to her customary welcome speech. She began routinely asking the less-ill presenting patients, "Do you have a regular primary doctor with our larger practice?" At least 10 to 20 percent of the time, the patients answered that they did. In these circumstances, in full view of the patient, the receptionist immediately made a phone call to the patient's primary doctor's office. They were then advised to go directly to this doctor's office housed in the same building or one just five miles down the road so that their own physician could see them then and there.

She explained in a clear and gentle manner, "Your doctor has saved emergency appointments in his schedule just for the purpose of seeing patients like you when unexpected medical problems come up. In the future, if you find yourself in a similar situation, it is OK to call your doctor's office first before you come to urgent care. Most of the time, they can see you in half the time we do here, and they know you much better." This new protocol also significantly unloaded the patient volume on the urgent care staff and shortened the wait time for the urgent care patients.

This urgent care scenario demonstrates that, for continuity of care to work, the existing policies and protocols must often be reimagined and implemented in new ways. It is also critical that continuity of care be funded properly, beginning at the primary care level, so that health problems can be accurately diagnosed and treated by health professionals who know the patients best. This avoids both the catastrophic illnesses that place patients like Evelyn in expensive hospital care facilities for weeks and the delay of appropriate treatment for days in patients like Johnny. Promoting prevention of illness and disease through continuous and accessible primary care also costs far less money over a patient's lifetime than allowing them to become sicker without such primary services. Healthcare reform policymakers and leaders must stop giving lip service to the continuity-of-care paradigm and urgently need to commit their efforts and money to their currently empty "buzz phrase" words. We would all be the ultimate beneficiaries.

ADDRESSING A POOR BUSINESS MODEL

After decades on the frontlines, I would argue that healthcare in the United States does not fit the economic paradigms of other businesses. A more appropriate model to apply to healthcare reform is that of a business founded upon trust and loyalty, the loss of which risks dragging the entire business into a downward spiral. The ACA indeed expanded access to healthcare and stands as a welcome improvement to the more exclusionary policies of the managed care models. We may thus be one giant step closer to our goals, but as the picture I painted in Chapter 7 portrays, we have overconcentrated on the economics of healthcare, painfully ignoring and eroding the patient-physician relationship more than ever. And at what cost? What happens when the trust between our people and their health professionals is severely strained?

I believe the answers lie in the dismal economic outcomes and loss of lives we endured with the COVID-19 pandemic, despite our technological prowess and vast material resources. Viewing American healthcare through a microscope designed to see only the money ignores our American values and aspirations of providing both meaningful and effective health services. These values are exemplified by the medical achievements that enabled many of my patients, including Gilbert Tremain with Tetralogy of Fallot, to enjoy long and meaningful lives. At their core, these values motivate our health professionals, scientists, educators, and policymakers to strive for technological exceptionalism without ignoring the need for equitable access to such high-quality services for everyone. This struggle in healthcare is nothing less than a microcosm of the yet-unfulfilled American quest for the highest form of democracy—one that equally benefits all our people and thus demonstrates the best aspects of our character to the world.

The latest example of this innately American philosophy centers around the COVID-19 vaccine,[47] the development of which I conclude was a historic and tremendous achievement involving many nations, initially backed by American resources in the Western world. However,

---

47 Klobucista, Claire, "A Guide to Global COVID-19 Vaccine Efforts, Council on Foreign Relations, Dec. 5, 2022 (online), https://www.cfr.org/backgrounder/guide-global-covid-19-vaccine-efforts.

as the Biden administration has stressed,[48] a vaccine on the shelf does no good. It must be delivered sensibly and equitably to everyone if we are to eradicate the viral source of this pandemic once and for all. All the world's leading virus and epidemiology experts agree that the virus is nonpartisan in its choice of victims. Stopping short of achieving such mass vaccination levels only perpetuates this pandemic through the evolution of ever more dangerous SARS-CoV-2 variants.

This means that the United States cannot successfully combat any pandemic by delivering and administering the vaccines and treatments only within our nation's borders. We must lead a worldwide effort to provide treatments to our entire vulnerable species. Americans intuitively understand that in today's interconnected global environment such efforts, though initially costly, are essential to ensuring our own democracy and thus consistent with our value system. An analysis that focuses purely on the upfront finances not only oversimplifies the issues, it grossly ignores such core principles and threatens our freedoms.

I am not advocating a purely idealistic solution to our health system problems. I am well aware that there are actual economic issues plaguing us, but I sense that the financial decisions promoted by many administrators and policymakers ignore some fundamental realities and are ultimately both wasteful and ineffective. A prime example of this misguided approach is the assumption that most doctors' career goals are mainly money-driven. Anyone taking the time to sit down for five minutes and have a heart-to-heart conversation with any one of my hundreds of colleagues and students would soon be convinced otherwise. Any successful healthcare reform cannot ignore the pervasive and oppressive monetary stresses with which today's practicing physicians and future medical students can barely cope. Many physicians who remain focused upon their patients' care admit that they would

48 Miller, Zeke, "US to Swiftly Boost Global Vaccine Sharing, Biden Announces," *Associated Press*, June 3, 2021, https://apnews.com/article/biden-announces-international-covid-vaccine-sharing-plan-cc4630f1d45b379c573c55a2042026e0.

readily choose a lower salary if the cost of their livelihood could be made more affordable.

"I can't believe how little they pay you doctors in New York compared to Georgia, especially with such higher costs of living up here. Your salaries up here are almost one-third less than the South," bluntly stated a new medical director during one of our regular physician meetings.

"I'd like to stay and practice in the Northeast," confessed one of my medical students while I held an early morning teaching session. "I just can't see how I would pay back all my student loans and have any meaningful quality of life for my family without returning to the Midwest," she added.

So why does this wide variation in salaries based on geography, gender, and specialty[49] persist? Does it make good policy sense that the cost of medical education[50] and providing healthcare[51] are so dependent on geography? Aren't all doctors in the United States supposed to be trained and provide healthcare in pretty much the same way? As my senior colleague pointed out, it's baffling that a physician in the Northeast has to expend significantly more of their already relatively lower income[52] to keep up with the costs of running a practice than their peers in the Midwest or the South.

---

49 Nielsen, Dave, "Top 10 Highest-Paying States for Physicians in 2022," Weatherby Healthcare, July 7, 2022 (online), https://weatherbyhealthcare.com/blog/highest-paying-states-physicians.

50 Hanson, Melanie, "Average Medical School Debt," Education Data Initiative, Nov. 22, 2022 (online), https://educationdata.org/average-medical-school-debt.

51 Johnson, William C.; Fuglesten Biniek, Jean, "Sources of Geographic Variation in Health Care Spending Among Individuals With Employer Sponsored Insurance," *Med Care* Res Rev, 78 (5):548-560, Oct. 2021 (online), https://www.ncbi.nlm.nih.gov/pmc/articles/PMC8414822/.

52 Stewart, Heather, "Physician Salary Report 2022, Physician Income Rising Again," Weatherby Healthcare, Nov. 9, 2022 (online), https://weatherbyhealthcare.com/blog/annual-physician-salary-report.

It seems like every day I hear that a medical colleague of mine is moving from New York because they just can't keep up. "I would rather earn less, keep more, and be happier in Ohio than stay here, work myself to the bones, miss time with my family, and have only a little nest egg to show for it in the end," complained one of my exasperated pediatric colleagues during a phone call to discuss a mutual patient. Unless there are major reasons to stay in the Northeast, such as family ties, many medical professionals I know choose a situation with a lower salary if accompanied by a better quality of life.

Perhaps policymakers have not addressed physicians' lifestyle concerns in earnest because of the misconception that most physicians focus on higher salaries more than quality of life. On the contrary, and perhaps refreshingly, if I noted any dominant pattern in the recent trends of the priorities of my students and young physician cohort, it is that quality of life carries more weight than a high salary. Time and time again, this dynamic manifests in the discussions that the young candidate employees have with their potential employers.

"These young doctors do not want to work as hard as we did in 'our day,'" complained an almost 60-year-old obstetric friend of mine during a Friday night couples' dinner out.

His lawyer wife responded calmly, "Perhaps, dear, this is not actually a problem but the point—quality more than quantity is the focus of many of these new doctors. Maybe it is we who had our priorities wrong. How many of your colleagues ended their careers as divorcees, estranged from their kids, or became sick themselves just as they retired?"

I delicately but decisively joined in on the wife's theme. "Perhaps we should fully support this latest professional value system and understand that seeking a high quality of life should be as much of a goal for ourselves as we believe it is for our patients. Why can't happiness be the basis for the professional satisfaction of any honorable physician? We don't have to be rich, just legitimately fulfilled at home and work."

In the end, before dessert was served, we all agreed that it was simple and common sense that a satisfied physician will in turn more likely be an attentive and caring physician when they are themselves happy. These economic realities and their impacts on physician and healthcare professionals' career choices should factor into any meaningful healthcare reform strategy. It is my impression that, if the playing field for becoming a physician and practicing medicine were more equitable across the nation, many of the health access and quality disparities would be more effectively addressed. In the end, the system would be much more administratively and economically efficient if physicians did not have to struggle with the dilemmas of minimizing education debt and maximizing quality of personal and professional life.

It's time that we Americans are honest with ourselves and not try to pretend that the private health insurance companies are in business for anything but the money. Without some form of regulation, they will not willingly make the best use of their financial resources to provide the highest level of care to their clients. They want to keep as much of the money to themselves and their shareholders. As was outlined earlier in this chapter, the more the patient pays in copays and deductibles, the greater the employer portion of the costs, and the higher the premiums, the less the health insurance companies have to dole out for any claims. Until the ACA stepped in to regulate how much of the premiums were dedicated to patient care, the insurer's business model was a runaway train holding onto more and more of our money. Even worse, I feel that they made many unwise business decisions because they so severely restricted the scope of the benefits they offer that they risked losing clients.

If they truly intended to be in business for the long-term—perhaps even ignoring health outcomes altogether as an objective—then why have they excluded so many of the basic items that most beneficiaries hold to be vital and attractive? If, for example, an insurance package doesn't give someone the control to choose their own doctor or denies them a medication that they have successfully taken for years, why should they remain enrolled? It may initially save the insurance company money to control costs in this way, but eventually, there will not be enough people willing to pay the premiums to keep the health insurance company solvent. Their *modus operandi* betrays their true nature. The private health insurers focus only on the short-term or for as long as they can hold onto enough of the healthcare premiums to invest them elsewhere and create a huge profit for their CEOs and investors. Then they just abandon ship and are free to move on or merge with another entity to operate under a new name. Given the poor health outcomes that result from their tendencies to deny medical care more often than they approve or facilitate it, the health insurance industry can no longer feign to truly be dedicated to participating in meaningful healthcare reform.

The public has started to call out the health insurers for their hypocrisy. Enough is enough. Third-party payors can no longer be welcome into the honorable halls of healthcare if they are unwilling or unable to meet the same high standards as all other medical professionals. I believe in holding physicians to high ethical standards. I also am a strong advocate for an approach to health reform in which the financiers and medical professionals are guided not by profit but by the effectiveness of their resource utilization over the long term. The sustainable improvement of an individual's and the public's emotional and physical well-being must be the only true objective of our policies and efforts. Patients, healthcare professionals, and policymakers must consistently work together to set and maintain the goals and evidence-based health standards that we expect for this nation. Any entity that chooses to participate in the American healthcare system and fails to meet these benchmarks should be liable for remuneration costs just like a physician in a malpractice suit. If the provider of health insurance continues to cause harm or consistently does not meet the standards of care, like a physician who loses their license to practice, they too should no longer be allowed to participate in healthcare at any level. If, on the other hand, the insurer demonstrates that they are indeed helping to make society healthier, then, and only then, can they be allowed to reap some financial rewards.

ACCESS

Finally, a six-year-old Emaan from Pakistan arrived at my office. She was a petite, beautiful, but also frightened, cyanotic, and sickly, brown-eyed girl. She bravely and patiently bore the endless questions, examinations, and hour-long detailed echocardiogram study. Gradually, she warmed up to myself and the staff.

She began asking questions in her soft but clear voice. "Am I going to be OK? Will the operation hurt?" Her mother was an impressively bright young woman in her mid-30s with slightly bloodshot eyes from a combination of jet lag and tears. She was clearly shaken by her daughter's innocently direct questions that highlighted Emaan's fragile health. Her slow, deep breath before she spoke again belied her determination to be strong and proactive for her daughter. It was immediately apparent that she came prepared and knew a lot about Emaan's heart condition. She was thoroughly inquisitive about the many aspects of her daughter's complex heart defect and the possible options available to her here in the United States.

After two hours, at the end of this first of many visits, she saved the most important question for last. "We have come all this way because she has become so tired that she can no longer even play with the other children. Will Emaan ever be able to have a normal life?"

I sat down on my stool and rolled closer so that I sat directly across from mother and daughter. As I laid one hand on each of their shoulders, I responded in a calm and deliberate manner. "Emaan and

Mom, the surgery won't be easy, but yes, I believe that in the hands of our heart surgeon and hospital team, Emaan's chances of getting back to being a normal kid again are very good. I promise you won't be alone, and my team and I will be here for you 24-7 through the whole process. " As I finished speaking, I felt the tension fade from both of their bodies simultaneously, replaced by two beautiful smiles and some tears of relief.

Two days later, with the updated information gathered in my office, I presented Emaan's case to my medical and surgical colleagues at the Montefiore Children's Hospital in the Bronx. As we sat in the relatively small and comfortably crowded conference room, I told them her story and showed them all the information and images we gathered so far. To my relief, they were unanimously excited and optimistic about helping Emaan return to being an active child again.

My gifted surgical colleague, Dr. Samuel Weinstein, an energetic and warmhearted man in his early 40s whom I trained with at Columbia years before, spoke up. "She's about the same age as my own kids. You got her here just in time. She will need a cardiac catheterization to take more pictures and measure the hemodynamics of her heart before I operate, but yes, I am confident that I can recreate an effective blood flow to her lungs. Her oxygen levels should normalize, and I think she'll do great." I always liked a confident but honest surgeon, and Sam was both.

Over six months after her uncle first contacted me, the day arrived, and Emaan was wheeled into the operating room. During the five hours since her mother left the room—having imparted a long gentle kiss and tears on Emaan's forehead as her sleep gave into the anesthesia—the head surgical nurse came to the waiting room three times to give reassuring updates. Several hours later, a slightly tired but smiling Dr. Weinstein emerged and met with me and the family. Still dressed in his surgical scrubs with his mask and hairnet crumpled in his hands, he motioned for everyone to sit across from the small coffee table he used as a bench.

"Emaan is doing fine," he started. "The surgery went very well, and there were no complications. Her heart is still very strong, and her oxygen levels are now normal—actually probably higher than they have ever been throughout her life." Hugs and tears both flowed freely at that moment.

Over the next several days, Emaan continued to make a remarkable and smooth recovery. Within a week, she was discharged to her uncle's home. She remained there for the next two months and came regularly to my office for outpatient visits. On one such visit, with a cultural fondness and respect that grew out of our close and intense work together, Emaan freely bestowed upon me the honor of also being called "Uncle." She was thriving, and her physical and inner beauty shone through brighter than ever.

Every time we met, Emaan continued to be more and more remarkable. As we finally said our goodbyes in my office the day before her long plane ride back to Pakistan, there was a clear and unspoken realization that we established an invaluable and lifelong relationship. To this day, her mother sends me regular emails, wishing my team and family well on every holiday and, most importantly, updating us on the tremendous well-being of her daughter. Over the past six years, they continue to fly back to New York annually for a full heart assessment with me. I am thrilled to report that Emaan remains an active, healthy, and thriving young lady with a promising future. It is an immense compliment and point of pride for me that she wants to be a pediatric cardiologist someday.

It never ceases to amaze me how the boundaries between our two nations appear to have been permanently blurred for any of us who had the fortune to care for this special child. Simply put, Emaan has become a valued part of our own lives. We may have changed her life forever, but in so doing, we further reestablished and enforced our own sense of mission and purpose in our personal and professional stories.

My Montefiore colleagues were drawn to helping Emaan from Pakistan in large part because there was so much less red tape involved in providing her medical and surgical care than when US health insurance is involved. Emaan's access to care—the funding and the logistics—was pure and simple because each party involved had a vested interest in helping this child. The ground rules established by the Montefiore administration were based on what was medically and socially best for her, instead of what her insurance allowed. This access was more equitable because it depended solely on the combined charity of her family, the clinicians, and the tertiary medical institution, not the employment status of her parents or their particular health insurance package. Yes, in a sense, there were copay and deductibles that her family was ultimately responsible for, but the amount of these costs was set by a discussion between the care recipients and the care providers, not a distant, economically driven third party. The partnership between these two was defined by the primary goal of enabling Emaan to undergo a successful heart surgery.

From the start, my pediatric colleagues approach cases like Emaan's by tailoring them to the unique medical, financial, and logistic needs of the child. As Emaan's surgeon, Dr. Weinstein said at her presurgical conference, "If it looks like we can help her safely, and you can care for her in your outpatient office before and after surgery, we'll make it work. We'll make sure Emaan gets all the care she needs."

Emaan's story highlights the effectiveness of healthcare delivery when there are fewer intermediaries between the clinicians and the patient. This pure and unadulterated access to care is so refreshing to providers because it is unencumbered by the typically complex logistics and financial restrictions of the current American system. I can honestly say that the constant excess paperwork and phone calls to assist an American patient of mine through heart surgery have become a costly and exhausting logistical nightmare. Even worse, for the patient and providers, the particulars of each domestic case in terms of access and finances depends on the patient's type of health insurance, which varies widely depending on the patient's socioeconomic status.

Though it may be hard to believe, the particulars of a patient's health insurance, not the quality of the healthcare available, often determines in which institution a patient ultimately finds care. Even if the best surgeon for a child's specific heart condition is at Hospital A, if they do not accept the patient's insurance, the patient must go to the less-qualified Hospital B. So much for the standards of care as a guiding principle. In Emaan's case, the socioeconomic walls that so often divide American patients were torn down. Emaan had full access to all the necessary resources at a level equal to a VIP patient. Everyone involved clinically in her care was free to focus all their efforts on creative solutions devoted solely to her medical needs.

Participation in charity-based endeavors like Emaan's is also emotionally and intellectually gratifying for many physicians and allied health professionals. As one of my pediatric colleagues recently so well summarized at the end of a long workweek, "I'm constantly clicking away at our EHRs in between 15-minute visits and repeatedly arguing with health insurance providers. I often feel more like a social worker or psychologist trying to overcome the hurdles to healthcare access for our patients. It's so easy to lose sight of our professional purpose."

Especially during times as stressful as the COVID-19 pandemic, healthcare providers need to be able to step back and reassess our career priorities. This explains why so many practitioners, including myself, take time away from our office-based or hospital-based work, often dragging along our families, to travel to underserved areas of our own nation and other countries to donate our clinical skills to those in need. Though I knew that each trip away from my office for several days meant several thousands of dollars of revenue lost, it was still worth it personally and professionally to visit underserved areas in New York City, the Dominican Republic, Central America, or Asia. These altruistic activities reinforce the all too easy to lose sense of pride in my profession and remind me once again, like drinking from the waters of a rejuvenating mountain spring, why I became a doctor in the first place. If our healthcare system is to have true value and once again prove to be exceptional, it must regain, sustain, and expand upon this sense of purpose—this mission of physicians to serve everyone to the best of our abilities—that was the original democratic foundation for our nation's healthcare system.

I understand why it would be easy for many readers to dismiss stories like Emaan's as an exception to the norm and unrealistic to hold up as a template for the American healthcare system. After all, wasn't she just another charity case who was fortunate to have her family and the American medical team agree to cover a large part of her healthcare costs? I would argue quite the contrary. In a country with an unmatched abundance of human and material resources, Emaan's story should be held up as a very achievable vision—the ideal behind a truly patient-centered healthcare system. If we boldly address the real problems through healthcare reform, everyone should be able to afford and access healthcare on an equal playing field. Currently in the United States, because of varying employment and socioeconomic conditions, there exists an extreme range of health insurance coverage amongst our people. In some fashion or other, because of this widening gap between the lower and upper extremes of health insurance benefits, we distribute the financial burden of increasing inequities to access and quality of healthcare amongst all our people. Those among us who are less fortunate become the domestic charity-cases of our own healthcare system. Emaan's dependence on others to achieve the best healthcare available is not the exception to the rule—it is a prime example of what has become the norm here at home.

In the end, it all boils down to a fairly basic issue. The whole US healthcare system is exorbitantly expensive to operate, and we cannot sustain the *status quo*, even if we continue to allow the "haves" to pay for the "have nots." As I endeavored to demonstrate so far in this book, one of the main reasons for the runaway costs of our healthcare is that too many outside entities have pushed themselves into the once-sacrosanct patient-physician relationship. They promoted a bureaucracy that at its heart is nothing more than a cover for their true money-centered agenda. They seek to get their hands into the money pot that should be protected and dedicated exclusively for public and individual patient health services.

The COVID-19 pandemic clearly showed that the increasing operational complexity of the US health system is ineffective in serving the health needs of all our people. Those who have gotten fat off the spoils of the healthcare industry sit in their box seats, sheltered within an unwieldy and massive stadium. As long as there is a profit to be made, they have little interest in the individuals playing on the field or the outcome of the game. The patient should return to the center of focus for anyone requesting a seat around the field of US healthcare.

We can no longer afford to tolerate this BS. We spend too much money to administrate the unnecessarily complex healthcare infrastructure and receive unacceptably poor quality-of-health returns on our investment. The excessive profits of the health insurers, hospitals, and biomedical industries should be reallocated to patient care. We can and should simplify the current paradigm by removing the numerous intermediaries that incur additional costs and interfere with patients' access to their doctors. Those who care more about their shareholders than patients—the rightful beneficiaries of medical care—should not be welcome to this house of medicine we call the American healthcare system. If we strive to eliminate all the BS, we can and will make Emaan's legacy the story for all patients in our system.

CHAPTER 9

ANSWERS OUTSIDE OUR BORDERS

The valve that Dr. Humphries created for Gilbert during his last surgery worked wonders and never caused him any problems. After Dr. Malm patched the hole in his heart, Gilbert proudly boasted, "My circulatory system worked somewhere near correctly, at almost 90 percent of normal capacity. I may have tired a little more easily than some people, but not by much. There was also a time that if something unmovable had to be moved, people knew to call for me because I was a bit stronger than most other people." Gilbert always believed that much of his strength was due to pure willpower.

During his young life—admittedly somewhat passive-aggressively in response to his mother's constant reminders that he had a "bad heart" and should "take it easy"—he always pushed himself harder. During one of our most memorable conversations at the opening celebration of my new office building, sitting back and enjoying the attention of a small group of mesmerized students and patients, he reflected, "Throughout my life, I have done some crazy things. I pushed myself to extremes a few times, but it did not hurt me. That might very well be a large part of the reason that I am still here today. I did not let 'you've got a bad heart' stand in my way."

Remarkably, between the age of 35 to 60 years, Gilbert did not see a cardiologist. As far as he was concerned, his heart was fixed. If it wasn't seriously broken now, then it didn't need to be fixed again. He certainly didn't want any doctors "meddling" and end up creating a new problem. He just figured that he would get it fixed when and if it ever broke. Otherwise, just leave it alone. His logic was very clear. "To me, there is no use of trying to do something for a maybe. Maybe just doesn't cut it with me. However, if there is a very good reason for doing something, then I am all for it."

In his 60s, he started to experience shoulder pain, and his orthopedic surgeon initially thought it was due to a torn rotator cuff. However, upon reviewing X-rays, together doctor and patient both knew immediately where the problem lay. Gilbert, having seen dozens of his own X-rays since the age of nine, looked over the doctor's shoulder and proudly said, "Oh, boy, there's a little piece of broken calcium floating near my shoulder joint right next to the bone. Must be what's causing my pain." The amused and impressed surgeon agreed and indicated that, during the operation, he would explore the rotator cuff and planned to grind the calcium off. Gilbert prepared himself for yet another operation. A date was set, and everything was a go.

In the end, however, the operation never took place. The day before the operation was supposed to happen, Gilbert went to his PCP's office to obtain medical clearance for surgery and anesthesia. His regular doctor was away, so another physician was scheduled to give him his final checkup before the surgery. As Gilbert sat on the examining table, talking to his wife about the details of going to the hospital the next morning for the operation, the new doctor came in.

After examining Gilbert, she turned to husband and wife and indicated that she could not clear him for the surgery until he was seen by a cardiologist. Gilbert vividly remembered his reaction to this news. "Sorry to say, but this new doctor quickly saw the worst side of me. She even stepped out at one point to get another nurse to come into the room just to make sure I didn't get out of control. I can usually control my temper, but when something ticks me off, I tend to get very vocal." Gilbert realized later that he spent a very long time mentally and emotionally preparing for an operation that deep down he did not believe he needed in the first place. He was scared about taking unnecessary risks that might affect his heart. When the doctor would not clear him and his orthopedist rescheduled the operation, she took the brunt of Gilbert's frustration.

In the end, the new doctor reclaimed Gilbert's respect when she quickly scheduled him an appointment with a cardiologist in Newburgh where he could have a stress test and echocardiogram done. To Gilbert's dismay, the stress test showed some inadequate blood supply to his heart, so the cardiologist advised that he should start some new medication. To add salt to the wound, he also told Gilbert that he needed to see a pediatrician for an accurate echocardiogram. When Gilbert questioned why he had to see a pediatrician, despite being over 60 years old, the adult cardiologist admitted honestly that he could not pretend to know what he was looking at on the echocardiogram when it came to congenital heart defects like Tetralogy of Fallot. He explained that he only dealt with old-age heart problems like high cholesterol and hypertension. At that point, with no small sense of irony, Gilbert figured out that he had to see a pediatric cardiologist.

Miraculously, one week later, Gilbert took a tumble as he tried to lift something into his truck. He landed up against the open door of the truck and suddenly heard a pop, followed immediately by brief horrible pain in his bad shoulder. A couple days later, having forgotten about the fall, he noticed that unlike in the recent past, his shoulder did not hurt at all while doing some yard work. He chuckled as he recounted to me, "It turns out that when I hit my truck, little pieces of the calcium in my shoulder broke off. The accident actually helped make my arm better. I immediately called the surgeon and told him that I did not need the surgery anymore because I fixed it myself." The next day, after an examination and reviewing repeated X-rays of Gilbert's shoulder, the surgeon agreed and called off the operation once and for all. Because he did not need surgery anymore, Gilbert decided to cancel the echocardiogram with the pediatric cardiologist. The fates dictated that Gilbert's journey back into the world of pediatric cardiology and his first encounter with me would have to wait.

OUR NEIGHBORS TO THE NORTH

The Canadian Health Act of 1984[53] established a "single-payer" system in Canada, in which their government funds health insurance using taxpayer monies. This allowed Canada to achieve universal healthcare coverage for all of its people. Canadian citizens only need private health insurance if they seek nonessential health services, such as dentistry or cosmetic surgery. Even in such a socialized healthcare system, all of the physicians and hospitals actually remain private and are not owned by the government. Fifty percent of the Canadian physicians are dedicated to primary care services, compared to 33 percent in the United States.

Contrary to the political rhetoric and folklore tales regarding the healthcare status of our northern neighbors, Canadian citizens are not all dropping dead on the streets waiting in line for lifesaving medical tests or treatments. On the other hand, it is an accurate assessment that, relative to the United States, wait times[54] for health services are a point of contention in the Canadian health system.[55] Many US policymakers use these lengthy weight times as a political weapon to portray the downside of the socialization of healthcare in Canada. Their goal is to dissuade the US voting public from seriously considering

53 "US vs. Canadian Healthcare: What is The Difference," Ross University School of Medicine, May 11, 2021 (online), https://medical.rossu.edu/about/blog/us-vs-canadian-healthcare.

54 Barua, Bacchus, "While Politicians Dither, Patients Die," *Alaska Highway News*, Fraser Institute (2023), https://www.fraserinstitute.org/article/while-politicians-dither-patients-die.

55 Barua, Bacchus and Moir, Mackenzie, "Waiting Your Turn: Wait Times for Health Care in Canada, 2020 Report," Fraser Institute, Dec. 10, 2020, https://www.fraserinstitute.org/studies/waiting-your-turn-wait-times-for-health-care-in-canada-2020.

any candidate for political office who supports transitioning the USA to a similar universal or single-payer healthcare system.

These politicians warn against anyone waving the banner of "socialism," hoping that American voters will run to the loyal capitalists for protection from the virtually communist monster from the north. Examples of this rhetoric have been touted by our former president and are typified by a quote from one of his "Make America Great" rallies in Kentucky, where he criticized the Democrats' proposal known as "Medicare for All" by responding, "By the way, it ("socialist" healthcare) doesn't work anywhere in the world. It is good if you don't mind waiting for like five weeks to see a doctor. They come [to the USA] from socialist countries—frankly, they come from Canada."[56]

While in Canada on vacation in 2018, Viyada and I were surprised to see how generally well-appearing Canadians were. As we explored the fall harvests in the local orchards and farms and wandered the markets and sites of the charming cities and towns from Montreal to Quebec, we noted that Canadians were generally eating healthy food and being very physically active. During a two-hour guided historical tour of the ancient sections of Quebec City, the sun shining brightly as the ocean breezes freshened the air, we started chatting with a friendly Canadian couple. As we finished our organized exploration, now relaxed and a bit hungry, the wife of the couple introduced herself as Mary and graciously invited us to join them at an outside café for a pre-dinner snack and local cider.

The satisfying drinks and food soon helped open up the conversation, and we learned that Mary was a nurse administrator from a community hospital in western Canada. Mary was a jovial, well-spoken, middle-aged woman who reminded me of several of the dedicated

56 Gomez, Amanda Michelle, "Trump Lies About Medicare for All. Says Universal Health Care Doesn't Work Anywhere in the World," ThinkProgress, Oct. 14, 2028 (online), https://archive.thinkprogress.org/trump-lies-about-medicare-for-all-says-universal-health-care-doesnt-work-anywhere-in-the-world-ed3d37dabe4d/.

nurses back in New York. Her husband, Max, was retired, warm-spirited, but more reserved. We never learned what he did for a living, but he appeared content to let Mary mingle with some American medical professional counterparts. As the second round of ciders began, she was clearly very open to sharing her perspectives of working for and living within Canada's socialized healthcare system. Feeling more welcome to share my own views, I proceeded to agree wholeheartedly with Mary that nurses are actually the ones who run healthcare in both of our countries. The ice was now completely broken, allowing the conversation to flow freely.

As the sun began to set, across the wooden picnic table filled with plates and tall, half-filled glasses of amber cider, we discussed and shared the experiences of our respective healthcare systems. We approached our conversation not as purported authorities on healthcare policy but rather as clinicians who have practiced our craft in one of two neighboring nations for a combination of almost 10 decades. Mary, Viyada, and I had in common that we have all been medical workers on the frontline—the factory floor.

Like me, Mary also had administrative experience. There was a consensus that, due to excessive administrative burdens—including privacy protections, electronic records implementation, malpractice insurance, billing services, preauthorizations, copays, and deductibles—the expenses trickled down, and individual US citizens are personally paying significantly more for the cost of healthcare than Canadians. Every Canadian citizen or physician does not deal with these processes under the universally covered government insurance known as Canadian Medicare.

"You're right," Viyada piped in. "All too often, American patients find themselves stuck standing outside emergency room doors, struggling with the concern that if they go inside to have their medical problem attended to, they may be stuck with a huge bill they can't afford."

"That's so sad," responded Mary. She explained proudly that the Canadian patient does not pay a dime to the doctors or hospitals for these services. They therefore do not hesitate to seek out healthcare services fearing that they may not be able to pay. Mary emphatically pointed out, "So, my dear American doctor friends, contrary to the common portrayal, we three can agree that in large part, it is US citizens, not Canadians, who significantly ration healthcare access on the basis of ability to pay." She clarified that medications are not universally covered by the Canadian government-based single-payer system. She looked around thoughtfully and boasted, "Though the other provinces do not pay nearly as much for medications as US patients, here where we now sit, the province of Quebec even extended government coverage to all medications."

I chimed in, "You know, in the United States, insurance companies basically use copays and deductibles to pass on the exorbitant cost of conducting business to patients or employers. This is just an accounting maneuver of moving some costs from one column to another so they can maintain a profit for their executives and shareholders."

Mary wondered if this coverup failed to address the most relevant issue. "The elephant in the room appears to be that the total cost to run the US health system may be too high because of an intrinsically cumbersome system."

Mary is right. Internationally maintained statistics reveal that above and beyond its "private payer" insurance system, the US government's Medicare insurance—designed specifically to cover the population greater than 65 years old—still costs the United States significantly more *per capita* than the Canadian system pays *per capita* to insure its entire population.

According to Mary, "One of the ways we streamline the system and save money in Canada may be too obvious. It is the single-payer concept itself. Because all medical care providers are paid through the same system, clinicians and hospitals are not as motivated to compete against each other for patient business."

This basic fact clarified to us at the table why excessive marketing costs are deemed critical to the survival of large hospital and physician corporations or mega-groups in the United States and serve no purpose in the Canadian system. Our mutual discovery further uncovered that reduced overhead costs allow the single or small practice to still survive in Canada, whereas the excess costs in the United States led to the few remaining small-sized practices persisting essentially as historic relics.

Our discussion soon focused on other financial strains to the US care providers. Mary inquired, "Is it true that when a patient in the United States has no insurance or is underinsured, the costs are essentially swallowed by the hospitals or doctors?"

Viyada clarified, "Yes, American doctors are ethically bound to provide care to all comers and often legally concerned about denying someone needing medical care."

We eventually all came to the conclusion that there were several other common sources of significant waste in both systems. Mary displayed her full nursing-administration hat by commenting, "It appears that, in both our countries, nurses and physicians needed to step up and play a major role in making the day-to-day flow of patients more efficient." As with her nursing counterparts in the United States, Mary stated that she spent a large part of her day trying to communicate with the physicians to clarify their plans for hospitalized patients.

In either system, when it came to admissions to the hospitals, whether the payor was the government in Canada or the private insurers in the United States, there was an impetus to keep the patients in the hospital for as short a time as possible. As experienced clinicians, we all learned that, because patients ultimately consistently recover better and remain at the lowest risk for complications and exposure to strong hospital-based infections the sooner they return to their own homes, the hospital was not necessarily the best place for patients to stay beyond their critical care.

I concurred. "I essentially teach all my student physicians that they need to be adept at planning discharge requirements and expectations as part of the admission process itself." I expanded this concept by recognizing that this usually meant a patient required some home-based services, which I assumed could take a while to set up in either country. I finished by adding, "If such services are not initiated until one or two days before discharge, the patient regretfully often stays in the hospital longer than necessary. Given the odds, the longer you stay, then the longer you stay because of complications as well. It's a wasteful, vicious cycle." Everyone, including Max, nodded in unison.

Mary shed some light on an important difference between our countries regarding hospitalizations. In her experience, in the Canadian system, she has seen that fewer patients actually end up in the hospital in the first place. Mary believed that this is because, unlike their US counterparts, Canadians have a tendency to see their physicians more frequently in any given year for outpatient visits. Thus, it is more likely that a problem is recognized before it becomes severe enough to require hospitalization.

Feeling somewhat despondent about how our US health system was stacking up to the Canadian version, Viyada and I had a brief, pleasant surprise. It appeared that our Canadian colleague was less satisfied with the home-based outpatient resources, social services, and rehabilitation programs in her country than we were in the United States.

"You may be shocked to learn that the Canadian universal health insurance system does not cover rehabilitation and home-based services," admitted Mary. She wondered aloud why these services were covered differently in each province and by varying degrees of private insurance or self-pay. In the end, it appeared that both nations had not maximized the opportunity to get patients home sooner and keep them from returning to the hospital. Apparently, this remains an important area that needs more work.

Mary expressed the same concerns for over-testing and prescribing medications in Canada as we did in the United States. We all agreed that this was because of a combination of medico-legal factors, as well as patients' misguided expectations. In both countries, there seems to be a pattern of physicians ordering tests as a medico-legal defensive strategy instead of because these tests are clearly or necessarily indicated.

Mary spoke without hesitation. "So it looks like in both our countries, the doctors practice the art of 'covering your ass,' instead of practicing according to their education and the best evidence-based standards for each patient." Despite the efforts of the government in Canada and the insurance companies in the United States, even with the guidance of their respective leading medical authorities and attempts to codify clear indications for testing in any particular situation, the pattern of over-testing and over-treating remained a shared problematic issue.

Mary sighed, "The one consolation in Canada is, again, that the medications and diagnostic tests are much less expensive than they are in the United States." Mary informed us that she was working on solutions to this excessive use of tests and medications in her own community. She concentrated her efforts on better patient education and making sure there was more continuity of care at the primary physician level. She remained hopeful that this would reduce the pattern of jumping from one doctor to another. Mary warned, "This patient behavior of wandering between different primary doctors or urgent care facilities results in no single physician being able to truly know any particular patient very well."

We all agreed that when a patient and doctor relationship is strong, there is intrinsically more trust. In this scenario, doctors are less likely to require testing or medications to reassure the patient that they are well or not in danger. Even more poignantly, in our experience, the number of mistakes and injuries is definitely reduced.

Viyada wondered, "Have you guys adopted an inpatient-focused physician coverage system known as a hospitalist?"

"Yes, over the past few years, hospitalist positions exploded where I work. Some of these doctors are great, and it is definitely helpful to have someone in the hospital at all times available to care for the admitted patients. But I think that this whole approach still needs a lot of improvement."

We all expressed similar concerns. Hospitalists are clearly not a surrogate for a good primary physician-patient relationship. In many ways, hospitalists have been relegated to functioning more as housekeepers and record keepers than clinicians. There is a constant burden on them to move the patient along quickly through their hospital care and get them back home as soon as possible. They are often clearly overwhelmed by the high numbers of patients they cover, many of whom are also clearly quite ill. Compared to just a few decades ago, when such patients were cared for in the urban centers, now in the community hospitals, their medical situations are more complex. We all witnessed the impact of modern medicine in both countries, which allowed a lot of medical conditions to be managed as an outpatient. Today, only the sicker patients end up in any hospital.

Mary succinctly summarized our opinions about hospitalists. "A good collaboration between the primary outpatient physician and the inpatient hospitalist can be an effective approach, but the communication has to be consistent to avoid excessive testing, over-treatment, medication errors, and frequent repeat hospitalizations."

Mary ultimately dispelled one of what she called the biggest misconceptions about Canada's healthcare. She paused as she sipped her last drop of cider and then looked directly at Viyada and me. "I know the rumor that you Americans have been passing around for decades about us. It's not true that if a patient needs a possibly lifesaving diagnostic test urgently, they may die waiting for this test in Canada. In an emergency situation, no time restrictions apply, and all tests absolutely can be done rapidly."

She qualified her point by admitting that there are indeed fewer testing centers and facilities available in Canada for any geographic region than the United States. These relatively more limited resources are therefore necessarily scheduled on an elective basis in Canada, and the population does not have the expectation of same-day testing or even testing within a week, as do Americans. Thus, in the outpatient settings in Canada, diagnostic testing, such as CT scans and MRIs, are rationed according to need and specific clinical indications and in turn do not tend to be as overused as in the United States.

I admitted, "Truth be told, we noted a similar trend in the United States under a different guise. Over the past decade, our insurance companies more routinely require a step called preauthorizations for most non-urgent diagnostic testing. Only in emergency situations, which are admittedly rare in the outpatient situation, will these tests be approved immediately." I confessed to Mary that in my own experience, similar to their Canadian counterparts, my patients can often wait two to four weeks for specialized tests such as pediatric cardiac MRIs. This is because such diagnostic tests are not only specialized but also concentrated in a handful of tertiary medical centers, analogous to the overall less prevalent tests in the Canadian system. As in Canada, I have no patients who died because of this wait. In both countries, if the physician believes the test is needed urgently, the test will be done.

As the streetlights illuminated the ancient cobblestone alleyways, over an hour since we first sat down for this memorable exchange between kindred spirits, we finally reached the heart of the matter. Mary sighed, "I wish both our countries were much better at making healthcare available equitably for all our citizens. We still have too many disparities of care quality and access, and this is ultimately hurting every one of us."

I was somewhat surprised to hear this from her, given my understanding that, in the Canadian system, payment for healthcare was not based on financial ability or insurance, and even the poor and unemployed benefited from coverage. Though this was true, Mary clarified that the way healthcare was delivered in Canada varied between provinces and, in particular, the ethnic backgrounds of the patients.

This latter factor appeared to upset Mary as she told us, "It's a shameful fact here. The Canadian indigenous population, for example, has a much lower health standard, quality of life, and life expectation than other Canadian inhabitants. As with your American minority populations, our own indigenous people, access to healthcare for these people is much lower than the rest of the population."

I was so intrigued by this issue of racial disparity in Canada, that evening I conducted some of my own research at our hotel. I learned that lately the solution to this deficit has become a matter of pride in the Canadian healthcare system. There is now a concerted effort to fill in these gaps and cover all of its inhabitants equitably. The socioeconomic impediments and disparities in their indigenous peoples are seen by many Canadians as a point of frustration and embarrassment. Overall, they seem to want better for these valued people and struggle to address the issues creating these problems.

Given our recent dismal experience with COVID-19, which our discussion with Mary foreshadowed so poignantly, it seems to me that the United States still has a long way to go before we too all feel that such disparities are a poor reflection on us as a people and not just a thorn in our side to be used as political fodder between candidates. Hopefully, we can learn to emulate the empathy that drives the Canadian people to seek 100-percent equitable coverage in healthcare for everyone as a matter of national pride. Only with such a common goal can any nation hope to achieve this landmark.

The comparison of the Canadian and US healthcare systems has recently become of increasing practical and intellectual interest. It has also been picked up by many of our conservative American politicians as a political bludgeon to warn voters to stay away from anything that smacks of the socialization of our healthcare. In many ways, healthcare assumed the mantle for debates regarding socialism formerly occupied by the US Social Security benefits system. In 2016 and 2020, politicians, including presidential candidates Bernie Sanders and Elizabeth Warren, proposed models for a universal healthcare system in America as a major component of their campaigns. Like our picnic-table discussion in Quebec with nurse Mary, these leaders see the value in exploring elements of other nations' healthcare policies that may prove beneficial to their constituents. There are abundant and reputable sources of information backing up their rationale.

Several international and domestic authorities keep close tabs on the outcomes and status of the decades-old and ever-evolving Canadian Health Act as it compares to the United States' fledgling ACA. These authorities come from entities such as the Organization for Economic Co-operation and Development (OECD), the Fraser Institute, the Commonwealth Fund, and, recently in 2018, even the *Journal of the American Medical Association*. These and other experts maintain statistics on the North American healthcare systems and compare them to each other and their economic peers in other developed nations.

When all is said and done, the analyses often come down to subtle but important differences. We compare entities that have more in common than separates them. Naysayers regarding the value to the United States of incorporating elements of the Canadian healthcare system will argue that such an exercise is futile because our respective systems are too different—apples versus oranges. However, I remain more optimistic. I feel strongly that we should all take solace in the fact that we are still comparing systems that share the same foundations—a fruit to another fruit. We need to take a collaborative, not divisive, approach when forming our own health policies. We should analytically—free of the biases of politics—look at elements of each other's systems to clarify which aspects may or may not help all of our respective nation's people to be healthier.

In reviewing the reports and analysis of the data about healthcare standards, access, and economics from the experts in institutions such as the OECD, the bottom line correlates well with what Mary from Canada concluded during our evening conversation. The United States pays much more for healthcare at all levels than Canada and many other countries in the world. The figures are staggering. Switzerland, for example, is number two in healthcare expenditure at 12.7 percent of their gross domestic product (GDP) and ranked internationally as almost equal to the United States in overall quality of the healthcare system at 33rd. The United States by comparison spends almost 17 percent of our GDP on healthcare and ranks as 32nd. Canada, proudly, can boast that it only spends 9 percent of their GDP on healthcare and ranks 25th overall internationally. Given these worldwide statistics, it is understandable that Canada and the United States both strive for the same objective—the ultimate *trifecta* of reducing costs, covering as many people as possible, and improving the overall quality of healthcare for their nations. If Canada is already doing so much better in this effort, shouldn't we ask ourselves how and why? Do we have to be stubborn and create our own wheel at such exorbitant costs while so much of the US population remains underserved?

What do the American people want? I remain concerned that we have not spent sufficient energy on this crucial introspective analysis. Given our relatively poor healthcare standards when considering our abundant material and human resources, we need to step back and collectively answer this fundamental question before we can take any meaningful steps forward. We need a solid framework to hold the details together, or else we risk chaos and frustration. Lately, the public debate regarding healthcare reform in the United States has become very unclear in terms of these big picture goals. It seems that we repeatedly allow political forces to take sides and define these issues for us. We are thus destined to change directions to a significant degree with each new political administration. As a citizen and practicing physician, I prefer a more consistent long-term vision to build upon. Like others before me, I advocate for the ideal of a separation of health and state.

Perhaps this could be achieved by establishing a common nonpartisan body of individuals analogous to the concept of the Supreme Court. The members of this US Healthcare Advisory Panel—including medical experts, our Surgeon General, laypeople, and academic and private industry representatives—would coordinate our collective wishes and continue to build upon former precedent as our society evolves. Along the way, we must also determine how important it is for us to focus upon healthcare policy apart from, but not ignorant of, infrastructure, environment, immigration policies, and other social issues. I would in fact argue that the success and resilience of these other issues are dependent upon a healthy society supported by a secure and consistent healthcare approach. Like others before me addressing government intrusion into healthcare,[57] I advocate for the ideal of a separation of health and state.

On the one hand, diving into social media and even more credible public news sources, and reading thoughtful works such as *Dying of Whiteness*[58] by Jonathan M. Metzl, I fear we are still too torn apart by hatred and prejudice to find this essential commonality of vision

57 Romano, Michael, "Separation of Health, State," *Modern Healthcare*, Oct. 26, 2003 (online), https://www.modernhealthcare.com/article/20031027/NEWS/310270313/separation-of-health-state.

58 Metzel, Jonathan M., *Dying Of Whiteness: How The Politics of Racial Resentment Is Killing America's Heartland*, Basic Books, May 2020.

in our healthcare policies. Can we overcome this divisiveness so that, like Canada and other countries, we may strive to cover 100 percent of our population with equitable healthcare for all? I certainly hope so. Are our values so different from our neighbors and peer nations?

On the other hand, recent polls indicate that across the United States, the one thing that all people agree upon, regardless of political persuasion, is that improving healthcare for the United States is a priority. This gives me hope. This shared vision is very good starting ground for a common approach. It is a ray of light that provides a contrast to the present tendency to use healthcare policy as a political wedge.

What about the American medical profession itself? Are medical professionals sufficiently in sync with each other on our objectives that we can help lead the way forward toward true population health? As a physician, I hope that my colleagues are not honestly accepting that the extreme variation in healthcare quality—so dependent upon social and economic conditions—is a valid endpoint for our nation. This clearly contrasts with the ethics of our medical profession, which cannot and should not provide different levels of necessary care to people depending on any number of socioeconomic factors. Essentially, like the financial aid programs in many universities, medical professionals and policymakers should advocate for a "needs blind" approach when dealing with any particular patient. Can we agree on these principles?

I have participated in a community-based health screening program advocating for and addressing the prevention of sudden cardiac arrest in the young for over 10 years. As the medical director, I oversee the clinical guidelines and administration of the program, along with the remarkable founders of these advocacy groups, many wonderful families touched by sudden cardiac arrest personally, and other health professionals. I attend each of three to six screening events annually as a medical volunteer and help guide the clinical decision-making. At a recent screening in Long Island, New York, several of my physician colleagues entered into a political discussion regarding the effect of the

Trump administration on our healthcare system. It was a respectful and interesting debate, or so I thought.

One of my colleagues asked me furiously, "How has the Trump administration affected or hurt your personal medical practices? You are still doing OK economically, aren't you?"

Somewhat taken aback by the abruptness of the change in tone of the discussion, I reflexively and later on somewhat regretfully shot back at him, "The current political environment deeply affects many of my patients, especially immigrants and people of color. Therefore, it does affect me."

"Come on. You don't really believe that, do you?" my colleague retorted dismissively. "Your bottom line is more secure with this administration than the liberal one before, isn't it?"

It was clear to everyone engaged that our interaction was about to turn from collegial to confrontational. So no one responded—conversation over. As I excused myself, I realized that I felt shaken and resentful that this colleague, who I knew to be bright and caring, held such opinions. His social, political, and economic priorities triumphed over our profession's principles, which saddened and deeply disturbed me. I did not have an eloquent response to overcome his biases. Still, I was angry with myself for staying silent.

As I drove home, I couldn't stop thinking about the conversation. This interaction conjured the repugnant vision of physicians as a people from an entitled privileged class—not recognizing how fortunate they are to have a steady income and the means to send their children to fancy colleges. This view ignores that others with fewer means work just as hard in favor of the concept that doctors "deserve" to be well off. My own parents worked tirelessly for years so that my sister and I could be the beneficiaries of a better life than them. My goals as a physician—which I try to share daily with my students—are not driven primarily by selfish personal or economic influences. On the contrary, I chose to be a physician to serve others in need of biological and psychological healing. I simply want to help people be as healthy as possible. The fact that I make a secure and reasonable living doing so has always been the icing on the cake for me.

When American society as a whole allows any thought leaders to infect us with division, prejudice, violence, selfishness, and greed, my colleagues and I, as American physicians, must contend with much more illness. In this corrosive environment,[59] I find it hard to promote healthcare as a human right according to my intrinsic vision of medicine as a vital component of democracy. When our people are not well psychologically, socially, morally, and biologically, then I believe that my profession is failing.

After some time to reflect about an appropriate response to my colleague's question—"How has this hurt you professionally?"—I can attest that I am professionally poorer as a direct consequence of the current non-inclusive and polarizing political environment that threatens to slam its doors on those most in need while shouting, "You don't deserve it. You must earn it." My morale and moral compass are both challenged by the current attack on our American value system's mission of reaching for a level playing field for all comers. It may be an ideal that is still out of our reach, but I resent the current political discourse that even suggests that they might deny me the right to keep reaching.

Medicine is by nature a social endeavor not promoted by polarization for the benefit of a few but rather by socialization that unites everyone equitably. The rhetoric of "us versus them" espoused by our politicians cannot help but affect me as a doctor. I see my colleagues burning out, leaving their careers prematurely, or becoming ill themselves—even taking their own lives under the mental health burdens of trying to provide care in a dehumanized system. Like my screening colleague who

---

59 C.K., "The Partisan Divide in America Is Widening," *The Economist*, Nov. 22, 2017 (online), https://www.economist.com/democracy-in-america/2017/11/22/the-partisan-divide-in-america-is-widening.

posed the question, they have become lost. To practice as if medicine is purely an economic commodity, rather than an honorable calling, is not sustainable for physicians or patients alike.

In 1903, a poem by Emma Lazarus was mounted on a bronze plaque on the Statue of Liberty. During a visit to the statue after the attack on New York on 9-11, I took a picture of this plaque and refer to it regularly. The second stanza of the poem, *The New Colossus*, in the voice of the Mother of Exiles, reads in part:

> Give me your tired, your poor,
> Your huddled masses, yearning to breathe free,
> The wretched refuse of your teeming shore.
> Send these, the homeless, tempest-tost to me,
> I lift my lamp beside the golden door!

We are a country of immigrants. We claim to be a caring people who welcome others, regardless of race, religion, gender, sexual orientation, or socioeconomic status. The tired and poor coming to America, some of whom are ill and in need of emotional and physical attention, should be welcomed with open arms. As one of many physicians and medical professionals, I was on the front lines of caring for the sick and downtrodden, even before the COVID-19 pandemic. Lady Liberty's lamplight holds the promise of well-being for all. Anything that threatens to extinguish it threatens my ability to reach with her—to be an American physician.

A SOBERING LOOK IN THE MIRROR

As we strive to improve our own healthcare system, we need to look to other models for insights and comparisons. As we do so, it is so important for policymakers to realize the limitations of isolating themselves behind closed doors and looking at tons of cold data in a vacuum. I learned the hard way that statistics are just processed data that still require thoughtful analyses. It is negligent at best and harmful at the worst to jump to conclusions that form our policies based upon superficial information. They are not necessarily always valid representations of the current reality that people face daily, and more often than not, they certainly do not provide a clear understanding of the motives and factors impacting peoples' health-related choices and actions. If we are to truly understand the relevant strengths and weaknesses of the existing and proposed healthcare systems, all advocates for meaningful reform need to actively engage with the people on the ground. Only then can they truly understand their deepest needs and concerns.

When we compare the numbers for problems such as obesity, poverty, life expectancy, infant mortality, and other similar criteria, we must look well below the surface to understand how a particular community or society as a whole came to find themselves in this situation in the first place. Any one of these statistical values belies a complex set of circumstances unique to our respective histories, cultures, and values. If we refuse to look honestly at these factors, we are stubbornly superficial—dare I say, lazy—and the solutions that we create based on numbers alone will inherently be fragile and transient as well.

Factors such as socioeconomics, geography, and racial biases all come into play, and we should not pretend otherwise. By analyzing the forces behind any given healthcare statistic amongst different countries, we may better see our commonalities and our unique country-specific differences. We should not use these statistics simplistically as a report card to make ourselves feel better or worse than other nations or, domestically, pit one state or city against another. These forces are dynamic factors that clearly underlie what we all share as part of the human equation. With this constructive and honest approach, many sincere and dedicated people have shown that we can learn far more working together than apart. We should thus urge our politicians in earnest to stop using each other's healthcare systems as political fodder and weapons against their political rivals. If we work collaboratively for the common good of our people—stop knocking others down for short-term personal gains—we have a much higher chance of long-term global success. The pandemics and natural disasters of our planet shout more loudly than ever that we need to work together if we are to survive as a species.

An example of the divisive propaganda is the portrayal of the Canadian healthcare system as being virtually extremely inaccessible to the people when they most need it. This well-worn propaganda[60] portrays the Canadians as people forced to cross the border into the United States to procure health services that are either lacking or delayed in Canada. In the full light of day, the political biases and agenda behind this oversimplified negative depiction of the Canadian *status quo* as hordes of people waiting in never-ending lines of bureaucracy can be more honestly exposed.

The reality is that many Canadians live and work in the United States, and their Canadian health insurance coverage extends to their needed services while here. These individuals are not coming here specifically for healthcare but rather simply visiting the doctor or emergency room in the middle of their work time just as any American working and living in another country would do. It may be true that the more economically fortunate Canadian individuals come to the United States to seek medical procedures or evaluations by some of our best physicians or medical centers, but this is not unique to the wealthy of Canada.

As discussed in a review of the February 2017 CNN political debate for the US presidency between opposing candidates—Democrat Bernie Sanders and Republican Ted Cruz—this wealthy outmigration for medical services actually only accounts for less than 0.5 percent of all Canadians. Many millionaires cross state and country lines to obtain the best medical care possible for themselves and their loved ones.

---

60 Aronczyk, Amanda, "Why Americans Have Been Deceived About Canada's Health Care System," *NPR News*, Nov. 6, 2020 (online), https://www.npr.org/2020/11/06/931990578/why-americans-have-been-deceived-about-canadas-health-care-system.

Every year, medical tourism leads to over 750,000 Americans seeking healthcare outside US borders.[61] This is an issue of economics involving a small subset of the Canadian population,[62] not a general trend of Canadians running *en masse* into the United States for health services.

It is also important to note that the Canadian government aggressively recognized specific areas of low resources. Therefore, some of the Canadian patients cared for in the United States were intentionally sent here by their own government in recognition of certain temporary deficits such as new cancer therapies. This has been an open, collaborative effort between our nations focused on patient care, not some under-the-rug arrangement. In the interim, Canada is expanding many of their resources to meet the medical needs within their own borders within the foreseeable future.

The irony of this exchange of medical services is that a counterbalancing trend to this socioeconomic pattern recently developed. Medical resources from other countries are being procured not by wealthy Americans but actually by the less economically well-to-do. This situation is best exemplified by the purchase of prescription medications by US citizens from Canadian pharmacies, where the costs of these medications are significantly lower. Many US health insurance policies do not adequately cover the exorbitant costs of medications coming from US-based pharmacies. Rather than choose food over taking necessary medications, Americans discovered that these medications are much more affordable in countries such as Canada and China.

This scenario is in itself enigmatic because, as highlighted earlier, one of the main and most contentious "holes" in the Canadian universal health program that impacts their citizens is that many of their

---

61 "Medical Tourism: Travel to Another Country for Medical Care," *Center for Disease Control and Prevention*, June 1, 2023 (online), https://wwwnc.cdc.gov/travel/page/medical-tourism.

62 Druzin, Randi, "Crossing the Border for Care," *U.S. News & World Report*, August 3, 2016 (online), https://www.usnews.com/news/best-countries/articles/2016-08-03/canadians-increasingly-come-to-us-for-health-care.

provinces do not cover any of the costs of medications. Recently, the province of Quebec elected not to exclude medication coverage, but this decision is still left to the individual provinces. They for the most part rely on keeping medication costs low enough that, hopefully, most people can afford to pay for them on their own.

Canadians as a whole are actually much more upset about the lack of universal medication coverage than they are with wait times to access medical care or tests. Historically, when Canadian public pressures forced elected politicians to officially support broad measures granting Canadian citizens the ability to access limited diagnostic medical tests and procedures outside the country, to everyone's surprise, very few people ultimately availed themselves of these opportunities to cross into the United States. Some actually expressed a distrust of the safety and motives of US healthcare services. They chose to wait until they could receive the services at home in Canada. This is clearly an example of how perceived political views do not always align with practical common sense and behaviors when policies are ultimately put to the test.

Both the United States and Canada are vulnerable to mistaking political agendas as a surrogate for the true motives of their citizens' healthcare-related choices and behaviors. Ultimately, a person's medical decisions are based upon specific practical issues such as economics and trust of their clinicians and medical institutions, not a politician's often misguided agenda.

Another often forwarded misconception when comparing the American to the Canadian healthcare system is that, unlike American medical services, Canadian services are much more rationed, limited, and restricted. The essence of the party line can be summarized as, "Everyone knows that Canadians are not free to choose their own doctors like we are in the States." Actually, Canada does not have limits regarding who an individual can choose as their regular provider or hospital, as long as the provider is within the province where the patient lives. Within these parameters, there are no barriers such as copays, annual deductibles, preauthorization, and requirements for chosen doctors to be in-plan. Administrative approval for out-of-network medical services and limitations as to whom an individual can choose in terms of hospitals or physician groups are nonexistent.

On the contrary, the reality in the United States is that our healthcare is clearly and harshly rationed and controlled by the third-party payors themselves. In very few medical insurance plans are individuals or families openly "free to choose" their physician. For decades, each insurance company has designated and controlled which clinicians and facilities are included in their plans. They also created tiers of coverage within these already limited systems by changing the levels of copays and deductibles in the different silver, gold, and platinum packages. If one looks further behind the Wizard of Oz's curtain, we can also see that our government actually pulls a lot of the levers on the system by indirectly and directly influencing the government and private payors. When Medicare restricts or lowers the reimbursement for medical services, the other payors traditionally used this as a green card for them to follow suit.

In Canada, the hospitals and care providers are all reimbursed by their federal government at a uniform level comparable to their provincial peers. They are actually not paid much less than their US counterparts. The honest truth is that American PCPs and surgeons earn more than most of their Western country counterparts, but they accrue much higher administrative and operational costs. Other countries have far fewer extraneous expenses and administrative "red tape" to deal with, such as the very high-priced US malpractice coverage, licensing, billing, and education-related costs. One of the often-not-publicized advantages of this simpler Canadian system is that, within one's own province, there is virtually no need for medical entities and providers to compete with each other for access to patients. The ubiquitous, confusing, and often disingenuous US healthcare advertising practices are not a priority and therefore less prevalent amongst the providers in other countries such as Canada. The whole system is much simpler and less expensive. It thus comes down to the basic economic premise—it's not what you make that matters; it's what you keep.

One of the most important issues that Americans in the United States must face is that 20 percent of citizens and residents are completely uninsured when it comes to healthcare coverage. Many more are "underinsured." This lack of coverage falls far short of other socioeconomically equivalent countries such as Canada, whose continued efforts have achieved virtually 100-percent healthcare coverage. This lack of health insurance coverage in the United States has been identified for decades as an unsustainable economic situation.

Because medical facilities and clinicians are not able to ethically refuse anyone in need of health services, the costs created by the insufficiently insured patients are essentially diverted elsewhere and spread out amongst the insured patients or swallowed by the providers. This situation has significant consequences. To remain solvent or pay dividends to their shareholders, the third-party payors repeatedly increase the beneficiaries' healthcare insurance premiums. Even more concerning, this imbalanced distribution of premiums, which relies on the adequately insured to carry the burden of the less insured, strains the operations of medical facilities. They increasingly struggle to cover operational costs, particularly in socioeconomically depressed areas. Many have closed, thus widening the socioeconomically based inequities of healthcare access and quality.

As discussed with my Canadian nurse acquaintance, Mary, behind the curtains, we are simply moving these costs from one column to another on the ledger of our healthcare budget. In our evening discussion, Mary warned, "Americans should not pretend that these costs are somehow magically disappearing. This game of charades with healthcare-related dollars now teeters dangerously on the edge of being unsustainable."

I agreed and added, "Because US healthcare expenditures are already near 20 percent of our GDP, these 'hidden costs' now constantly threaten the whole US economic system itself."

In the end, the fundamental lesson I learned in my comparison of the United States to other developed countries' healthcare policies is that a system's sustainability and level of quality is proportionate to the percentage of people with appropriate health insurance. The COVID-19 pandemic further emphasized this fact by adding that we are all intrinsically connected to each other's well-being. One of the main results of the ACA was that it reduced the level of medically uninsured Americans from nearly 20 to 9 percent, but sadly, this level returned to 16 percent with the slow dismantling of the ACA under the federal administration in charge between 2016 and 2020.

This constant fluctuation of the portion of people with adequate health insurance is a salient example of how US healthcare evolved into a huge political football over the past two decades. This lack of resiliency of coverage necessitates that we pay close attention to the truth behind our politicians tossing this "hot potato" amongst themselves and their constituents. When it comes down to it, what good is it to have some of the best medical resources in the world if we do not have a health system that allows all our people to equitably access these services?

There are many disparate factors that explain why the US health system costs more in absolute dollar amount than any other in the world. Even more disconcerting is that, when we drill down to look at our healthcare accounting ledger in more detail, we also spend disproportionately higher for comparable materials and services than all other nations. The factors that contribute to this include, but are not limited to the following: high physician education-related debts;

relatively higher physician salaries; excessive administrative burdens; nonuniform and user-unfriendly electronic medical records systems; exorbitant pharmaceutical and diagnostic equipment costs; competitive advertising-related expenditures; unique and highly prevalent complex socioeconomic issues; medicolegal liability practices; the relatively much higher charges for diagnostic tests; over-testing and over-treating practice patterns; convoluted billing services and regulations that rival the tax codes and which providers must strictly follow to be reimbursed for their services rendered; and, regrettably, even downright fraud.[63] Understandably, most of my doctor colleagues despise the bureaucracy of medical billing and never wanted to put fees between themselves and their patients in any fashion.

Many of these excessive costs are also directly related to our support for and often blind belief in the uniquely American free-market system. It is argued that this supply-and-demand-based system best stimulates innovations in medical care, whereas the socialism-based systems of other countries stifle the potential of such advancements. This argument takes its full form when applied to the American private-sector pharmaceutical companies who spend a significant amount of money on research and development to create new and "better" drugs for humanity. They conclude that because of the free-market system, the United States is the world's greatest supplier of the amazing medications used to combat all of the major illnesses facing our species. These proponents of the benefits of this capitalist approach conclude that other countries are in fact "leeching" off our system when they ultimately purchase or eventually "copy" these discoveries.

Though the rationale is convincing on the surface, the actual business practices of these pharmaceutical industries are in direct conflict with several traditionally maintained values of our American health system. The most fundamental of these values dictates that physicians

63 Simon, Gilbert, *Ripped Off!: Overtested, Overtreated and Overcharged: The American Healthcare Mess*, Paper Raven Books, Feb 27, 2020.

are clearly trained and ultimately legally and ethically bound not to have conflicts of interest when it comes to choosing medications or treatments for their patients. According to this principle, a doctor should only prescribe or order a particular medication for their patients based on scientifically derived evidence, not on the influence of the manufacturer.

However, over the past two decades, these pharmaceutical companies had to be legally reined in from their natural free-market tendency to "buy off" doctors with gifts to convince them to prescribe their newest or most lucrative medications. It is regretful that this same restriction is not as vehemently reinforced when it comes to these same companies financially supporting political candidates. In fact, many of the largest and most politically powerful special interest groups include these very same pharmaceutical companies. Perhaps, despite facing such unethical violations, this backdoor political clout further emboldened many of these pharmaceutical companies who recently were caught red-handed paying off less reputable physicians to prescribe some of the newest opiate medications.

This behavior occurred right in the midst of our generation's greatest healthcare crisis—the opiate epidemic. Our ignorance of this conflict of interest and leverage by these behemoth private companies within our free-market system played a significant part in creating and maintaining this historic opiate crisis. Yes, due to significant fiscal and intellectual investments applied within the framework of our free-market system, we may have created many more remarkable painkilling medications. All the same, this does not justify their unscrupulous marketing and coercion to have doctors prescribe as many of them as possible. Even more heinous, when a pharmaceutical company does not find a domestic market for a medication on which they spent a lot of time or money, or if the medication does not meet the strong American standards for approval, all too often, the company will market the medication to another country with fewer resources and standards.

Imagine the moral and professional backlash if physicians practiced healthcare this way.

The largest pharmaceutical entities also created such a monopoly and domination over the market that many smaller companies found it necessary to leave the country to create their own medications. This explains why many relocate or start up their new operations in countries such as China. Ironically, most of these small startup companies ultimately hope to "cash out" and have their discoveries bought out by the giants of the US industry. It also cannot be overstressed how much of an influence is created by the fact that the pharmaceutical companies constantly answer to their shareholders. They are thus not actually focused on using the free-market system to financially stimulate their employed researchers to discover new wonder drugs but rather bent on implementing capitalism to make outside investors wealthier.

Sadly, it appears that some of our politicians who were given the very role of "reforming" our health system forgot the most fundamental ethical principles of this system. They forget or willfully ignore that doctors are supposed to adhere to higher professional and ethical standards than those that govern the free market. On a positive note, the recent successful lawsuits against some of the large companies involved in the opiate crisis give one hope that we may not have completely abandoned our morals.

The absolute reliance on the free-market system as the best vehicle for innovation also flies in the face of reality when we review some of the most enduring and influential medical innovations of the last century. Alexander Fleming was an academic scientist in Scotland when he discovered the world's first antibiotic, Penicillin G, in 1928, for which he was awarded the Nobel Prize in 1945. Jonas Salk was an academic physician researcher funded by the nonprofit precursor organization to the March of Dimes, the National Foundation for Infantile Paralysis—established by President Franklin D. Roosevelt—when he successfully tackled one of the world's greatest public health problems by creating the polio virus vaccine in 1955. The list of such non-privately funded major and earth-shattering discoveries supported by public or academic entities is extensive and has been most recently manifested in the fight against cancer. In October 2018, another academic American doctor, Dr. James P. Allison from the University of Texas, and a Japanese researcher, Dr. Tasuku Honjo of Kyoto University, were both awarded the Nobel Prize for their research on cancer immunotherapy. This novel treatment modality is touted as possibly the greatest breakthrough ever in the field of cancer.

It would be naive to imply that there is no role for private industry in medical research. Rather, in such a complex country as the United States and in the world at large today, there is no one solution to our greatest problems. This diversity in approaching our challenges is not a weakness when it comes to America—it is our greatest strength. We must remain cognizant of any special economic interest groups or political power biases that threaten to cloud our judgment—create adversaries, instead of allies—when we pursue these challenges. Support and maintenance of a hybrid system that combines the best tools of the private pharmaceutical and medical instrument companies, universities, nonprofit-funded research grants, and international cooperatives provides the highest potential for success.

As discussed with my Canadian nurse acquaintance, the most culturally important remaining problems in common within our health systems are the significant disparities in healthcare access based upon race. Only by working together can we ever hope to address the racism and prejudices that directly conflict with our shared core ethics which claim to equally value all human life. As discussed by Paul Starr in his Pulitzer Prize-awarded treatise, *The Social Transformation of American Medicine: The Rise of a Sovereign Profession and the Making of a Vast*

Industry, refugees, immigrants, and those politically less represented in our country intrinsically remain under the influence of the "authority" of the US health system.

He explains that this is because they essentially have no other choice if they are to access any of our medical services:

> When poor and working-class people encounter professionals… they are more likely to be guarded in their communication and to feel alien and hostile. Many of their contacts with professionals are involuntary or take place in public institutions, and they do not have control. Under these conditions… individuals from the lower and working classes may comply, if at all, more for reasons of dependence than for reasons of belief. They may simply have few alternatives.[64]

In my own experience, they are indeed often afraid to speak out or challenge this authority for fear of being negatively identified or sent back to whence they came.

Manuel was almost four years old when he was first referred by the local community health clinic to see me. His family emigrated from Mexico two years prior. They followed his father, who journeyed to our upstate New York area as one of many seasonal migrants seeking work in the local farm fields. At that time, Manuel was an only child, and his mother did not speak any English. Manuel's new pediatrician recently noted a significant change in his physical examination. About one week prior, a new heart sound, a "swooshing" signifying turbulent blood flow and known as a murmur, was appreciated by this doctor. Manuel was a strikingly handsome and shy boy with large brown eyes and a bowl-style haircut bestowed upon him by his adoring mother.

My medical assessment of the source of his murmur revealed that he was born with a large hole in the wall of the top chamber of his

---

64 Starr, Paul, *The Social Transformation of American Medicine: The Rise of a Sovereign Profession and the Making of a Vast Industry*, Basic Books, 1982.

heart. He was in need of elective surgery within the next few months to close this hole, known as an atrial septal defect. I had seen Manuel with his mother but had never actually met his father. After I explained the issue in detail to his mother in my best broken Spanish and with the aid of drawings, I scheduled the surgery for one to two months.

Almost one year later, we were still unable to schedule the surgery at the recommended urban tertiary medical center. After many attempts to reschedule the surgery, I learned that the father was hesitant to sign the consent for surgery. I therefore arranged for the father to meet me one weekend in the office before he started work. I soon learned that he worked off the books in a small grocery or bodega in town as an illegal immigrant. His employer was very strict and threatened to fire anyone who did not show up for work. The father was torn between losing his job—possibly being arrested or deported back to Mexico—and his need to care for his son's heart if he took too much time off from work to attend his son's surgery. He also expressed a fear of being seen in public in the big city medical center where his son needed the surgery.

In the end, I decided to call the father's employer. I threatened to report him for hiring illegal immigrants and creating an abusive work environment. I used this threat as leverage to firmly direct the employer to give the father five days off to attend to his son and allow this employee to return to work after the surgery without fear of any reprisals. He reluctantly agreed, and the child finally had the surgery over one year after I initially met him.

The United States was historically a unique society in regards to our foundation as a culturally diverse nation. However, many other countries have since seen a significant increase in their diversity due to immigration, refugees, and the adoption of protections similar to those originally founded in America. In all of these nations, the forces of economics, healthcare, migration, race, and authority are intertwined. However, the United States remains unique amongst nations in regards to the level of authority and autonomy that the health system maintains relative to the other power brokers in government, education, and private industry. With this power comes the proverbial "great responsibility" of American healthcare leaders to enable equitable access to medical care for all.

As a Bosnian refugee patient of mine stated bluntly, "Though our hospitals in Bosnia are barely standing with rubble all around from the bombings of the wars, we are still all treated respectfully as equals when we go there as patients. To our surprise, now that we are in the United States, when we seek medical attention in the very sturdy and beautiful buildings in New York City, because of the way the staff treats us in the clinics and emergency rooms, we always feel undeniably like second- or third-class citizens."

They longingly missed the kind way they were treated in their homeland. They had to tolerate being treated as a number—not a person—because it was politically and physically too dangerous to return to their beloved war-torn homeland. If we are still determined to hold the torch of freedom and refuge to all those who come to our shores, we must ensure that those granted authority in our health system do not carelessly blow out this torch and instead enable it to burn brighter.

It has been my professional experience that universal healthcare systems, such as that of my British-trained medical mentors, are much more prevention-oriented than the US system. I first became fully aware of this difference when a British physician, Dr. Lindsey Allan, was recruited to Columbia University to introduce and train my colleagues in the modality of fetal echocardiography—a novel means of assessing a fetal patient's heart for possible problems before they are born using ultrasound-derived images. As one of the main founders of fetal echocardiography, Dr. Allan discovered that the American medical system was initially hesitant to implement this technology because the health insurance companies were not reimbursing for this procedure.

In their proverbial wisdom, the insurers determined that the immediate, short-term cost savings and the ultimate change in health outcomes for the fetus did not appear to justify the utility of fetal echocardiography. Unlike her experience in the United Kingdom, the American insurance payors did not address factors such as improved timeliness of medical care delivery, downstream cost savings, long-term improved health outcomes, or emotional support of the families. The US health system's sights were limited to what they could see immediately in front of them economically and not how this new technology could change the big picture of newborn acute cardiac care as a whole. I always sensed that her frustration with this myopic view played no small part in her decision to eventually return to the UK professionally.

Over 20 years later, her approach has won the day worldwide—including the United States—and is now considered the standard of care in assessing a patient's heart for potential cardiac disease many weeks before the baby sees daylight. I am thankful that communication technology allows the unfettered exchange of medical literature and research amongst colleagues, but I would have preferred for Dr. Allan to remain in the States to continue her work and teaching. However, given the recent continued debate over the value of Planned Parenthood, I am not sure that the United States is any more inclined to provide forward-minded care than we were when she taught me and my colleagues in the late 1990s.

We remain focused on short-term costs and politically motivated biases, rather than trying to understand the power of providing those most in need amongst us with evidence-based preventative care and education. Can anyone be more vulnerable than a single, underinsured, pregnant young woman in need of guidance and prenatal care for her and her baby? Who among us stands to lose the most if this care is not provided? If we look only to the immediate timeframe and not beyond to the course of her unborn child's whole life—to the implications for the welfare of the community they will live and work in—we are destined to lose not just economically, but morally.

Daily, I challenge myself, colleagues, and students to become seriously engaged in these issues as we decide what form our US health system will take. We would clearly benefit from the examples of our peers in other countries who made these issues a priority. There are many models to draw from, including hybrid systems that combine universal socialized healthcare with private healthcare. The political banter must be replaced by coherent action if we are to avoid completely losing our way. As a long-time practicing physician and educator, I am convinced that where our healthcare system goes, so goes our society.

CHAPTER 10

THE SYNERGY OF COMMUNITY MEDICINE AND GREAT INSTITUTIONS

Though Gilbert's shoulder surgery was no longer necessary, his PCP, Dr. Laura Samuelson, insisted that he undergo an appropriate echocardiogram with a pediatric cardiologist familiar with Tetralogy of Fallot. After several months, he still had not scheduled this test. Finally, after a routine checkup, Dr. Samuleson approached him with a soft smile and a twinkle in her deep blue eyes as Gilbert was about to exit the exam room.

She spoke gently but firmly. "Please stop at the back desk before you leave. I have left a script for you and an appointment confirmation for a long-overdue test I really want you to have." Gilbert reluctantly agreed to follow the guidance of this paperwork. To his amusement, it turned out to be an appointment for a pediatric cardiologist.

Gilbert fondly recalls that first of many phone calls from my office. Over the years, he repeatedly boasted to anyone within earshot, "Dr. Fethke's receptionist wanted to know if I was Gilbert's father. I chuckled and informed her that actually I was Gilbert. She sounded somewhat confused, but nonetheless, she confirmed my appointment."

One crisp, early spring day in 2011, Gilbert finally crossed the threshold of our pediatric cardiology office for the first time. He later recounted his memory of the moment to one of my medical students. "Everyone just stood there and stared at me. I was in my 60s at the time. They were trying to figure out what was going on. Dr. Fethke himself was a pretty kind soul. He told me that I needed an echocardiogram, but he also wanted to put me on a Holter monitor to check for any irregular cardiac activity. I was put on the Holter monitor that day, and then I came back a few days later for my echocardiogram."

Thus began a routine of annual checkups and very fond visits between Gilbert and me. After completing the professional and technical part of the encounter, we spent another few minutes catching up. We talked about our families, and he always made a point to share his philosophy about what makes good healthcare.

At one particular visit, he latched onto some good news with a dose of selective memory, which he later recalled to a student. "The only significant comment Dr. Fethke ever made about the progression of my heart condition was about three years ago. He held up the most recent echocardiogram and compared it to the ones over the prior years. He told me that these images showed that my heart was actually getting stronger, not weaker, with age. What do you think about that?"

At 1 p.m. sharp, on a late spring day in 2012, Gilbert approached the front desk receptionist of my office with his usual jovial banter mixed with a small dose of flirtation. "Hello there, young lady. I'm here for my regular visit with Dr. Fethke."

The receptionist smiled politely, knowing well that Gilbert would be interested in what she was about to tell him. She proudly replied, "Dr. Fethke is running a bit late with starting afternoon patients because an hour ago he was called urgently to the delivery of the first new baby with Tetralogy of Fallot to be born at the local medical center."

Gilbert's thoughts harkened back decades before in a different era to his own family's experiences as he waited anxiously for my return. Thirty minutes later, as I ushered Gilbert into an exam room, before I even closed the door, Gilbert blurted out, "How's the baby, Doc?"

Given his apparent concern, one would think this baby was a member of his own family. I calmly filled him in on the events of the baby's arrival. "The baby is fine, as I hoped and expected by our prenatal evaluations over the past six months. I did not anticipate any problems, but because this was the first time a baby with a known complex heart condition was scheduled to be delivered at the new hospital, I went over there to make sure everything was alright."

Gilbert reacted to the news with a mixed sense of reflection and joy. "Just like my mother. She initially thought she had lost her baby during the third month of pregnancy. Then the rest of the pregnancy appeared to go fine. She didn't know I had the Tetralogy of Fallot until after I was born. You have to feel sorry for that new mother today, knowing all this scary information about her unborn child while pregnant and being unable to do anything to help for all those months. How is the mother doing? She must have been on pins and needles."

That day, I suddenly understood the depth of Gilbert's own emotions regarding his heart condition. It was clear why he was so driven to emphasize that healthcare should be delivered not simply as technology but with compassion. I gained a much deeper and more meaningful insight into the emotions of the families that came to me during pregnancy because their unborn child might have a heart condition. I so wanted to let him know that he made a profound difference in how I delivered care to all these babies and their families.

I responded, "It's a good thing you came in today. After I examined the brand-new baby and told the parents that everything was fine, I had the opportunity to tell them that I had to return to the office to see another 'Tet' patient, only he's 75 years old. When they heard this, I could immediately see six months of stress and strain drain out of the mother's face."

Gilbert's wide smile was only further accentuated by the soft tears rolling down his rosy cheeks.

LOCAL CARE STEPS IN TO FILL THE GAPS

Much transpired in my medical practice and regional pediatric care since that cold and damp early spring morning when the young, cocaine-overdosed, and pregnant Tanya was found in labor lying in a street ditch. Twelve years ago, I gave the ambulance crew the directive to urgently transport her to Columbia while in active labor.

I matured as a physician, and the cadre of locally available pediatric care services expanded significantly. My efforts had borne fruit. Hundreds of children could remain in their own communities to receive pediatric specialty care, including visits and testing. Compared to the decade earlier, far fewer young patients were transferred away to the urban centers because we now cared for them locally. This was both because we could identify impending medical problems before they rose to the level of an emergency and also because most of the children's conditions could be managed in the community outpatient or hospital settings.

One late September evening, as I sat down at my office desk to prepare for a practice meeting about further expansion of medical services, my eye caught a glimpse of a child's framed photo hanging on the wall directly in front of me. The adoptive parents of this child gave this portrait to me as a gift before the whole family was re-stationed elsewhere for military duty. The essence of the accompanying text was their gratefulness and recognition of my brief role at giving this child a chance for a full life. The warm, deep brown eyes of this toddler looking back at me were those of his mother, Tanya, and the memories of his first day of life brought me back to that early March day.

Tanya's baby was born naturally within minutes after arriving at Columbia's doors and barely one hour after the ambulance departed from the streets of Newburgh. They just made it. Within 30 minutes of Trayvon's birth, I received a phone call from one of my pediatric cardiology colleagues at Columbia.

The kind, familiar voice of this doctor emanated clearly through my car speakers. "Eric, it's Karen. I know that you must be worried about Tanya's baby, so I wanted to call you as soon as he was born and stable. The little fighter came through so much and is actually doing great. Tanya named him Trayvon."

The strain of worry that I carried all day melted away. My colleague thoroughly reviewed the baby's status. Fortunately, as I anticipated, the baby's oxygen levels were only mildly lower than normal, and he was doing remarkably well. He was transferred for monitoring to their neonatal intensive care unit, where he was monitored for 24 to 48 hours. I notified the local medical team that the baby was doing well, and 48 hours later, I drove down to Columbia. He was very cute, extremely comfortable, and seemingly healthy—almost begging us with his wide-open, inquisitive eyes to explain all the fuss.

I contacted Dr. Kay to arrange for Trayvon to be transferred back to the St. Luke's NICU for a few days before he went home with his mother. Everyone at Columbia and St. Luke's agreed that this was a reasonable plan. I walked down the hallway confidently hoping to tell Tanya the good news—her baby was well and could go back closer to home the next day.

As I walked to the obstetric ward, a worried-looking clerk stopped me outside Tanya's room. In an agitated whisper, she gave me the bad news. "Tanya asked to go out for some fresh air last night. Since she didn't have a C-section, she didn't need anyone to accompany her. Security searched for her after Nursing found her room still empty over one hour later. She apparently left the hospital on her own without telling anyone. It looks for all the world like Tanya abandoned the baby."

I was in shock with this additional hurdle now thrown into Trayvon's story. Though her home phone was disconnected and no one could reach her, we went ahead with the plan to transfer Trayvon back to St. Luke's NICU. He arrived there uneventfully and continued to do well for several weeks, an orphan of this unit. Social Services became involved to determine where and with whom this baby would leave the hospital. The situation was very bleak and frustrating. Nobody wanted this baby from the streets with a broken heart.

Then a miracle happened. A NICU nurse who had been caring for Trayvon since his arrival at St. Luke's offered to take him home. Mary Schmidt was a seasoned Irish-German nurse in her mid-40s with light brown, wavy hair, jade-green eyes, and a warm smile. Over the years, she and her career military husband, Michael—a strong, rugged soldier in his early 50s with a chiseled physique and face complemented by his huge soft heart—opened their home with three of their own biological children to foster several children of different races.

Along the way, they adopted and raised four of these orphans, thus creating a large and loving mixed-race family. Though the Schmidts weren't sure if they could adopt Trayvon, they were committed to fostering and caring for him over the next three years while he underwent a series of at least two complex heart surgeries. Dr. Kay and I agreed to watch him closely and remain his physicians throughout this process. The child welfare team approved of this plan and were actually very excited that so many of his medical professionals, including Mary, were involved in caring for him. Someone was watching out for the bright-eyed Trayvon. We never heard from Tanya again.

Over the first five years of Trayvon's life, the Schmidts brought him to regular local outpatient visits with me and to Columbia, where he underwent three complex heart surgeries by one of the best heart surgeons in the country. He did remarkably well and grew to be a robust and thriving child. In response to the unconditional love of Mary's wonderful family, Trayvon also became a very affectionate little man with a warm and charming personality. It was so easy to become attached to him. Everyone adored him. Because Michael was in the military, the family often traveled to different states and countries. Thus, the young Trayvon had the opportunity to see the world, experiencing other cultures and environments.

When Trayvon was five years old, his successful third surgery now comfortably two years behind him, his foster family had an important and difficult decision to make. Mary and Michael were now entering retirement and had successfully raised and funded college for seven children, all while fostering a dozen more, with whom they still kept in touch. Given the realities of their now older age, they were concerned that they would not be the best forever family for the young and vibrant Trayvon. By the time he would be ready for college, they would be approaching their 70s. Over several very highly emotional discussions in my office, the family became convinced that Trayvon's best future opportunities would be ensured with a younger adoptive family. He had now fortunately come to the point where he was both psychologically and physically well, with a medical horizon that was far less complex than when he came into their lives. They decided to search for an adoptive family.

It didn't take long for them to find one. Through Michael's military network, the Agnellos, another military couple in their early thirties, with one girl toddler, literally jumped at the opportunity to have a son. Like Michael, the father, Andrew, was a career military professional with a bright future. He was soft-spoken, tall, and lean with Cary Grant-like features. His olive skin and warm, dark brown eyes reflected his southern Italian heritage. His wife, Roseanne, an elementary school teacher, was her husband's opposite in almost every way. She was openly talkative and gregarious with lightly freckled, fair-skinned cheeks. Her sky-blue eyes sparkled with an inner light whenever she talked about Trayvon and her daughter.

Though initially somewhat alarmed by her tremendously positive energy, Trayvon quickly warmed up to her. Mary's warm tears, a combination of relief, joy, and sadness, signaled that she approved of them both from the moment she met them. Over several months, the Agnellos came along with the Schmidts to Trayvon's doctor visits and gradually attended his school and family activities. On one miraculous afternoon filled with love, I participated in the final and official handoff of Tanya's beautiful young child from one family to the next.

Trayvon's forever family, the Agnellos, continued to bring him to regular medical visits with me for the next six years. When he was 11, after I confirmed that he was doing very well from a heart health standpoint, they accepted an offer to move to another country where Andrew was commissioned. I spent several days organizing all of his medical records in one file for them and contacting my physician counterpart in Germany to verbally sign out both the medical details and the remarkable social story behind this child. Trayvon had grown into a strapping, healthy, tall preteen with his whole life ahead of him. The last I heard, he was applying to college and was doing very well. Of course he was—angels were watching over him.

The truth was that I couldn't be 100 percent certain that Trayvon would be perfectly well right after birth. Despite two decades of experience and training since then, I still don't fool myself into a false sense of security that I can fully predict the outcome of all my patients. Any clinician who claims to do so is deluding themselves. I remain confident that the combination of my training and best intentions on behalf of my patients were in play at that time and have been since. I followed my personal and professional ethics—my heart—along with my mind. My focus was on protecting Trayvon, not protecting myself from lawsuits. In so doing, Tanya and Trayvon's experience professionally liberated me for years to come. Henceforth, I could legitimately practice my craft with conviction, rather than from the vantage point of shallow, liability-fearing medicine.

My interactions with Tanya and Trayvon, and all who cared for them, also opened the doors to my belief in the power of local medical care and further convinced me that I made the right choice to leave full-time academia and stay in my community after all. At that point in my career, I knew that I would dedicate my efforts to improving local medical and healthcare. Through Trayvon's story, the vision became a fundamental reality. Witnessing Trayvon thrive because of the synergistic efforts of a tertiary medical institution like Columbia and the medical professionals and families in my community was transformative. I swallowed the Kool-Aid and changed my mission from a slogan on behalf of Columbia to my true *raison d'être*.

With this new and revitalized attitude, it was no surprise that I became preoccupied with teaching pediatrics to anyone who showed interest or worked for me. Over the next two decades, I participated in a frenzy of education. I put whiteboards in all my exam rooms to teach my patients about their conditions using multicolored markers. I held regularly scheduled continuing education sessions with my nurses, medical assistants, and technicians. I gave multiple grand-round lectures to nurses and doctors in the community and at the local hospitals.

Whether it was an elementary school or college, private or public, I conducted multiple classes for school coaches and nurses. I was invited to be a guest speaker at local community organizations, including the ambulance corps, the YMCA, and the local chapter of the American Heart Association. When the new hospital opened, it made more sense than ever to me that we should expand the pediatric services in this new facility. I therefore coordinated a team of subspecialists who could teach the hospital staff about inpatient pediatric care and thus create a more comfortable environment for caretakers and patients alike.

Everywhere I went, I found people excited to learn about children's heart issues and ways to keep their children healthy. When a local orthopedic surgeon proposed that we take the opportunity to start a second campus in our area for the first new medical school to open in New York in 30 years, I signed up immediately. After helping to establish the pediatric subspecialty curriculum for the arriving students, I sat proudly in the audience at the inauguration ceremonies of Touro

University's second and largest brick-and-mortar campus—the College of Osteopathic Medicine in Middletown, New York. My mind was abuzz with excitement and anticipation for all the places we could go together as a community.

SCHOOLS WITHOUT WALLS

Through the nineteenth and early twentieth century, like other aspects of higher education, the process of becoming a physician was intrinsically elitist. Certain well-established academic centers, where only wealthy students with high society connections could afford to attend, were the exclusive source of medical education. However, the lack of consistent national standards became a public health concern. The American Medical Association responded in 1910 by establishing a clear set of standards through the Flexner Report.[65] This effort standardized the process of becoming a practicing physician in the United States so that a student had to successfully complete the sequence of four years of premedical training at an undergraduate level, followed by four years of medical school at an accredited institution. Only then could an individual pursue a US graduate medical education (GME), which entailed an internship followed by several years of residency. Upon graduating from this GME level, and only after passing the medical field-appropriate board exam, could an individual receive a license to actually perform direct patient care independently. Many like me then chose to pursue further fellowship training to become a medical specialist.

Though these standards proved to be discriminatory to women and US minorities, they functioned as the rule of the day into the twenty-first century. However, as the twentieth century came to a

65 Allen, Chequeta, "An Historical Overview of How Non-U.S. International Medical Graduates (IMGs) Entered the Practice of Medicine in the U.S.," ResearchGate, Sept 2014 (online), https://www.researchgate.net/publication/326208245_An_Historical_Overview_of_How_Non-US_International_Medical_Graduates_IMGs_Entered_the_Practice_of_Medicine_in_the_US.

close, the issue of national standards for medical education was again challenged by a large influx of medical students who graduated from undergraduate premedical programs outside of the United States. From the 1950s, when the migration of these students first began, through the 1990s, these international medical graduates (IMGs)—both US and non-US citizens—were able to enter US-GME programs to pursue internships and residency programs as equals to students who successfully completed premedical education and medical school from US-based institutions.

As I grew up in suburban America through the 1970s, I witnessed the nation's largest influx ever of IMGs into communities like mine. My own beloved pediatrician was a wonderful man born and trained in the Middle East. The national response by the United States in 1998, just as I began my independent career in my hometown, was an aggressive attempt by the National Board of Medical Examiners to decrease the number of IMGs seeking entry into US GME programs.

The required post-medical-school education exam (the computer-based medical licensing exam) became more rigorous and computer-based for everyone. They specifically targeted the non-US IMGs by exclusively requiring them to additionally pass a clinical skills assessment supervised by the Education Commission on Foreign Medical Graduates. The non-US IMGs, who were under a J-1 visa, were also not allowed to remain in the United States directly after completing their GME and were required to return to their home nation for at least two years before being allowed to return.

Through a program known as the Conrad State 30 and Physician Access Act,[66] many non-US IMG physicians, like my neonatal colleague Dr. Kay, were given the option to avert this process if they committed to practicing in medically underserved areas such as Newburgh, New

66 Sen. Klobuchar, Amy, "S.1189-Conrad State 30 and Physician Access Act," congress.gov, 114th Congress, May 5, 2015, https://www.congress.gov/bill/114th-congress/senate-bill/1189.

York. To the surprise of many, even after a huge number of IMG applicants raced to enroll in US-GME programs, by 2005, the non-US IMGs were successfully certified through this new process at a level equal to the US trained medical students.[67] To this day, it is the US citizens who went to foreign medical schools (US IMGs) who have the most difficulty meeting these criteria.

The COVID-19 pandemic highlighted a well-known but sadly ignored fact that many areas of the United States remain medically underserved. Rural and inner city poor neighborhoods, typically serviced by Medicaid-funded clinics, remain in desperate need of primary medical services. This has historically been where IMG physicians, who now make up 25 percent of all licensed physicians[68] in the United States, filled the gaps. Even if the non-US IMGs meet the same credentialing standards as the doctors coming from the US GME pipeline, they face many obstacles in the underserved communities in which they tend to settle.

The typical Medicaid clinic is far from a desirable place to work or seek care. The doctors and their clinical colleagues try to care for large numbers of patients in understaffed facilities whose infrastructure is often less updated. They typically have less access to testing and therapeutic modalities than the private facilities. The standard of care in these settings is often variable and not as good as in the facilities and institutions where the American medical graduates are based. This created a longstanding intrinsic disparity in the provision of healthcare geographically and socioeconomically, which was further blown wide open by the COVID-19 pandemic.

---

67 Boulet, John R. *et al.*, "The International Medical Graduate Pipeline: Recent Trends in Certification and Residency Training," NIH, *PubMed*, Mar.-Apr; 25(2):469-77, https://pubmed.ncbi.nlm.nih.gov/16522588/.

68 Staff News Writer, "How IMGs Have Changed the Face of American Medicine," American Medical Association, Oct. 19, 2021 (online), https://www.ama-assn.org/education/international-medical-education/how-imgs-have-changed-face-american-medicine.

When I grew up, the urban trained doctors wanted to remain in or near New York City. They did not want to come to the suburbs of the Hudson Valley, where there was so little advanced infrastructure. This is why my family's doctors during my childhood were mainly non-US IMGs. The lack of pediatric specialty services in my hometown as of 1998 was precisely why Dr. Kay and I were recruited to return to the Hudson Valley after finishing our specialty training.

However, through the first decades of the twenty-first century, there remain huge geographic areas of the Hudson Valley designated as medical deserts. To address this issue, the state encouraged the creation of additional medical schools and GME programs outside the typical confines of the city. To my surprise, a new medical school was opened in my own county. Until 2014, when the Touro College of Osteopathic Medicine opened its campus doors in the then-abandoned community Horton Hospital, where I started my local career, I never even thought that this was possible.

Over the past 10 years, 18 new medical schools were created nationally. This effort primarily focused on addressing the forecast increase in the deficit of PCPs[69] from the current level of 7,300 to 43,100 by 2030. Even with IMGs filling a significant portion of the primary care gap in the United States, it was determined that the new medical schools needed to produce more US graduates to enter primary care GME positions.

Like Touro University's medical school, many of these new medical schools started as "schools without walls." The first-year and second-year students gathered in classrooms and lecture halls for didactic training but often did not have consistent medical facilities to expose them to actual patients in their third-year and final fourth-year clinical rotations.

69 Duvivier, Robert J.; Wiley, Elizabeth, & Boulet, John R., "Supply, Distribution and Characteristics of International Medical Graduates in Family Medicine in the United States: a Cross Sectional Study," *BMC Family Practice*, 20 (47), 2019, https://bmcprimcare.biomedcentral.com/articles/10.1186/s12875-019-0933-8.

For my experience at Columbia, it was implicitly understood that my and my fellow students' practical experience with real patients would occur within the walls of Columbia's iconic Presbyterian Hospital system. The main hospital and the medical school where I trained were literally all within a couple city blocks and often physically connected to each other architecturally. The clinical rotations for Touro medical students are spread out over miles and several counties to access multiple collaborating smaller medical practices and community hospitals. When Touro repurposed our empty old hospital building for student dorms, classrooms, lecture halls, and laboratories, this was a huge leap for them in establishing a large brick-and-mortar home base of 110,000 square feet compared to their first 75,000-square-foot Harlem campus.

Initially, my colleagues and I had concerns about the quality of the education for the physicians at our local new medical school. Like the concerns of the AMA in the early 1900s, we wondered if their academic curriculum would be up to snuff. More importantly, many were concerned that our community hospitals and medical practices could not maintain the necessary level of consistent patient exposure during their practical training. Before coming to the Hudson Valley, they relied upon less-organized education from nonacademic practicing physicians who were understandably very busy trying to survive the challenges of the private practice world today. These clinicians were not necessarily inclined to spend their valuable time with these high-maintenance students.

After completing their training, most immediately entered practice and never even taught using any consistent curriculum. Over the past eight years of growing pains, we identified those local physicians truly interested in teaching. Together with the school administration, we chipped in many hours to help, and the standard of education and the quality of the students entering and leaving the school steadily improved. At this point in time, I can honestly say that I enjoy the opportunity to spend time with these students. Many of them have enriched my practice and career.

No one is deluding themselves at this point into believing that the current status of the new medical school is equivalent to that of the broad base of long-standing medical education centers like Columbia. To the contrary, we are realistic that these new schools are designed to serve the specific role of producing graduates who can fill the primary care void in local communities. Their merit and potential lies in their ability to create a strong community presence of medical providers who will complement the services of the more advanced medical centers. If they remain focused on the mission of their foundation, these schools can become a vital part of a network of medical care and education with the potential to significantly improve the public's health.

As a child and young man who returned to the Hudson Valley through my college years, I never sensed that I received poor healthcare from the overwhelming majority of my physicians trained at foreign medical schools. I still fondly remember my Middle Eastern pediatrician, Dr. Amin, as one of the best physicians I ever encountered. He was bright and funny and involved in many of the community's musical and dramatic productions.

On one particular prekindergarten visit, in his office on the ground floor of his two-story home, he turned to me and my mother, speaking softly with a warm smile, "Eric, do you like ice cream?"

I perked up and answered, "Yes. My favorite flavor is chocolate with sprinkles."

"Very good," he replied. "Show me how you lick a pretend chocolate ice cream in a cone."

As I mimicked his request, he looked across the room to my mom. "I heard his speech pattern, and I thought something was up. Monique, Eric is mildly tongue-tied. He can't stick his tongue out fully. I can fix this right here and now, if you want."

My mother trusted Dr. Amin implicitly and consented verbally. He asked me to trust him and explained in detail that he would numb the area under my tongue with some medicine from a needle. "It will sting just a bit, but then you will feel nothing. I know that you are a brave boy. So is that OK with you?"

I too consented, and within two minutes, as I stood up facing him, I barely felt a thing as he cut the thin strand of tissue that tethered my tongue since birth. He then reached into his pocket and pulled out some money. "Here you go, Eric. Take this to buy an ice cream tomorrow on me for being so brave. I'm proud of you."

To this day, I can still remember my pride as I reached out farther than ever with my tongue to lick the best-tasting chocolate cone ever. Of course, this is the recollection through the eyes of a child, and if I had then been a physician, I may have seen the situation differently. Today, it is virtually unheard of for a doctor to perform this procedure, a frenectomy, in a non-newborn standing up in an outpatient setting such as Dr. Amin's office. Dr. Amin knew me well enough to make the judgment that I would comply with the procedure this way. Today, most kids are sent to a facility with a procedure room and sedation available at many times the cost. Back then, the patient-physician relationship was typically strong, before rampant malpractice suits.

Trayvon and many more patients since I met him have done well because of all the changes in healthcare policy that brought the strengths of a high-powered medical center together with enhanced local medical care and education. The Touro College also vitally emphasized training minority physicians to establish an ethnically and racially diverse population of tomorrow's physicians. My experience convinced me that there is no "one way" to address the medical needs of our people.

As with most problems and challenges in America, the best solutions are multidimensional. This approach best reflects who we are at our core—a hodgepodge of diverse individuals. To meet the healthcare needs of this beautiful quilt that I so love and respect, I suggest we refrain from being exclusionary and recruit all comers. Bring on the full force of the combined foreign IMGs and US citizen medical school graduates from both the traditional and the new medical schools. Complement this with a cadre of other medical professionals, including nurses, public health workers, psychologists, physician assistants, and nurse practitioners. All the while, work together to maintain and advance our standards of care on behalf of those we serve—our patients, not the almighty dollar or any political agenda.

With such a team, I cannot help but look upon our COVID-19 experience and chuckle that the most effective solution to this and other crises we face may best be reached by tearing down the walls that historically created the silos that divide these different healthcare professionals from each other. This division regretfully weakened and often crippled us from achieving our full potential to prevent and treat the illnesses and diseases that see no geographical or societal boundaries. Bring on the outside minds and hearts from foreign lands because they too share our suffering as a species. Invite the new schools and ways of learning and thinking so that we may always stay one step ahead of the true enemy—stagnation and prejudice. We don't need walls. We need bridges.

REFLECTIONS ON THE ROLE OF MEDICAL INSTITUTIONS

One of the more philosophically provocative and intellectually pleasantly unexpected experiences for me has been my work with the newly established local medical school under the Touro College and University System. Unlike my traditional medical training through the allopathic medical system, in which a Doctorate of Medicine (MD) degree is earned, Touro's medical school is for osteopathic medicine, where a student obtains a Doctorate of Osteopathic Medicine (DO) degree. Osteopaths' diagnostic and treatment principles were founded mainly upon the manipulation of joints and bones. They initially were designated to the general physician fields and did not specialize or perform surgery. Allopaths or MDs implemented the use of medications and interventions such as surgery based on evidence derived from public health and biomedical disciplines.

Historically, until the middle of the twentieth century, the allopathic system was portrayed as the more reputable and mainstream approach, thus fostering an inherent tendency of allopathic physicians to look down upon the osteopathic graduates as relatively less legitimate. I must openly admit that I was, until recently, one of those MD snobs.

The truth is that the training methods of these two disciplines have become so similar lately that it is hard for even a stouthearted proponent and student of allopathy like me to differentiate the two. Graduates of both systems now enter subspecialty and surgical fields. However, I witnessed the constant uphill and often unjust battles confronting the regional osteopathic medical schools. The fact that initially the new Touro Medical School did not come along with a fully designated brick-and-mortar hospital or medical practice facility on its home campus only heightened any preexisting biases. From the outset, because the students of any given class or rotation could be physically quite far apart, the Touro Medical School incorporated the Internet to coordinate its didactics.

During the COVID-19 pandemic, when isolation was required, this electronic approach was a major strength and asset that kept the school running while others temporarily shut their doors. However, initially, this need to use tele-education highlighted their lack of a fully centralized campus and was seen as a major weakness of their program. Furthermore, any hands-on patient training in the third and fourth years was only possible through the concerted efforts of Touro's leaders. The curriculum coordinators worked tirelessly, calling in favors and using their influence to scrounge up any opportunities for students to join alongside the MD students in clinical rotations. Their DO students were initially only accepted at some of the less-competitive and thus less-reputable clinical training centers. They were spread thin throughout the region and initially developed the reputation of being subpar and even a burden to the other training programs. This only served to further exacerbate their inferior reputation.

The establishment of a second and larger physical campus in the Hudson Valley was strategically necessary for the Touro medical school to begin to overcome its image handicap. Their stated mission to address the physician shortage and primary care deficits of our community and the underserved surrounding regions was honorable and hard to openly criticize. For decades, the MD programs never came to the table to sufficiently address these healthcare deficits. Collaborations like the one between NYPH and GHVHS systems that brought an allopathic physician such as me to the region were short-lived at best. These tertiary medical centers remained predominantly urban-based and hours away from our growing community. Unlike the intentions of the Touro program, they never promoted or established a solid primary care base in our communities.

Instead of acknowledging the osteopathic system's important role in filling our area's healthcare gap, the urban allopathic programs dug in their heels against the osteopathic programs even further. The prevailing attitude of the MD schools became one of protecting their turf in this very competitive, economic environment for medical schools. Simply stated, they did everything in their power to prevent the osteopathic students from accessing any of the clinical rotation spots in their established medical facilities.

However, by the 2010s, it was already too late to turn back the tide of opinion in favor of the osteopathic programs. Policymakers and healthcare leaders in our region were more confident in their local institutions' healthcare abilities. Given this sense of self-reliance, they focused more than ever on keeping their market share of patients from migrating to the city for medical needs.

As one of the local doctors involved in promoting the local Touro Medical School bluntly stated at a hospital planning meeting, "Eric, you and I both came from greater MD programs like Columbia. However, we are now onto them. We don't want or need these urban allopathic programs to keep siphoning off a significant portion of the southern New York medical marketplace. If they want our sicker patients, they need to support the improvement of the local healthcare or get out." The combination of a local DO school and increasing physician autonomy in our community thus posed a significant potential threat to the allopathic tertiary medical centers.

Many of the well-respected local physicians came from osteopathic training programs. To my sobering amusement, I could not differentiate any one of my colleague's osteopathic versus allopathic training backgrounds by reviewing their practice patterns. The allopathic and osteopathic doctors all seemed to merge together in practical terms, and their reputations were based more upon their ability to meet the needs of their patients than where they trained. In other words, the monopoly on healthcare that existed for the allopathic programs in the city simply did not exist in the community settings. Even more importantly, the more rural areas surrounding our suburban communities were characterized by a lower socioeconomic status and were significantly more medically underserved than my local towns. They were in dire need of any type of physician dedicated to their community and were in no way specifically aligned with one group or the other. These medical deserts were hungry for any type of medical presence that could improve the health access for their residents. The osteopathic Touro Medical School program in our own community fit the bill.

Historically, organized modern allopathic medicine in America formed in the late nineteenth and early twentieth century when the urban populations began to grow. A captive market developed within the cities, which became more reliant upon a structured healthcare service as a commodity. Prior to this, the more rural areas were fairly self-sufficient in regards to healthcare needs, with an approach based mainly upon a maternal or a home nursing model. If you were particularly sick, a doctor might make a home visit to attend to you and offer your mother some guidance. If a patient was sick enough that they could not stay home, they had to make the stressful decision of whether or not to travel far away to the few city hospitals.

The concept of a community hospital would not come to fruition until the mid-twentieth century. Thus healthcare became intrinsically divided, not only along socioeconomic lines but between rural and urban settings. Because of the urban centers' denser populations, it was natural for physicians to train, organize, and live in the cities, rather than in rural areas. This also lent credence to the belief that physicians were not only themselves from a more elite element of our society. They also appeared to focus more on caring for the elite city dweller.

It is true that many of the hospitals and the physicians that served them in the cities provided medical care to the less privileged, often through charitable organizations. However, history is very clear that many of these urban poor received a different type of healthcare than their wealthy counterparts. Many new procedures and experimental therapies originated in poor and minority communities before they were accepted and applied to the wealthy. The history of vaccination itself, beginning in the 1700s with the practice of smallpox inoculation[70] from a black slave in Boston, remains a salient example of this practice.

At this time, there were no such entities as review boards to guide medical research or ethics boards to consider the appropriateness of these endeavors, which unabashedly risked the lives of minorities, the

70 Blakemore, Erin, "How an Enslaved African Man in Boston Helped Save Generations from Smallpox," history.com, *A&E Television Networks*, April 8, 2021, https://www.history.com/news/smallpox-vaccine-onesimus-slave-cotton-mather.

poor, and orphans. The more self-reliant rural communities remained distant from this type of healthcare and understandably somewhat reticent to use it. Because they were not a big part of the nation's medical economics, more suburban or rural areas simply did not factor into the equation for early organized medicine.

It was not until after the World Wars, when suburban areas became attractive to a large portion of the middle class, that organized healthcare first turned their sights beyond the cities. As I grew up in my suburban community in the 1960s through the 1980s, community hospitals were still considered by my neighbors as far inferior to the large academic city hospitals. They simply did not have adequate human or material resources to address complex medical conditions. Despite this, there appeared to be a strong psychological divide between the suburban and rural inhabitants when it came to actually going down to the city. Many of the suburbanites and a majority of rural inhabitants were very reluctant to make it to the city. In situations such as cancer or complex medical problems, exceptions were made, and some people traveled at least two hours to medical institutions such as Columbia or Sloan Kettering to meet world experts familiar with these medical conditions. To this day, traveling to the city hospitals is very psychologically and economically disruptive to the family life of non-city dwellers.

I remember my own experience with this reluctance when my only sister, Karen, developed chest pain that the local pediatricians could not explain. Concern was raised that she might have some underlying serious cardiac problem. The only pediatric cardiology program within commuting distance was at Columbia University. At the time, these doctors did not have any satellite offices in our community. My parents planned ahead.

My mother explained, "Eric, your sister is going to be fine, but we have to be ready for the possibility that we may need to spend a couple days in the city. You're coming with us and will have to take a short time off from school. We have asked your teachers to give you some classwork so that you won't fall behind."

Three days later, we found ourselves all seated tightly together in a private doctor's office in the biggest hospital I had ever seen. We were greeted by a very kind, middle-aged nurse who informed us, "Please wait a moment here, and I will let Dr. Gersony know that you are ready."

One hour later, after a detailed questioning of Karen's health history and a thorough physical examination, the tall and well-groomed Dr. Gersony impressed my family with his soft, confident approach. As he sat down at his desk across from all four of us, he stated reassuringly, "Karen's heart is normal and very healthy. Her chest pain is coming from outside her heart in the chest wall itself. She will be absolutely fine with the tincture of time. You don't have to come back unless she gets worse, and I will send a full letter to her home pediatrician."

I could see tears of relief in my parents' eyes. Karen and I just wanted to explore the city a bit more. Years later, I would learn that this doctor was the very same chairman and founder of the pediatric cardiology department, and he would ultimately become my esteemed mentor during my pediatric cardiology training. What a small world after all.

Even when I returned to my community after training at Columbia, my community pediatric colleagues initially viewed me as an inherently elitist physician. After my first introductory pediatric meeting, one of the older pediatricians stopped me in the hall.

With a very accusatory tone, this obviously very bright doctor told me, "I know your kind. You think you are better than us. You've been sent here from the big university to judge the quality and competency of us local docs."

This was not the welcome I expected. I was stunned by the candor of such verbal concerns regarding my presence. This negative urban-suburban dynamic would prove to be an unforeseen impediment to beginning my career in this region. I knew I had to gain their trust. I reassured them that I was here to become a supportive part of the healthcare community and did not intend in any way to threaten them. It took at least five years of hard work to convince them that I was sincere in this goal before I truly felt accepted.

A decade and a half later, I recalled my promise to not come across as elitist, when I initially found myself unable to shake my own biases regarding the new Touro osteopathic program coming to town. Fortunately, my favorable attitudes toward the allopathic programs had already begun to erode. With the advent of EMRs and the growing influence of corporate economics, I started to notice that my allopathic students at the university medical centers were far less patient-oriented than their predecessors. I became concerned that the quality of MD students was more variable. On occasion, I even wondered how certain trainees were allowed to graduate with full credentials. There were clearly many reasons that explained this growing variation in student competency, but the bottom line in my opinion was that the MD programs were on shakier ground than ever.

My reality convinced me that their claim as the only legitimate standard-bearers for medical training was not necessarily fully justified. Because I practiced extensively in both academic city-based tertiary centers as well as the suburban community setting, I developed a unique perspective on this issue. It became quite obvious to me that many of my allopathic colleagues and students in the university setting were very knowledgeable about the science of medicine. However, they often lacked the practical "knowhow" and necessary sensitivities when it came to delivering this healthcare to patients from outside the city.

They appeared to overlook the disruptive implications of serious illness for those families who often had no choice but to leave home, work, and school to travel down to the city. Basic assumptions—expecting that the family would easily return to the city for follow-up care, the special medications would be available locally, or the local pediatrician would smoothly take over care after the hospitalization—were problematic, to say the least. These assumptions often left patients in limbo and feeling fragile after a hospitalization that was already traumatic.

It gradually became my unspoken and accepted role to help with the transitions between the community and the city tertiary center. Years later, I realized that I unwittingly developed a unique skill set as I negotiated these transitions. It was one thing for the patient to undergo the correct operation or procedure at the tertiary center but often a whole other venture to bring them back home and reintroduce them to community life. It was in no small part due to my active role in this dynamic that I eventually earned the trust of the patients and their local doctors that I had not been granted when I first arrived in the region.

As the osteopathic medical education program in our community has grown over the past eight years, while staying true to my commitment to remaining open-minded, it became even clearer to me that neither the allopathic nor osteopathic physicians are superior to the other. Their roles in our larger healthcare system are inherently complementary, and I noticed that they are learning from each other. If anything is true, I often found many of the MD students to be more entitled in their behavior than their humbler DO counterparts. This may be because many of the DO students actually started their medical education later in life, having initially had other careers, economic constraints, or real-life experiences. Many of them come from other cultures and minority groups, which are often not as widely represented in the allopathic programs.

As one of my DO students succinctly explained to me, "Not all of us have connections or the finances to go to Harvard. In fact, there is a strong selection bias against us inherent in the process from early on in our education." My DO students explained to me that, in many ways, the osteopathic programs are far more democratic in their acceptance and education than the allopathic programs. They believe that this characteristic naturally leads the DO students to medical practices in underserved nonurban community settings. What could be more American?

Historically, after World War II, much of the healthcare in hometown communities such as mine was provided by the IMGs. These medical students and physicians from other countries chose not to compete in the more stressful urban areas. Therefore, our area developed the reputation of being served by foreign medical students who often did not share the same cultural background as their American suburban and rural patients. Over the years, this reality became part of the medical care dynamic, and most of my neighbors openly accepted their doctors were likely not to have been trained in the United States. As the rules and requirements for foreign physicians to set up shop locally became deliberately more complex and prohibitive toward the end of the twentieth century, many of these IMGs found it increasingly difficult to follow the pattern of their predecessors in similar underserved or nonurban communities.

So that they could remain in the United States, many IMGs opted to base their livelihood back in the cities where they worked as ancillary staff to licensed physicians. I saw this dynamic firsthand when I worked in the clinics and hospitals in the northern Manhattan community of Washington Heights. I still fondly recall that many of these foreign-trained clinicians were not only very skilled but also extremely compassionate. They exhibited a refreshing sense of humbleness that I did not sense in their often cocky supervising allopathic physicians.

One very busy winter day in the community practice aptly named Pediatrics 2000, I respectfully asked Dr. Juan Tapia, the clinic's energetic and charismatic founder-director, "Why don't any of these very good, foreign-trained doctors work in the suburban or rural areas of the Hudson Valley not far from here? The cost of living is cheaper up there, and people in my hometown could really use their services."

Dr. Tapia replied thoughtfully, "Maybe someday, but for now, clinics such as this are their entry into a very complex and bureaucratic system. Even if they were fully and well-trained in their own countries, it is now almost impossible to meet the requirements to become a licensed physician in the United States. It was much easier just a few years ago when I came to the States. For now, these skilled surgeons and pediatricians are needed where their own people live and trust them."

It was this very same outmigration of foreign-trained physicians in our suburban communities that allowed the gap to develop and which then fostered the need for the osteopathic physician programs like Touro. As mentioned, many of my osteopathic students believe that their education process is truly democratic and thus made them uniquely inclined to provide more socioeconomically balanced care than that of their city-trained MD peers. They take pride in the fact that they are less elitist and see this as a strength.

Today, in the midst of a healthcare system that has become so confusing and complex, it is probable that a strong undertone of trust between patients and physicians started to return because of the increased infusion of these more approachable DO physicians. The authority of allopathic physicians based solely upon a monopolized claim to possess the keys to biomedical knowledge does not appear sufficient to replace any loss of trust between patients and doctors. If anything, the widening economic gap between all citizens—with physicians typically amongst the wealthier—makes this mistrust even worse. Enter the osteopathic physicians, who seamlessly become a part of the suburban and rural community in no small part because their training is also in the same communities they serve.

I noticed that the caliber of many of the students began to rival that of their MD counterparts that I taught. As importantly, the students live, shop, and raise their families in the same communities as their patients. We already see the benefits of this as they graduate and start their professional careers in the local hospitals and practices. The relationship with their patients and trust are often more natural and real. We have come full circle again, from the IMGs to the osteopaths, in search of a fundamentally trustworthy patient-physician dynamic.

Only time will tell if this new medical institution will become a vital part of our American communities' healthcare reform. Many of the new DO physicians and students have also begun to question the *status quo* of physician allegiances in our area. They dislike the recent tendency of physicians to become hospital employees or to join large business conglomerates that contract out physician services to hospitals or large practices. They are more inclined to resist the accepted and pessimistic attitudes of some of their seniors and mentors, which imply that doctors today have no other options. They do not want to just accept the orders and constraints regarding practice patterns dictated by large entities dominated by allopathic medicine. This spark of rebellion is refreshing and encouraging to witness. I must admit that I openly encourage such notions as an optimistic window into our profession's future.

THE DISSEMINATION OF HIGH STANDARDS

After two decades of my concerted efforts, I finally realized why everything I did to fulfill Columbia's original mission to enhance the pediatric services in my hometown area felt so deeply personal. The last straw was Mr. Batson's decision to relieve me from my directorship duties, and this hurt me profoundly. But why? I had run into many other obstacles along the way to promoting a better level of regional pediatric care. The answer was that I felt betrayed by the institutions that groomed me and I so revered. The administrators from Columbia, Montefiore, and the local hospitals made short-sighted, politically and economically based decisions that ignored my character and best intentions. My honorable motives were founded on a cause to which they no longer appeared to commit. They literally left me high and dry.

But how could these institutional leaders see the effects of their decisions if I did not see it myself? The cause of my initial distress in response to being relieved of my local administrative duties was glaringly obvious. I based my entire professional self-worth upon my value to the institutional leadership, who reassured me with the words, "You are a great doctor who will be an asset to your community." I now understood.

I was hopelessly biased from the start of my career because I had been entrusted by Columbia—the institution I so revered—with a mission to serve the community in which I was raised. This combination of deep loyalty and love for both the values of this institution and what they could mean for my own home community became a powerful driving force in my medical career. My very sense of purpose as a physician was linked to this mission.

If these institutions no longer supported my role in program development for my community after Mr. Batson dismissed me, they were then essentially contradicting his feigned attempt to reassure me, "You're still a great doctor. No one can take that away from you." I was misled by the notion that confining myself to my office to see patients would deter me from fulfilling this higher purpose. I thought that I had to perpetually run my practice in parallel with my administrative roles, treating them as two separate entities—one serving economic realities and the other a loftier ideal. As I concentrated back on my practice, I found renewed professional purpose. I now knew that my patient practice and administrative roles were always two sides of the same coin. Either would serve me equally well in my pursuits to leave a better healthcare status than when I started for the children.

Yes, I still wanted to be a doctor, even after all the ups and downs I experienced, because the core of my motivation remained intact. After almost a quarter century, I was reminded that our practice filled in a unique and much-needed niche in our area. It served the community well with a consistent culture and value system indebted to the care of the children. Our legacy of passionate community-based care of children with complex heart conditions turned the previous paradigms around 180 degrees. More babies and children now remained at home for their care than ever before. We became the region's new benchmark for such community care.

The new reality also indicated that our relationship with the tertiary pediatric medical centers and the community hospitals could and should be a symbiotic relationship and not one of master to servant. We all brought value to the table. Just as importantly, our practice influenced the medical education process. The next generation of physicians, nurse clinicians, physician assistants, and technicians were now our students passing daily through our practice halls in a fashion that had only been possible in the urban academic centers before we arrived.

We started the practice and my hospital work by incorporating the values of my Columbia mentors as the foundation. This remains intact to this day. To this was added the decades of dedication to local pediatric care that my only true competitor and now colleagues, led by Dr. Gewitz, consistently maintained. Dr. Gewitz set the standard of local pediatric subspecialty care for me to emulate. His vision of leaving the pediatric world better than he found it keeps him still actively involved.

These founders entrusted us to take their legacies forward. With the Boston Children's umbrella now over us, we invited the nation's highest clinical standards for children to the region and adopted a shared clear mission to move forward into the future until "every child is well." We now stand on the shoulders of Dr. Gersony, Dr. Gewitz, and my original administrative welcome team—the three amigos, Jeff, Norm, Jay. I proudly and humbly accept that our practice evolved into a small institution in its own right, with a very keen eye toward future growth.

Anytime I pause to reflect on the role of my practice, I cannot help but hear Dr. Gersony's words ringing in my mind: "An institution is not the building. It is the people." He had been so right and clairvoyant about this when it came to the transitions of leadership at all of the institutions I encountered. When the leadership no longer valued and respected the people working with them, the institution itself headed for significant change. This occurred in my pediatric cardiology division at Columbia after the new dean relayed his message to us through Dr. Gersony's successor.

Likewise, our first era of growth in local pediatric care came to an end for GHVHS when the new NYPH network administrator decided that he alone should run the negotiations without any input from those who had been working locally on the ground level. Montefiore and the Hudson Valley hospitals' leadership underwent analogous changes in direction and loss of momentum in their community-based pediatric programs when they chose to compete with, rather than include, the local pediatricians regarding relevant policy decisions.

Despite my frustrations with the process, I maintain that it is the sole right of these institutions to define their own course of action in any venture such as a network of pediatric care. They too must learn from their successes and mistakes. What I noted is that those institutions who are most admired and successful during times of growth and transition are more likely to proceed with their clinical teams alongside them as valued assets.

My local hospital system went through significant changes during my own career. Even one of the main founding institutions for American medical education and a leader in academic medical care—Columbia—is constantly changing. Like the institution of marriage, which has evolved from a foundation based on economics to one of religious and romantic pursuits, I sense that the institutions of American healthcare need to strive for the moral value of their pursuits. As they evolve, we must identify and preserve the characteristics of the great institutions and their leaders, which we hold to as priorities as a society. These important principles should not ever be replaced or removed carelessly if we are to maintain the integrity of our healthcare institutions.

Dealing with institutions as they change over many years can become physically, mentally, and emotionally tiring. I endeavored to highlight my own experiences merely to illustrate what many physicians often face as they interact with institutions at various levels. They seem to have a momentum of their own—sometimes this aligns with a physician's own agenda, and at others it appears as an oppositional force.

However, amongst all of these frustrations and the seemingly pointless politics that I personally encountered in my institutional work, there clearly remain entities which, in my experience, continue to uphold the highest guiding principles. These organizations define at their core what great institutions represent to society at large and to those individuals that work for them in the service of others. It has been my privilege and fortune to work in some of these time-honored institutions and thus experience what it means to dedicate myself to noble causes such as the welfare of people of all backgrounds.

If an institution is to become and remain great, they must attract and support great individuals. The medical professional leaders with the greatest positive impact on the organization are the true source of the institutional profile, often remaining so long after they left. These giants impart their legacy to their younger colleagues by setting a clear example to emulate. I believe that Dr. Gersony remains one such giant, who placed an indelible stamp on the institutions of Columbia and pediatric cardiology itself. This is not to deny that he had his own quirks and imperfections like any mortal. His strengths came from his highly consistent value system that he worked tirelessly to impart upon his students and his patients.

Despite advancing age, he miraculously remains open to changing his assessments or opinions regarding the appropriate course of action. This is true whether the subject is patient therapy or an administrative course of action. This willingness to accept new possibilities is founded on his immutable commitment to evidence-based decision-making. Even before the COVID-19 pandemic struck, he warned that to depart from this eternal spring of rationality in favor of the opinion of the day is fraught with disaster. His leadership will endure long after he has left the institution as a guiding voice in our hearts and minds. "What would he do in this situation?" remains a common question for all of his disciples. The simple fact that he was so consistent in his approach to colleagues and patients alike speaks volumes and explains why we know the answer to this question even if he no longer stands directly by our sides.

"An institution like ours is akin to a great ship on the seas," he explained at our informal weekly teaching sessions with him. "Others will rely on it to take them forward through rough waters. Along the way, others may attempt to steer you off course with their own misguided agendas. As long as you believe that where you are heading is based on sound principles and evidence, maintain your steady course. You will always arrive safely and intact in the end, and others will thank you." He remains his students' reference, guide, compass, and anchor in these rough waters. He is nothing less than the personification of our institutional values. Any effort to determine in my mind whether the institution or he came first is futile and pointless—they are one and the same.

One of the most remarkable institutions that I encountered soon after I arrived in the Hudson Valley was the American Heart Association (AHA). Just before the spring of 1999, their local representative, Ms. Wallace, contacted me by phone at my office.

"Welcome to the neighborhood," she greeted me cheerily. "As you may know, the AHA's main fundraiser is our annual Heart Walk. Our walk here in Orange County is typically in May, and we would be delighted to have you join us. We have never had a full-time, local pediatric cardiologist among us, and we think the kids with heart conditions should be well represented in our event. I was born with a congenital heart defect myself, Tetralogy of Fallot, so this is actually very personal for me. We would be honored if your practice and some of your little patients considered joining us this year." I was thrilled for the invitation. My enthusiasm was further stoked when she went on to explain, "The timing of your arrival into our community couldn't be better. For the first time ever, the AHA decided to focus this year's entire campaign on formerly underrepresented subgroups of people with cardiovascular disease—targeting stroke, women, and, yes, even children."

Under Ms. Wallace's leadership, the local branch of the AHA wanted to be seen as an advocate for life-threatening cardiac problems in children, including congenital heart defects and inheritable diseases that could lead to sudden cardiac death. How could I refuse? My clinical team was invited to meet with Ms. Wallace's crew for three in-person planning discussions. At the second meeting, her marketing staff inquired if some of our practice's pediatric patients were willing to participate in a televised commercial to kick off and lead that year's AHA campaign.

We were honored at the thought that our children could be recognized as representing so many other patients with pediatric heart problems. It didn't take long before the families of 10 of my patients volunteered their kids to participate in recording a broadcast throughout the country. My team and I were so proud to see our patients contributing to this very important cause through an institution as revered as the AHA.

Starting in that first inaugural year, we continued to nominate one of our local children to lead us in the annual AHA's Heart Walk as a representative of all children with heart disease. The first nominee was Joseph Miller, a remarkable child with Hypoplastic Left Heart Syndrome—a birth defect in which the left half of his heart was essentially missing. His mother, a vibrant five-foot-two brunette in her early 30s, walked besides me at the head of our gathering of patients and families. As she walked effortlessly at a brisk pace, pushing a double stroller containing the almost five-year-old Joseph and his sleeping two-year-old sister, she shared Joseph's life story with me.

"During my pregnancy with Joseph, I was advised by many of the local pediatric cardiology groups that I should have an abortion because nothing short of the remote possibility of a heart transplant could save him after he was born. I didn't want to abort, so I decided to go to a world-class institution for an opinion. I made it to Boston Children's just as my time for a legal abortion was about to run out. They told me that my baby was a good candidate for a series of three operations over the first couple years of life that they helped pioneer and performed many times for other children. When they told my husband and I that Joseph would likely be able to run and play after this, we agreed to deliver Joseph in Boston and base his care there."

"He looks wonderful," I chimed in as I looked at this rosy-cheeked boy sleeping soundly in the seat behind his sister.

"Thanks. We think so too," she added. "He survived the three operations at Boston Children's Hospital—the most recent one over two years ago. But that's not the most important part," she said with a secretive smile. "We're so honored and lucky to even be here walking with you all today. Just two months ago, Joseph woke me up at 4 a.m. from a sound sleep. My husband is a trucker, and I was alone with the kids that weekend. Joseph looked me right in the eye and said he woke up because he smelled smoke. Wouldn't you know it, he was right. The whole apartment smelled like something was burning. I told him to get his sister, walk her down to the first floor, and wake up one of our neighbors to let her know about the smoke too. I knocked on my neighbors' doors on our floor, and within 10 minutes, all the people in our building stood in the parking lot in their PJs and bathrobes, watching our entire two-story building burn to the ground. It happened so fast, the firemen couldn't even stop it."

I was so mesmerized by this incredible story that I hadn't noticed we neared the end of the walk. "I guess Joseph's a heart survivor and a hero too. You must be so proud of him," I offered.

"You bet we are. Just makes you think what would have happened to all those people in my building if we had never gone to Boston and instead chose to abort him, doesn't it?"

It was through these initial interactions with the AHA that I first sensed I may be able to promote some of my professional goals through an institution right in my own community. I was not completely ready to let go of my urban university roots, but it felt good to know that I could develop meaningful associations with local credible and honorable institutions.

Typical of my impatience, I initially hoped that my work with groups such as GHVHS, the community medical centers, Medicaid clinics, and the AHA would expedite our ability to build a solid infrastructure dedicated to pediatric healthcare. However, in retrospect, I acknowledge that timing is everything. It is highly likely that the local pediatric services in our practice and at the hospitals would not have been on a sufficiently strong foundation if they blossomed too soon.

Despite the fact that, over the years, much of the daunting local politics and economically driven agendas contributed to my frustration, I remain able to step back and realize that, during this time, our children have benefitted from the services and dedication of community-based institutions, including the AHA and several parent advocacy groups. Our growing clinical team remains humbled to have been invited to play a small part in promoting these local efforts.

I now also realize that we created something unforeseen but equally satisfying. We have written our own story. My uncertain venture from the port of Manhattan's NewYork-Presbyterian Medical Center to the shores of the Hudson Valley evolved from a practice with a small file cabinet in Horton Hospital to the region's largest full-time source of multidisciplinary pediatric care in a suburban community. As we continue our work in alliance with our new colleagues from Boston Children's Health Physicians, we have made a significant impact on the welfare of our local children that now extends to the children from more remote communities even farther away from the city institutions.

In other words, our local community-based program is now a recognized and legitimate regional authority in maternal-child care in its own right. Parents like Joseph Miller's no longer have to travel out of their home communities to find the best standards of pediatric care. Medical students can now learn about pediatrics within a couple miles of their new campus in our community. As a nidus for such specialized care, we continue to see not only children from the surrounding communities, but we also attract pediatric physicians and medical professionals from the larger city institutions themselves.

After 9-11 and during the COVID-19 pandemic, they are attracted to the potential for a good quality of life away from the crowded cities. Doctors, nurses, physician assistants, and technicians are willing and interested in becoming part of our community's child health efforts. Before we established our own foundation locally, both the community and the tertiary physicians were not certain they could trust the care of their pediatric patients in our hands. Because of our persistence—with a slow, measured, and thoughtful pace—our clinical services for children earned the trust of the community and the respect of many of the greater medical institutions themselves. Though we understandably feel very good about our accomplishments, we still feel we have much work to do. We are just getting started.

FINAL THOUGHTS

In December 2017, I had the opportunity to return to my *alma mater* for Columbia's annual pediatric cardiology day-long conference dedicated to a pioneer in the field—Dr. Sylvia Griffiths. One November evening during a dinner of Thanksgiving leftovers, I mentioned to my wife, "You know, it's been eight years since I've seen many of my colleagues from Columbia. I was thinking that some of my professors are not getting any younger, and it would be good to see them again. I got a notice about the Sylvia Griffiths Teaching Day coming up in December, and I was thinking of going. I might not have another chance to hear them speak."

She replied with a sense of nostalgia, "You're right. You should go. It's important to not lose connections with our best teachers. It reminds us where we came from."

I took the day off and drove down the Palisades Parkway to my old stomping grounds. Though the academic portion of the program was excellent, my main memories of the day center around my conversations with my mentors in between the formal talks. One of these mentors was the founder of my department—Dr. Gersony—who originally attended to my sister so many years ago. The other was his senior colleague—Dr. Silvia Griffiths—in whose name this Teaching Day program was dedicated in perpetuity since 1996. Many of the attendees regularly returned every year to this program because of the immense part that she played in pioneering the very foundation of our field in the mid-twentieth century. After graduating from Yale University as one of seven women in the medical school class of 1948, she completed her fellowship in pediatric cardiology in 1955. She then joined the Columbia College of Physicians and Surgeons medical school faculty and went on to be recognized in 1960 as one of the founding members of the Subspecialty Board of Pediatric Cardiology.

Only with the fortune of hindsight do I now fully appreciate the valuable role these particular two pioneers played in my professional life. I am convinced that they are amongst the few legitimate "giants" in the field of medicine. They embody every sense of what enables an institution to become prestigious. Without their work, there would be no enduring substance to such institutions as Columbia and the field of pediatric cardiology. To this day, they continue to represent professionals of the highest compassion and serve the most arduous role of standard-bearers for our field. Their resilience is even more remarkable in the current era where standards are threatened daily in favor of economics and politics.

They are amongst a handful of my teachers who remain a constant guiding voice in my mind decades after I officially left their formal teachings behind. Returning to this conference to see them was like returning home to touch base with one's own foundation and morals. They provide the home-cooked food of my medical education childhood. In many ways, this visit rejuvenated me and still continues to serve as a resource for my ongoing work. I have no doubt that I will return again to this well for sustenance. I am extremely fortunate to see, the world of medicine through their eyes and would have it no other way.

If an organization is to be successful enough to become an institution of merit, the people who work there have two options. These individuals must either band together in unity behind a worthy cause, fully devoting their talents and resources, or be guided by an individual of great stature who becomes a reference in perpetuity for the institution—the voice in all of our minds and souls. This collective voice espouses a shared vision and value system for the greater good of those the institution serves. In this sense, American society itself—with all its complexities—has at times risen to the level of an institution. It is therefore logical to deduce that Columbia's status as a prominent founder of the American medical education system did not arise from a vacuum but rather out of the furnace of American ideals.

It is with this lineage in mind that I urge that we as Americans need to consciously designate which of our institutions we are most proud of. Which ones do we most admire and why? What are the value systems that these institutions perpetuate, and do they best represent us as a people? If they meet our stringent criteria, should they not serve as our standard-bearers to the world at large? One of my main goals in writing this book is to stimulate a conversation regarding how the values and standards embodied in our most respected institutions function within our American society at large.

An institution itself consists of a combination of such standards, mutual trust, hard work, and compassion. It clearly needs to be important and of value to those it serves. As my own experience demonstrates, these entities can easily get caught up in turf and power struggles that cause them to lose their focus and risk their reputation. Even longstanding institutions can lose their time-honored place in society very quickly if distracted from their core purpose by such corruptive forces. I continue to learn from both the negative and positive interactions with institutions and—after two decades within the school of hard knocks—I finally recognize that all institutions are inherently vulnerable human enterprises tasked with pursuing lofty goals.

As long as they continue to strive forward in these pursuits, they will endure. If they lose their way or regress, they will likely become part of our society's history and end up replaced by newer institutions. The success and longevity of our medical institutions in particular demands that they remain open-minded and altruistic. I remain optimistic about the future role of these institutions in our healthcare given the guiding principles of those remarkable individuals who founded them and the legacy they passed on to America's physicians and medical students. We must always remember the lessons they taught us.

PART III

OUR FUTURE

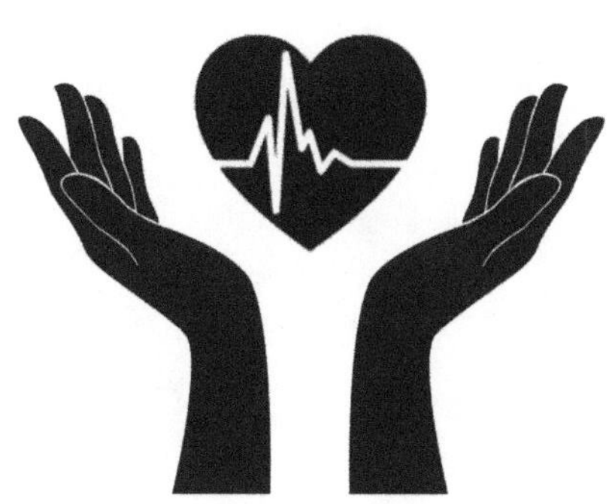

CHAPTER 11

WHAT SHOULD REAL HEALTHCARE REFORM LOOK LIKE?

"I did not know what to do. The situation felt so awkward." These are the continuing sentiments of Kerry-Ann, an immigrant from the "Islands," as she calls it, who also happens to be one of my most valued practice office managers. She was referring to her first experience as a hospital patient in the United States when she delivered her twin children. She worked for a visiting nurse service in New York that happened to have a contract with the very same hospital. She remembers a very nice room with two patient beds, a private bathroom, her own telephone, and a large television mounted on the wall. She essentially had her own private nurse and remembers feeling very special. This sentiment soon was challenged when another woman in the middle of labor was given the bed next to hers. The woman, who spoke only Spanish, was clearly in distress, disproportionate to her labor pains.

There were no other beds available on the floor, so this expectant mother was placed in this private room even though she was a clinic patient with Medicaid coverage. Kerry-Ann noticed that her roommate's television and telephone had not been activated. She did not have a cell phone and was clearly upset about not being able to notify any of her loved ones about her situation.

Kerry-Ann pulled back the curtain between their two beds and motioned that the woman was welcome to use her activated phone if she wished. The woman somehow managed to inform Kerry-Ann that her name was Anna. With gratitude, she accepted Kerry-Ann's offer and, in between contractions, excitedly informed her spouse that she had gone into early labor and was now admitted to the hospital. She smiled thankfully at her new friend as she hung up in time for her next contraction.

Within 15 minutes, Anna was informed in broken Spanish by the ward clerk that a bed opened up in a non-private room, and she would be moved out in about 10 minutes. Later, after both women delivered their babies, Kerry-Ann walked past Anna's room to wave hello to her old roommate. The room was slightly larger than her own, and there were at least six beds crammed into this space with very little privacy. One nurse scurried from bed to bed, apparently assigned to at least three or four mothers. Throughout the remainder of Kerry-Ann's five-day hospitalization, the second bed in her own private room remained empty, despite the fact that this multi-bed room was at full capacity and some expectant mothers waited for hours in the emergency room.

"I did not understand this system and somehow felt like I was not actually in America but instead back in my native country where resources were scarcer," Kerry-Ann recalls. This was the first of many times in her personal and professional life that she came face-to-face with the reality that, contrary to our billing as "the land of equality," there are at least two tiers of healthcare in the United States. Kerry-Ann's medical insurance provided by her nonprofit nursing agency was funded through these very same tax dollars that offered Medicaid coverage to Anna and the other women in the multi-bed room. Because her company used these federal and state monies to procure a private insurance plan and happened to have a contract with this hospital, she was treated much better.

"Somehow, even though I now understand some of the details behind this situation, it has never felt right to me. It is as if we immigrants were lied to." She sighs.

TAKE THE MONEY OUT OF MEDICINE

One of the most important skills of a competent and seasoned physician is to recognize when their patient is in grave danger because of a current or impending illness. Two decades of teaching and working in acute-care settings with patients with complex congenital heart defects, combined with my directing community-based pediatric care in hospitals and a large private practice, honed my triage skills to an almost instinctive level. My students taught me to be self-aware and crystal clear about my clinical thought processes and decisions.

Lately, the doctor in me cannot help but apply these same diagnostic skills to our current healthcare system. My conclusion is that this system is on the verge of a full life-threatening arrest. The good news is that my instincts also lead me to conclude that this is still avoidable if we address certain key details before it is too late, and we find ourselves deep in the midst of a full resuscitation effort. We cannot just cross our fingers and try to get away with it. To do so is risky at best and extremely irresponsible.

The architects of Obamacare understood this as well and thus strove to shore up the system before it collapsed. While it is true that the ACA is flawed, this does not negate the fact that it was a sound start to build from and reduced a significant amount of our system's blood loss. My clinical concern is that, since the passage of the ACA, we have all been standing or walking in circles, around the patient's—our nation's—bedside, when we should be moving forward to the next phase of treatment. I conclude that it is time to act, and we need to decide as a people what our next steps should be, or else we risk losing both our patient and ourselves while we watch idly by.

What are the possible courses of action we should consider? Should we accept the status quo that shook the spirit of Kerry-Ann when she saw the differential in healthcare dissemination amongst her patient peers on the baby delivery wards? Should we continue to accept such degrees of separation in our emergency rooms, outpatient practices, and communities at large? We need to decide.

Do we accept that healthcare is a public good and universal human right? If so, what does this universality actually mean when we look at it in detail? Is it restricted only to how healthcare is paid for through our government agencies and insurance companies? Listening to our presidential candidates throw around healthcare reform like a political football, one would think that the funding scheme is all that matters. Are they correct, or should universal coverage also extend to other areas, such as the way we deliver our medical care, standardization of screening, prevention, and treatment strategies, as well as pharmaceutical access and costs? We need to decide.

My own experience leads me to conclude that placing too much emphasis on money within the clinical sphere tends to create conflict and mistrust between doctors and patients, among doctors, and within healthcare institutions. The unions of the past fought to protect employees and their families from excessive costs associated with medical insurance coverage. They advocated for individuals against all-powerful crony capitalism. Now that unions have become far less effective, should we address this clear mismatch between David and Goliath? Is this another rationale supporting universal coverage? We need to decide.

Is capitalism truly the best model for healthcare? The tactic of placing a Starbucks or gas station on every corner may make sense in the food service and fuel industries, but this approach clearly impedes attempts by policymakers to achieve efficient care delivery in the medical field. In my own region of New York, the duplication of services leads to patient confusion, repeat diagnostic testing, and miscommunication, not to mention often-vicious public confrontations among the large medical practices and local hospitals. The scene is more consistent with survival of the fittest than an approach guided by true compassion and wisdom. Do we believe that capitalism applied in this way still makes sense for our healthcare system? We need to decide.

Capitalism is based upon profit. Most Americans can do the math and realize that their insurance premiums add up to much more than their doctors are billing. My single-parent employees typically pay at least $5,000 per year in premiums, deductibles, and copays. They rarely use more than $2,000 per year in services. Like with fire insurance, the extra money goes back into the insurance company's accounts for a potential disaster. The well-recognized truth is that the excess money generates profits as long as payouts are minimized. In addition, a good proportion of the excess premiums are invested by the company to generate further profits for its shareholders.

Should this whole funding scheme be returned to the insured in some way, such as reducing premium costs for employees and employers alike? Is this a strong argument for universal Medicaid and Medicare? This is not my area of expertise, but I sense that we need to think outside the box when it comes to funding our healthcare. The power brokers in the medical insurance industry would clearly feel threatened by the prospect of a more centralized funding process. Do we now dare to openly challenge their influence with such a centralized competitive option for our people? Should we give the insurers an opportunity to develop their own proposals to establish more of a middle ground? Our patient is still on the table, and the time to decide is now.

I have seen many examples of excessive and unnecessary financial waste in our healthcare system, all of which significantly contributed to the national economic burdens and social unrest we face today. This waste of resources occurs in broad daylight and compromises us all in one way or another. Even before the COVID-19 pandemic, our healthcare was in crisis. Our healthcare system suffers from multiple problems, including operational inefficiencies, a lack of primary care with an overemphasis on specialty medicine, the normalization of constant competitive advertising between medical entities, and the establishment of bureaucratic boundaries between the branches of public, mental, and medical health.

Many experts, including one of my senior colleagues from Columbia, Dr. Gilbert Simon,[71] argue convincingly that we must urgently reclaim this waste so we can then use it as a source of "found money" to support constructive and meaningful healthcare reform. Once rid of these inefficiencies, we can then harness our economic and human resources to focus on preventative health programs and address the many social problems, such as health access inequities, that continue to confront us. The solution lies in redirecting our profession's resource—time, intellect, and money—to addressing the gaping primary care problems in areas such as nutrition, education, housing, substance abuse, and poverty—all of which contributed substantially to the erosion of our people's health. Unless we make a united and concerted effort to maximize the health profession's potential, our nation will never achieve the goal of establishing a truly healthy population.

As with many serious problems, the answers often begin with taking a good look at ourselves before we start to blame others. This is a very uncomfortable and often controversial endeavor. It isn't easy to do. Nonetheless, if we are to be viewed as credible authorities, physicians need to publicly accept and admit that a part of the runaway healthcare costs in our nation are directly attributable to our own professional behavior patterns. These include the expectation of relatively high physician salaries, practicing medicolegally defensive medicine, and the excessive ordering of expensive diagnostic tests. As a physician, I understand very well why doctors adhere to these expectations. However, nothing will improve if physicians don't actively participate

71 Simon, Gilbert, *Ripped Off!: Overtested, Overtreated and Overcharged: the American Healthcare Mess*, Paper Raven Books, Feb 27, 2020.

in the healing of our system. Who better than the engineers to step up and lead the effort to stop this runaway train heading for a cliff?

Instead of accusing my colleagues, I tried to understand the motives for their practice patterns. Why do we operate one way or another? Why do we expect certain things to be part of our profession? My ongoing, decades-long, frontline analysis with colleagues and students has been revealing. The consistent sentiment amongst physicians is that the extensive time commitments and financial burdens incurred with our training are the major factors that justify a sense that doctors deserve to be well compensated.

As a recently graduated student resident of mine so well expressed, "Our peers in other fields have been out working years before us with far less tuition debt and better pay. We simply start our careers with a sense of needing to pay back and catch up."

No wonder many doctors who initially planned to pursue primary care careers change their minds, buckle down a couple more years, and choose a higher-paying specialty practice instead. It is simply a matter of common-sense accounting. With this in mind, the found money retrieved from wasteful practices should go to increasing the reimbursements for our understaffed primary care workforce. I suggest that, as in many countries, many more American physicians would accept the lower salaries of primary care if some of the administrative, medicolegal, and educational costs—compounded by excessive bureaucratic requirements—were removed from the system. Even specialists would be less inclined to expect high six-figure incomes if these burdens were removed.

Clinicians' experiences during the COVID-19 pandemic also reshaped the priorities of many physicians. A middle-aged primary care colleague of mine summed this sentiment up well over a recent evening bonfire. "After two years of struggling during COVID and seeing so many lose their lives and livelihood, I now realize that my personal time and mental space are valuable commodities that I would readily exchange for less take-home pay." In the end, even with a lower income, lowering budget items such as educational debt, practice management, and medical malpractice costs may actually add up to a net-neutral accounting of our bottom line personal and professional finances.

It's worth repeating Bernie Sanders's explanation to the nation in his proposals for healthcare reform, "It's not what you make. It's what you keep." A reduction in administrative and financial burdens would inevitably have the added benefit of improving the psychological health of our profession's members. How much is that worth?

I also seriously question the conventional wisdom of the payors. Is it actually wiser for all stakeholders that we adopt highly restrictive policies, or would more inclusive spending practices use our health-care-designated dollar more productively? Until now, the government and private health insurers have been implementing a very concerted campaign to reduce their costs by denying payments to hospitals and care providers through multiple means. These included direct measures such as reductions in the reimbursements for specific tests or medical care services, increasing the proportion of the bill that the patient pays, and outright denying any coverage for certain diagnoses. In a less direct and more subtle fashion, they also delayed payments by increasing the complexity of the billing process required of the physicians to receive payments.

Ironically, I am now convinced that limiting access to any form of health insurance may ultimately prove counterproductive economically to all parties—the payors, providers, and beneficiaries. Consider the make-believe model of a fast food street cart known for making the best French fries in town—Best Fries. They start out their business by openly welcoming all 10,000 of their community members to buy a serving of their fries at $3 each. Everyone is excited because they can afford this and plan to buy at least one serving per year, thus generating at least $30,000 annually for Best Fries. Then a new business entity comes to town and wants a piece of the action. Their idea is to offer their customers exclusive access to these incredible fries. This entity proposes to act as negotiator—a third-party payor—between a select group of privileged and hand-picked customers and Best Fries.

These customers will thus benefit from exclusive access to these coveted fries. The third-party company proposes to pay Best Fries $10 per serving to guarantee this exclusivity, and the vendor, seeing the potential to make significantly more money, readily agrees. In exchange for guaranteeing this exclusivity, the third-party payor requires a relatively small additional fee from their members—a premium—to create a pool of money to support these operations. They will pay Best Fries on behalf of their member customers, who are free to order at the cart without needing to pay Best Fries directly. To ensure that this business model is not only solvent but profitable, the third party carefully selects who is allowed in this limited beneficiary pool. The select members must be both highly reliable to pay the premiums and unlikely to order too many servings of fries. They thus initially are very conservative and restrict their exclusive customer base to 1,000 wealthy individuals and restrict each of them to one purchase of French fries annually. Alas, in this make-believe example, only 10 percent of the community are given the exclusive buying power by the entity holding the purse strings, thus limiting Best Fries's earning potential to a maximum of $10,000 per year. The other potential customers who can only afford $3 using their own money have been completely denied access to the fries on the basis of multiple inclusion and exclusion criteria established by this deal. Best Fries's hands are tied.

One day, a twist to the whole French fry operation is thrown into the community. Outside government regulators come to town and deem the member restrictions imposed by the payor as unethical and too restrictive. The regulators insist that Best Fries now has to serve all 10,000 community members. They impose a policy that requires the prior excluded 9,000 people must be funded by a newly appointed third-party payor who will only provide $1 per serving of fries. Best Fries is prohibited from charging any of these additional customers more than this amount. This means that instead of helping the situation, the additional customers are now a financial burden to Best Fries.

The new regulations create a gap of $18,000 because at $1 a head, the 9,000 additional customers can generate only an additional $9,000, instead of the potential $27,000 if the vendor was free to reset the market price back to the original $3 per serving. Because Best Fries now has to cover the operating costs of providing at least 9,000 more servings of fries, they turn to the original exclusive third-party payor and demand that they help close the $18,000 gap.

In the end, to stay in business, the original payor agrees to pass a portion of the gap expenses onto their original 1,000 elite customers by increasing their individual annual premiums by $5. The payor also agrees to contribute an additional $5 per member. Even still, this closes the $18,000 gap by only $10,000. Best Fries can barely keep their French fry operations solvent. For the original 1,000 customers to maintain any access to the fries, they now find themselves forced to help cover the costs for the 9,000 new customers. They become understandably resentful.

Ultimately, everyone loses or pays more in this analogy. The 1,000 original customers cover the costs for those 9,000 who were restricted to paying only $1, and the cart vendor loses $8,000 a year. A short time later, the cost of potatoes increases a tiny amount and pushes Best Fries into a losing proposition. They ultimately can no longer stay in business. All 10,000 customers lose their access to these great French fries. The original third-party payor is no longer needed and is forced to close operations.

This fabricated French fry story summarizes almost a century of the US experience with health insurance, starting with the creation of Blue Cross Blue Shield after the Great Depression in the 1930s. Whether a small medical practice or a large corporate hospital system, many of these vendors had to close their doors because the reimbursement model just does not sustain the provision of their medical services. When a significant proportion of people are excluded from any insurance or have insufficient insurance coverage to pay for medical care, the hospitals, physicians, and their high-premium elite patients are all placed into an equally ridiculous and unsustainable position as the French fry analogy.

For the past several years, the United States has teetered on the edge of complete virtual financial ruin of the American healthcare system because of this economic model. The majority of Americans, the medical profession, and institutions would be willing to have more patients with insurance coverage, but the third-party payors have been allowed to actively limit and deny coverage to millions. Because we were distracted by political shenanigans, to date, we have not achieved or guaranteed medical coverage for all our people through private or public insurance. Given the economic fragility of the current model, proposals for universal healthcare coverage, such as those included in the ACA, are no longer topics for theoretical debates. They are practical and necessary to avoid the entire system from collapsing.

Like the Best Fries analogy, an up-close, honest, and logical look at the current funding of our healthcare services supports an expansion of the paying customer base, not exponentially increasing restrictions. However, I admit that there is a clear flaw in applying this French fry analogy to the current US paradigm for funding healthcare. The recognition of this flaw is not a problem—it is the point.

It is of paramount importance that we shine full light on this critical difference between the analogy and reality if we are to ever get ourselves out of this mess. It is the key to identifying the design problem which impedes our progress toward expanding coverage to more people. The issue is right in front of us if we would only dare open our eyes and hearts. The economic model of the health insurance companies and other third-party payors is in direct conflict with the fiscal model of those providing the health services.

Insurers are motivated to keep as much of their money for as long as possible. The less they spend from the pool of insurance premiums paid by their exclusive customers, the greater their profit for themselves and their shareholders. Like all other insurance businesses, this profit-based objective leads them to cherry-pick those customers who are least likely to use their accumulated funds—buy too many French fries. Using complex algorithms, they thus identify this "low-risk" pool. They then deny or restrict coverage to those 9,000 at "high risk," the hungriest amongst us, because they represent the group most likely to demand the insurance company's funds just to eat.

Those directly providing the health services—clinicians, hospitals, vendors, as well as the patients who contributed funds to the payors—require and support a very different funding paradigm. They are motivated to increase access to healthcare—the French fries—to as many people as possible. In the process, they would be more productive if they could spread the wealth and enable more people to pay for the health services rendered. Like the Best Fries analogy, the providers cannot remain in business if only a fraction of the patients can pay for the healthcare provided to all comers. Those paying customers too are not thrilled with their increasing premiums required to sustain the whole system.

An increasing number of medical care providers decided to no longer tolerate these controlling purse strings to neglect a large base of people denied any coverage while the insurance system makes a huge profit. At a college alumni meeting I attended in the late fall of 2020 to discuss new student candidates, Dr. Mark Lewis, a 40-something, tertiary-center-trained orthopedist from New York City, addressed this issue directly.

"I no longer accept any type of insurance for my services. I set my own fees and take direct payments from my patients. I found that, when I got rid of the overhead and the cumbersome burdens to process my bills for my patient care, my reimbursements actually allow me to achieve a substantially greater net profit than when I worked through the insurers. Not only can I now pass some of the savings to all my patients, I can provide free care to many indigent people. I actually ended up turning no one away." With obvious passion and excitement, he went on to extrapolate how the success of his business model shaped his views on the current healthcare reform debate. "I never would have believed it, but I actually now strongly support a universal healthcare model over the current insurance system that has failed so many. If universal coverage was in place, I am convinced that my current model would only be enhanced further. Everyone could contribute something, and I still would not have to turn anyone away."

I chimed in with interest, "Would you go as far as to give up your private-pay system and take a cut in profit?"

Dr. Lewis paused for a moment and then replied thoughtfully, "That depends on which procedures I need to provide for any given patient. If I could justify the overhead, I would certainly think about it."

Later that evening, Dr. Lewis and I sat for a beer together after everyone else left. As we talked, we realized that, though we both trained in conventional FFS models, we shared a passion for something better. Our ideas flowed like an excited stream of consciousness. We discussed several benefits of a more equitable and less profit-driven means of covering the costs of healthcare. We both agreed that universal coverage has the potential to save money downstream by leveraging some health-promoting influence on the lifestyle patterns of those covered.

Properly organized, the system has the potential to encourage good health behaviors such as seeking better nutrition. Some funds could be specifically designated as incentives for buying more fresh fruits and vegetables, rather than processed food. Attendance at regular maintenance and screening visits could be required for an individual to participate in universal coverage. This approach could identify diseases in early stages before they fester and become critically dangerous and ultimately more costly. We concluded that copays and high deductibles only lead to a sicker population by denying or discouraging routine care. In the end, we realized we shared the belief that a universal healthcare funding model without such patient disincentives enables the whole population to become healthier, and the system thus gradually would find itself spending less.

A couple weeks after my discussion with Dr. Lewis, I was literally blown away by a phone conversation with a physician representative from one of the largest private third-party health insurance companies. This faceless doctor on the phone expressed many of the same sentiments regarding the need for a more universal healthcare system. Lately, the insurance companies increasingly require that physicians step aside from their patient responsibilities to speak to such medical professionals to obtain the "authorization" from the company to perform any number of diagnostic tests that we may order. It has become blatantly clear that many denials for such services are just another means of the companies not paying for care and thus increasing their profits.

In any given week, I may be required to have at least five such phone conversations. Typically, these discussions are fairly dry and all business, lasting less than five minutes. After 10 minutes of my navigating through the automated options on the phone to request authorization to perform a cardiac ultrasound study on an unborn child with suspected heart problems, a woman's voice identified herself as one of the doctors from the insurance company. Surprisingly, she demonstrated a genuine interest and concern regarding the situation of the family of my fetal patient. She explained that she remains an active obstetrician in her community and often interacts with high-risk obstetricians and pediatric cardiologists such as myself.

After 15 minutes of a very stimulating exchange, during which we thoroughly reviewed the medical details of the pregnancy in question, she literally apologized for any disrespect in wasting my time with the authorization process. "You should be spending time with your patients and their families, instead of being stuck on the phone with me for such foolishness. This is just one of the reasons why I actually believe that a universal healthcare system is preferable to our current system."

Was I hearing correctly? Had she been eavesdropping on my recent conversation with Dr. Lewis? Was a major gatekeeper in one the largest health insurance companies openly admitting that the system was dysfunctional? It was obvious that more physicians support a broad and radical change in our current healthcare system than I previously suspected. Given this turning of the tides, I pondered—who is actually left still advocating against a universal healthcare option for the United States? With a moderate dose of cynicism, I concluded that any such holdouts must have a significant financial stake in the current, overly bureaucratic, and dysfunctional system to contradict the trend that even some of the major third-party payors are beginning to support.

"Dr. Fethke, the biggest problem that prospective doctors face today is the struggle to pay for college and medical school. We are so behind the eight ball before we even get started with our careers, and it takes years before we see any hope of coming out from under all the debt."

This is one of the most consistent sentiments that my students raise on a weekly basis. They love what they learn and are excited about becoming a doctor, but they are also frightened to death of the financial burden they will incur. They know that this education-related cost is not unique to medicine. However, unlike many other professional careers, the path to becoming a doctor is by definition significantly longer than analogous disciplines in law, business, or journalism. This delay in their ability to take a reasonable paycheck home inevitably drives the students to choose positions that give them some reasonable chance to pay off their debts and catch up for the years of lost income.

My wife and I were in our early 40s by the time we made our final medical school loan payments. It's hard to imagine, but the average medical student today faces an even greater debt burden than we did. Before they see their first patient as an officially independent physician, the majority of my student doctors are forced to consider economics over any sense of commitment to a higher calling. Instead of choosing to dedicate their professional lives to the underserved or in primary care, such as pediatrics, family, or internal medicine, they are drawn to further training to become a medical specialist.

Many of them now choose to enter non-physician allied industries such as pharmaceuticals or medical technology, which provide more realistic opportunities for economic security to these once-altruistic aspiring physicians. The inclination to become a subspecialist takes place even in the relatively new education programs strategically designed to promote an increase in the number of general practice physicians as a solution to the current shortage of PCPs. This is in direct conflict with the goals of the policymakers, who argue that healthcare reform should be based upon a platform of increasing the workforce of generalists while decreasing the number of costly subspecialists. Perhaps these same policymakers, if they truly want success in their endeavors, should be more conscious of the financial impediments incurred by their intended future general physicians during their medical school education.

It was understandable that Johnny always wanted to be a doctor. He essentially grew up in the Midwest spending his free time in the private medical office where his grandfather and father worked together as pediatricians. Just when he accepted an offer to a prestigious college, where he intended to pursue a premedical education, his grandfather became ill and took an early retirement. This left his father with all the financial responsibilities to both run the practice and serve as the main physician provider. His father hired a nurse practitioner to assist him, but the resulting insurance reimbursements did not make up for the loss of his grandfather's income potential as a full physician.

Johnny's father took out a loan for the practice just to survive. Johnny and his father were therefore also forced to take out an education loan to fund his college. By the time Johnny finished four years of college and was accepted to medical school, he was $50,000 in debt. Because he continued his education, he postponed this loan for four more years. By the time he finished medical school and entered the next level of his training as a pediatric intern and resident, young Dr. Johnny's debt principal was $120,000 with interest due. He was now required to begin some routine payments back to the loan agencies, which changed hands at least three times with increasing interest rates since he first accepted the college loan. These payments significantly impacted any ability to save money on his current annual training stipend of $50,000. This was particularly the case because his training hospital was based in an urban area with a relatively high cost of living for even basics such as groceries.

When he finally finished his residency training and joined his proud father as a junior partner, they were both in significant debt. Sadly, they could not afford to keep the nurse practitioner. After two years of trying to dig out from this debt, Johnny proposed that they hire another pediatrician and he return to training to become a pediatric specialist. He could scrape a living on an education stipend for the next three years and would return to the practice with a much greater earning level than a general pediatrician. His father agreed, and this plan went into effect just over three years later.

Johnny was now 34 years old. His 64-year-old father looked at his own retirement in the mirror, but because of their financial situation, the father delayed retirement until he was 70 years old. Johnny finally paid off the family's medical education and business loans by age 45. Upon his father's retirement, he and the other pediatrician agreed to merge the practice with a larger hospital-based program and become employees. For the first time in their careers, they began to set some money aside for retirement in their new hospital employer's 401K program. They both accepted that they would have to work until at least 70 years old to save enough retirement savings. Only 25 more years to go.

Doctor Mary lives in an alternate reality from Johnny. Like Dr. Johnny, she always aspired to be a physician since her single nurse mother encouraged her to reach farther in her education than a nursing degree. In Mary's world, a college education is funded by multiple sources that guarantee she will not finish school with significant debt. When she entered medical school, she owed $10,000, the maximum debt possible upon receiving her undergraduate degree set by the policymakers. By the time she finished medical school, she added an additional $40,000, which is the cap for a graduate degree. She thus began her postgraduate training as a physician intern with a total debt of $50,000 at a fixed, low interest rate specific to education loans.

As an incentive for her to choose a career in primary care, she was given the opportunity to reduce her total loan by 50 percent. To do so, she agreed to work in a medically underserved geographic area after completing two years of residency training in family practice. Now three years after completing medical school, Mary began working with a total debt of only $25,000. Free of any significant financial burdens, Mary liked her job in the underserved community so much that she decided to stay in the area and continue to work at the local clinic. Over the years, she also started a private practice with some of her local colleagues.

Because she was not burdened by significant debt, Mary accepted an offer to teach at her local medical school for a minimal additional salary. In Mary's universe, the costs of education were thus further reduced by encouraging the physician alumni to return to academia as part-time teachers at a minimal cost to the school. In return, the doctors shared in other university benefits, including reduced health insurance costs, retirement savings investments, college tuition reductions for children, low-cost malpractice insurance, and free continuing education programs. These benefits provided significant value and reduced the business overhead costs for the physicians in Mary's community and private practice.

Over the next decades, Mary and her colleagues made a major positive impact on the health status of this originally underserved community. With the reduction in several originally prevalent conditions such as premature deliveries, obesity, diabetes, and heart disease, the cost savings to the region and health insurance companies were in the millions. A portion of these savings were returned back to the college and medical education programs to keep the tuition costs down for the next generation of students. Mary finished her very fulfilling and productive medical career by age 60 with sufficient savings for retirement. Today, Mary frequently travels and conducts volunteer medical work in remote parts of the country and the world.

The situation for most of today's physicians is best depicted by the fictitious story of Dr. Johnny. However, Mary's version of a health career is not entirely a fairy tale. Many of the components of her story were implemented over the years by health education reformers, only to be later abandoned. Education loan debt reductions for those electing to work in underserved areas were in vogue in the New York metropolitan area as we entered the twenty-first century.

When I started my work as a junior attending Columbia University, the college education benefits for my future children were still in place, though at a significantly reduced level compared to my mentors only 10 to 20 years ahead of me. This was clearly at odds with the fact that the cost of university and medical school education became several folds higher since the time my senior colleagues' children graduated. Other creative financial incentives included subsidies for the expensive CME requirements made mandatory for physicians by hospitals and medical licensing agencies. The cost of these CME credits is often quite prohibitive, especially when one considers the loss of patient visit productivity while away attending several days of courses. Concerted attempts to provide CME benefits at low cost or for free through individual private institutions served as a way of enticing physicians to join them. Recently, a few, select private institutions made efforts to reduce medical education costs using their substantial endowments to guarantee debt-free undergraduate and graduate education. In August 2018, NYU made headlines by announcing that their medical school would now be tuition-free for all accepted students.

What limits our ability to create a Dr. Mary-type scenario for all medical students—starting with education funding—is the lack of a comprehensive national program to equitably support the careers of physicians and allied healthcare professionals. At this time, the economic solutions are left to the local governments and the many private colleges that function as profit-oriented businesses. Many institutions have now realized that there is a lot of money to be made if they start a medical school or residency program through student tuition or government-funded subsidies.

As an example, I noted an exponential increase in the number of community hospitals with newly established medical training programs where the quality of the medical education appears to be less important than the quantity of students and trainees who bring in the money. The cost control of higher education in the United States has historically been left up to free-market competition. Under the capitalist system, institutions like NYU may indeed spark a trend of lowering tuition burdens at other medical schools who can also afford to attract the best and brightest students. However, they inadvertently foster a wider economic and intellectual gap between those institutions with the financial resources to offer free tuition and those who are less financially endowed.

If my own medical students are afforded the ability to study and work in a real world similar to that of our fictitious Dr. Mary, there would be no such division, and I believe that everyone—students, universities, medical institutions, society, and patients—would end up as the beneficiaries. There are indeed glimpses of Dr. Mary's fabled world just over the next horizon. If America is to succeed in attaining a universal and equitable approach to medical education, all stakeholders must remain determined to climb this hill together and not allow selfish profiteers who view medical education as a cash cow business to risk our collective progress.

DEFINE OUR PRIORITIES

As we work toward our common goals, we probably should agree on some rules of engagement. This should include a clear and conscious expectation that, for success, we cannot engage in destructive ridicule of others with whom we may not agree. The healthcare reform process should be based upon the mutual desire and freedom to constructively criticize our particular respective situations—locally, regionally, and nationally—as we strive to collectively pick ourselves up and aim for loftier common goals. Healthcare policies should be evidence-based and not driven by constantly changing and divisive politics. As an American physician-citizen, I believe that we should and can be much better at this process.

Both at home and abroad, the public persona that our policymakers currently demonstrate in regards to healthcare is at risk of eroding any sense that our priorities are clear or well-intended. Even before the COVID-19 pandemic, our collective behavior determined if the medical profession was trusted and respected. The horrendous losses to SARS-CoV-2 leave little doubt that we have a long way to go if we are to shore up any legitimate authority to guide our people's health.

I stress daily to my students that we, as physicians, need to make a concerted effort to openly serve all American citizens in a manner whereby they can become better informed about the issues and dynamics that influence the status of our unique health system. When physicians and other health professionals take ownership of this role to guide and educate our patients and community members, we empower those we serve to make better healthcare choices. They will be less likely to just accept a politician's or self-serving entrepreneur's statements at face value. Like any civil liberty, access to the best healthcare possible requires knowledge of and involvement in the process by the people themselves.

In the end, I sense that Bernie Sanders's repeated and consistent cries for urgent reform and his rising zeal are not due to his being a crazy liberal. He may simply now be getting older and thus more impatient than when he was younger about attaining his visions for a health system that he sincerely believes is in the best interest of his nation's people. Recent surveys indicate that he is not alone. More Americans than ever, as many as 60 percent, are now considering a single-payer system,[72] instead of today's complex and less effective situation. His vision was made even more possible when President Obama chose to tip the socioeconomic pyramid upside down, finally and rightfully placing the base of those less fortunate on the top. He thus realigned the administrative process to our health system in a fashion that was less dependent on having the wealth of the few trickle down to the rest of us. Many wise people joined Sanders and Obama in the sober assessment that the resources of the wealthiest have not uniformly or effectively made their way down the pyramid. Even though some people may argue that economics work best with a trickle-down theory, this paradigm simply does not work well for our healthcare system.

The system is much more effective if we address the healthcare of whole communities, rather than individuals. This phenomena clearly manifested when we faced the loss of health coverage for millions of our people during the Trump administration as he made repeated efforts to tear down the ACA without a clear alternative plan. These repeated attempts to repeal the ACA were thwarted by the very simple fact that there has been no viable counterproposal for healthcare reform. We cannot simply go back to something that was not working in the first place.

This scenario is analogous to the disastrous venture of Great Britain's Prime Minister, Boris Johnson, as he attempted to proceed with Brexit by separating from the European Union with no other deal in place from which to independently launch his nation's next phase of political and economic existence. This left the British people economically and psychologically in turmoil as they suffer through the largest turnover rate of leadership in their nation's history.

72 Jones, Bradley, "Increasing Share of Americans Favor a Single Government Program to Provide Health Care Coverage," Pew Research Center, Sept 29, 2020, https://www.pewresearch.org/fact-tank/2020/09/29/increasing-share-of-americans-favor-a-single-government-program-to-provide-health-care-coverage/.

It is paramount that we realize that the ACA was stimulated but not unilaterally designed by one man, President Obama. It is only through a political slant that anyone can deny that very smart people—his advisors—designed this initial proposal. The ACA stands as a sorely needed solid attempt to address and no longer ignore our need for a better health system for our nation. This program was never touted as the ultimate and final solution but as a starting point from which we could evolve together. Not just Mr. Sanders has been sensitive to this. Senator John McCain's historic vote shortly before his death on the Republican proposal that helped dismantle the ACA set the standard of placing national well-being above politics. He might not have agreed with all the specifics of the ACA, but he could see that it was at least a start in the right direction, and undoing it would take us many steps backward solely on the premise of political rivalry.

As we step forward in the evolution of our healthcare system, we need to actively evaluate and choose amongst certain finance models. For decades, medical professionals and institutions were reimbursed for their work on an FFS basis. This FFS approach essentially allows the care providers—hospitals or clinicians—to bill for each separate item or unit of service rendered during a particular patient's care. This is the "shopping list" approach to medical care reimbursement and is not significantly different from the billing approach used by any other service industry such as a local plumber.

To organize the massive list of items available on this medical shopping cart, we essentially created a huge catalog that attempts to be all-inclusive regarding what we can buy and sell. This document is uniquely American, known as the International Classification of Diseases or ICD, the 10th version of which was recently published. It assigns a code to each item or procedure, and the billing process requires that these codes link to medical problems or diagnoses, which are in turn given their own codes. This ICD-10 system grew exponentially to now include 68,000 codes, compared to 13,000 in the prior ICD-9 version. To describe this as unwieldy would be an understatement.

Many of my physician colleagues also agree that even this expansive version is incomplete and misrepresentative of what we actually do as physicians. To make matters worse, these codes are not only embedded into our electronic records platforms, they are also used by administrators at many levels to quantify physician productivity. "How many widgets did Dr. X sell last month compared to Dr. Y?" This comparison model, known as RVUs, also took on a life of its own, further bogging down physicians with quantity over quality.

A value-based care (VBC) system of financing grew out of cost-containment strategies to reduce the rate of hospital admissions and reimbursements. The fundamental principles of VBC originated from the 2008 Medicare Improvements for Patients and Providers Act and the 2010 ACA. Over the past decade, VBC has been proposed as an alternative to the FFS model. The VBC system focuses on the actual health outcomes of patients and uses these outcomes as the basis for physician and hospital reimbursements.

According to a *New England Journal of Medicine* article in January of 2017, "Under value-based care agreements, providers are rewarded for helping patients improve their health, reduce the effects and incidence of chronic disease, and live healthier lives in an evidence-based way."[73] In this paradigm, we essentially ask, "What are we getting for our time and money?" Though the transition from an FFS to a VBC system has been slow to catch on and onerous at best, it provides a conceptual model more in line with what "good medicine" should look like. It encourages a more global approach to how physicians function daily and emphasizes high-quality, scientifically evidence-based care

73 NEJM Catalyst,"What is Value-Based Healthcare?', January 2017 (online).

over sheer volume of services. It actually looks more like the medicine that professionals were trained and educated to provide.

As this more holistic approach gradually permeates our daily practices, certain encouraging outcomes that further support this model have started to manifest.

"I do not know why I am even here," gasped Alex, a 16-year-old patient brought in by his mother to see me one morning. He recently began experiencing several fainting episodes. At first, they occurred only at home but now occurred in the classroom and at track practice after school. Before he was allowed to return to either, the school and his pediatrician required that his heart health be fully assessed.

It would have been very easy for me to simply order several relatively expensive diagnostic medical tests, including an echocardiogram, cardiac home monitor, and a full exercise stress test, along with bloodwork. These tests would likely exclude any serious cardiac problem and also medicolegally "cover" me from the liability of missing a potentially life-threatening cardiac problem. The bill for these services would easily total over $3,000. Would this battery of tests actually find out what the underlying problem was and ultimately help him? Probably not.

A cheap and simple ECG test was normal. The details of the fainting episodes and his general personal and family health were non-alarming, and my thorough physical exam was almost completely normal. He was, however, strikingly underweight for an athlete of his reported caliber, with a very prominent rib cage and other bony landmarks. He also seemed quite defensive in his tone and demeanor. I therefore elected to break the ice with him and take a different approach.

"I try to run and do charity races at my age. Do you like running?" I inquired nonchalantly.

"Yeah, it's OK, I guess," he replied.

"What do you mean? You love running and have been doing it for years!" his mother suddenly and forcefully interjected.

Alex looked up at her almost with tears in his eyes, looking from me to his mother. "I used to like it, but not so much lately. The coach has been a jerk, and the other guys are assholes."

The ice broke, and the next 30 minutes opened a Pandora's box. I learned that Alex's mother and father recently underwent a nasty divorce process which started when Alex was 13 and he had just moved to his new school. His older sister was away in college, and he was the only child left at home with his now-single working mother. To complicate matters further, Alex had been somewhat overweight in the past and was now on a "health kick" to look better to fit in with his new friends. This included a newly announced boyfriend as Alex had only recently come out, declaring that he believed that he was gay. Over the past six months, he lost over 60 pounds. He exercised twice a day and took in on average under 700 calories daily. It was no wonder he fainted so much.

Over the next few months, Alex entered into counseling and followed a better nutritional program with a local sports expert. He put on increased weight and muscle mass, and the fainting episodes resolved completely. He was back to running competitively and was accepted to college with a track scholarship. On his final visit with me in the office, he and his mother looked much more relaxed and happy. I never ordered any of the expensive medical tests.

Once again, an emphasis on emotional intelligence skills over liability-driven, profit-generating testing proved invaluable. Such emotional IQ, or EQ, is strengthened by one's ability to recognize nonverbal and emotional cues from others and respond appropriately to address these signals. It takes time to develop and practice emotional intelligence. It cannot be well administered in a 10-minute doctor's visit such as that promoted by a high-pressure FFS environment.

Not surprisingly, emotional intelligence functions much better in a VBC approach. I only recently learned that I function and thrive in my daily patient care when I can apply my EQ as a therapeutic and diagnostic tool. The recent literature on VBC further supported approaches by physicians who incorporate a high EQ because they result in significantly improved health outcomes at a much lower cost.

Physicians are trained in medical school to recognize and appreciate such emotional signals from our patients. Over the past few decades, all too soon in our individual careers, these lessons have been abandoned during our residency and early practice years in favor of volume-based productivity. Is it any wonder that the costs of rendering our healthcare rose disproportionately to our good results? If I rushed my visit with Alex and hadn't deliberately applied my EQ, where would he be today? If we validate, emphasize, and support such approaches in every physician-patient encounter, our entire patient population and, ultimately, our society will benefit.

Because the US federal government presently spends more of our tax money per individual on health coverage than any other nation, we must soberly admit to ourselves that, for decades, we have essentially operated under a government-based health system model. We must call out the political distraction of derisively pointing to other countries who employ a socialist model of healthcare for what it truly is—a shameless attempt to cover up the fact that we Americans spend more on government-funded healthcare than most other equally developed nations.

In fact, the projected trend of our healthcare spending[74] is in the direction of increasing the portion of the healthcare dollar that our government pays for up to 50 percent, which equates to nearly $6

74 "Government Now Pays For Nearly 50 Percent Of Health Care Spending, An Increase Driven By Baby Boomers Shifting Into Medicare," *KFF Health News*, Feb. 21, 2019 (online), https://khn.org/morning-breakout/government-now-pays-for-nearly-50-percent-of-health-care-spending-an-increase-driven-by-baby-boomers-shifting-into-medicare/.

trillion. Like Canada, the United States is actually a hybrid system of government-supported healthcare combined with private insurance for medications, supplies, and ancillary services such as home care. Canada simply takes more ownership of the fact that their government tries to support healthcare for everyone, not just the poor or elderly.

During one of Viyada's college reunions in 2016, we attended several lectures by alumni who are national healthcare policy experts. One of the consistent themes that ran through these talks was the warning that, if America's efforts to reform healthcare are successful, we must avoid the tendency to hold onto the concept of dualities, in which the issues are portrayed as simply binary—black and white, on or off, all or nothing. These experts advised that we should make a concerted effort to stop taking philosophical sides in which we hold on so tightly to our respective paradigms that we are not able to meet in the middle. As I digested the concepts proposed by these pundits, I sensed the profound wisdom in their approach. Why would we ever believe that, in a nation which claims to be proud of the diversity of its people, our healthcare system should be rigidly two-sided? Dualities such as either entirely private or entirely public health insurance do not serve our people any better than we would expect two sizes of shoes to adequately fit everyone's feet. Such opposing concepts must give way to collaborative models that incorporate the best components of several models.

Even though a universal health funding system may be funded through the federal system, this does not imply that it should ignore the idiosyncrasies of its people and their communities. To do so risks perpetuating the inequity of healthcare delivery that plagues our nation and resulted in such poor outcomes during the COVID-19 pandemic. A community-oriented proposal naturally dictates that each of our 50 states chooses what works best for themselves. This is why the ACA proposed that medical care be carried out state by state with certain basic federally mandated requirements for equitable distributions.

As these state-based models develop, everyone can begin to tailor options that may work best for their particular situations. This state-based flexibility is in fact consistent with our overall sense of civic rights and may be more palatable to us than a universal federally distributed model. In pursuing individualized choice, some states or regions may choose a two-tiered or hybrid system with Medicaid and Medicare, combined with some private-sector components. In such hybrid systems, basic medical care may be accessed using the federal and state tax-based funds, while any medical care above this basic level is supported by private sources. Other states or communities may attempt a purely single-payer public or private system.

Over time and with full transparency, as we collect cost and health-care quality data in each of these models, we can better address several of today's most complex health issues. The different systems will learn from the other models around them to see what works well. For example, is it better to completely deny or should we simply limit access to medical care if an individual or their family does not adequately pay into the system in some way? Should those less fortunate still be required to make monetary contributions, or is it better for everyone if they are instead required to work as employees of the local health program in exchange for health insurance benefits? If we remain flexible through a local process, but universally consistent in our dedication to equitable access to care, we have an opportunity to address these issues and so much more.

DEFINE OUR NATIONAL HEALTHCARE PLATFORMS

Yes, we Americans are sick. Much sicker than a nation with our abundant resources should ever be. The COVID-19 pandemic—caused by a virus blind to race, gender, and economic status—took us all to our knees and struck us with the reality of the depth and breadth of our infirmities. This tragedy demands a response. Now is the time to get back up and do something to fix the systemic problems that continue to threaten us all.

If we prioritize public well-being, rather than capitalist-driven profits, as the driving force of our healthcare system, we may discover that our struggling health system is not actually irreparably broken. Too many of us succumbed to the cynicism and pessimism that now threatens to remove our hopes for a better healthcare system. I too sense the oppressive forces, both political and psychological, that threaten to stifle my own efforts to use my pen as a tool to unite others in the good fight. I choose to ignore these destructive voices and continue to write to provoke actions that will enable our healthcare system to reach its full potential to improve our lives.

Perhaps because I work with children, I personally refuse to be paralyzed by the naysayers who have already abandoned any aspirations for a better tomorrow. I write about this issue because, as a doctor, I sense that if healthcare reform is to work, physicians must become the lead activists dedicated to bringing people from all backgrounds and institutions together to create a united front to constructively address all the factors that make us unhealthy. Along with our co-citizens, we have to roll up our sleeves and remove the extensive clutter that has distracted us from establishing and defining our shared priorities. In this process of cleaning house, I remain convinced that we can rediscover our old principles and values, still fundamentally intact, upon which we founded our unique healthcare system in the first place.

An efficient healthcare reform process dictates that we should first focus on clarifying the big-picture issues so that we do not become entangled in the weeds by starting with the details. We should begin by defining and returning to our national priorities, rather than allowing our leaders to distract us with endless discussions and debates about items such as health insurance.

Though the wealthy and influential corporations that dominate medical technologies and how we pay for healthcare may protest, we should not allow them to be held up as the most important nut to crack in healthcare reform. We should not allow health insurance policies to take up all the oxygen in the room nor be as complicated as our tax codes. Health insurance should simply be a vehicle by which we enter the health system and access the evidence-based medical care that we choose for ourselves according to our predetermined ideals. Reforming our health insurance systems in isolation from our pervasive socioeconomic issues is futile and misguided.

Of course, much in the same way that each of Canada's provinces are different from each other, we are a different and perhaps more complex nation than many other countries. This seemingly daunting task of defining our healthcare reform according to our national and regional ideals should not be seen as frightening and stop us in our tracks. After defining our broader visions, we should gradually implement our policies regionally, with a clear pathway and timeline not repeatedly encumbered by the changes in the political wind.

Our pursuit of the ideal national healthcare system should also be nonpartisan. Despite all the ongoing flaws of the Canadian health system, the shared pride in their goal of universal 100-percent coverage is what allows them best to persist onward and upward together as their system evolves. We too should strive to protect our vision of healthcare as a mutually recognized branding of our best American character. Our health system is now, more than ever, in dire need of assured longevity and the legs to move forward with a clear focus on attaining universal access to equitable basic medical and public health services. Like any well-run household, our healthcare system needs a comprehensive business plan and a socially and politically well-balanced budget, not a political debate influenced by special interest groups. These groups are blatantly attempting to divert monies away from healthcare to other sectors such as military defense contracts and fossil fuel energy instead of our schools, family planning, affordable housing, and sustainable energy.

It seems that too many of America's human and material resources are presently spent on insurance and technologies such as medications and medical devices when they should be dedicated to the elephant in the room—our larger social problems. Many countries already set the example that solving public health issues is the key to improving a nation's health status. As physician leaders, we should proactively avoid accepting the notion that our social issues are separate from our health issues. Public health, after all, by definition includes the term "health." The reality is that these issues are intertwined, not mutually exclusive. Creating intellectual constructs that silo them from each other creates a dangerous artificial boundary that erodes our entire nation's well-being.

If we are to be consistent with the ideal that all aspects of health—biological and psychosocial—are interdependent, then we must erase the artificial boundaries between the fields of mental and biological illness. Non-psychiatric doctors should stand united in their refusal to support any construct that denies that psychological health problems are a major factor leading to a myriad of other health problems that our patients face.

It is dangerous to ignore psychological factors as we treat other medical conditions. The refusal of insurance companies to pay for psychiatric care in parity with other medical diagnoses is paramount to forcing an athlete to run a race without any legs. Our mental well-being is critical to any health maintenance or healing process. All of us doctors need to actively step into this debate and not push this off into the realm of our psychiatric and psychology colleagues as "not our problem." Substance abuse is a salient example of this interaction of social and psychiatric problems. As a public health problem, it is perhaps even more relevant because our profession's medication-prescribing patterns enable and support some of this abuse. Because we stand the best chance of making an impact in this drug abuse crisis, physicians need to aggressively and proactively step into this world of substance abuse, not isolate ourselves from it.

A big picture approach to healthcare reform reveals a strong need for us to define what we believe constitutes a healthy society. Once we do this, we can effectively take a step back to legitimately assess our current status in regards to this self-defined standard. Our current decades-long epidemic of gun violence is a good example of this need for self-analysis. Is America's uniquely high level of gun violence and mass shootings actually a manifestation—a disease or plague—of a very ill society? If so, is it really wise to address the solutions to this illness by focusing myopically on only certain features of the problem, or is it more logical to take a holistic approach? When we get lost in a debate that isolates poor gun control regulations from psychiatric illness as the major culprits leading to gun violence, we become very ineffective public health advocates.

Public health has always relied on two major weapons to combat any illness that affects a large portion of our population—primary and secondary prevention. Primary prevention attacks a health problem as early as possible in the chain of events that ultimately leads to the illness. Secondary prevention focuses later in the process by buffering or shielding the individuals from the illness when the pathogen—the disease-causing entity—attempts to attack them.

These prevention approaches are well characterized by our approach to malaria and Lyme disease. These are illnesses spread by a germ carried in the bodies of insects—the vectors—which eventually bite a person—the host—and inject the germ into their victim's bloodstreams. Once inside the body, if the germ overwhelms the individual's immune system, they then become ill. Primary prevention of such diseases involves eradicating the vectors by killing the insects or preventing them from procreating. Thus, chemicals that kill mosquitos or ticks are delivered to the geographic areas where these insects live and breed. Secondary prevention involves giving medications or vaccines to the hosts who live in areas where these insect vectors are plentiful before they are bitten. The goal is to help the host fight off the germs as they enter their bodies through the bite of the insects. Any truly successful program to fight malaria or Lyme disease combines both primary and secondary prevention.

If we apply this analogy of diseases requiring insect vectors to injure or kill the host to the problem of gun violence in America, the explanation for our present inability to eradicate this plague from our society becomes all too evident. The disease—gun violence—requires that a vector—the gun—delivers the germs—the bullets—into the body of the host—the victim. The political environment in which vector guns proliferate is our own society, which in fact provided a generous source of nutrition for these guns to grow and become stronger. From the days of the American Revolution, when we supported the possession of guns by individuals as a Constitutional right, these weapons morphed from single-bullet systems that required pausing and reloading in between rounds to awesome machines of war that deliver hundreds of rounds within seconds.

When psychiatrically ill people from the past only had knives or single-bullet-delivering guns, there was a limit to the number of people they could attack within a certain timeframe during episodes of violence. Today's enhanced gun vectors now guarantee to allow anyone of sound or unsound mind to effectively deliver huge doses of bullet germs in just minutes into many more host victims than before. It is noteworthy that in other countries today, without the sheer number or sophistication of guns that exist in America, even with similar prevalence of psychiatric illnesses in their societies, the numbers of hosts killed or maimed by bullets is magnitudes lower than in the United States. Without a powerful vector like the AR-15 rifle, neither a psychologically well nor ill person can kill so many people in just moments.

Mosquitos and ticks thrive in certain moist and wooded environments. The current American environment likewise has clearly fostered a greater degree of mental illness and promoted increasing socioeconomic disparities by not adequately preventing or addressing these problems over the past several decades. The psychosocial soil of our society has thus been primed for gun violence to proliferate. With the addition of increased availability of high-round delivering guns, this combination of factors has proved a lethal cocktail.

To eradicate gun violence once and for all, we need to apply both primary and secondary prevention public health strategies. To continue to neglect any component of this complex web of violence is paramount to medical negligence of our whole society. The disease of gun violence will definitely persist and continue to spread as a plague. Primary preventative measures need to address both the vectors—the sophisticated multiple-round guns of war—as well as the environments—psychiatric illness, socioeconomic stressors, and political forces such as the gun lobbies—that this disease leverages to wreak havoc on our nation. Secondary prevention also entails a large gamut of interventions, including public education, to recognize the warning signs of a potentially violent and troubled individual and improved background checks for gun purchasing.

As a veteran physician who daily diagnoses and effectively treats serious and complex medical conditions of multifactorial origin, I know that this approach to the analysis of gun violence should be implemented to appropriately address other grave chronic problems weakening America. To harness our full resources against conditions such as substance abuse, gender and domestic violence, and racism, we must begin by universally agreeing to identify these problems for what they truly are—diseases of our society. Once identified, we must hit such plagues with everything in our arsenal—primary and secondary prevention, as well as potent treatments for those adversely affected—to eradicate them from our midst. We have the resources and capabilities to succeed in this fight. Do we have the willpower to apply them all?

CHAPTER 12

ALL THE PLACES WE CAN GO

After several years of working with Gilbert Tremain, I started noting that the right-sided lower chamber of his heart showed signs of muscle fatigue from the decades of blood leaking back from the malformed valve that led to his lungs. Respecting Gilbert's inclination to leave things well enough alone until absolutely necessary, balanced by his insistence that he be made aware of every detail of his health, I broached the subject with him during a routine biannual visit.

"Gilbert, as we discussed, at some point we may need to consider replacing your pulmonary valve so that your heart does not become irreversibly weakened."

Gilbert responded thoughtfully, "Doc, Dr. Malm told me and my family that the X cut he made on top of my heart to open up the passageway where my deformed and blocked valve used to be was my last operation. I know things change with time, and God knows I probably lived longer than anyone anticipated, but I feel fine right now. Let's just wait a little longer."

I agreed as long as we could increase the visits to three times a year, and he promised to let me know if he felt even the slightest change in his health. We had a deal. Another year went by uneventfully. In the meantime, Harvard reported a very timely study which indicated that Gilbert was once again much more in tune with his health than most.

"I have some news that you probably will find amusing," I started during a late afternoon visit with him. "You seem to know what's going on before it's going on. Remember last year when we talked about replacing your pulmonary valve and you requested that we wait a while? Well, a recent study from this small institution up north, called Harvard, supports your claim. Their research with several adult patients with Tetralogy of Fallot who all have chronic leaky valves now suggests that it may indeed be more dangerous to perform surgery to replace the valve in people over 40 years old than to leave them alone. Their patients did much better with medication to strengthen the heart and limit any irregular heartbeats. They now advise this older group of people not to undergo surgery but instead receive a special pacemaker, called a defibrillator, to help stop any dangerous racing episodes of the heart, called ventricular tachycardia. If we see any signs of this in your heart, that's what we should do."

About two years later, Gilbert's heart indeed started showing brief moments of this ventricular tachycardia on a home monitor study called a Holter. Apparently, Gilbert didn't even notice these episodes because they were so short-lived.

He reassured me, "Doc, I know very well what a serious episode feels like. Remember, I stopped one of these myself right in front of my school teacher many years ago."

I responded with a seriousness and concern that I never had expressed before to Gilbert. "I remember, but you were a teenager then. Your heart is older and has been working against this leaky valve for years. I am worried that it would give out if you had an episode like that again without any way to stop it. You need a special pacemaker called a defibrillator to limit the chance of a life-threatening event, even in your sleep. It's like an insurance policy."

Gilbert drew much quieter than I had ever seen before he responded thoughtfully, "If I was asleep and it stopped, I would not be able to get it going like I did when I was awake and a kid. My wife would have to wake up next to a dead man. Let's look into it, Doc."

I arranged for Gilbert to consult with a colleague of mine who specializes in electrical problems of the heart and places defibrillators in those who could benefit from the added protection. He agreed that Gilbert was a very good candidate to receive this device. However, we ran into a very serious snag. Gilbert's health insurance did not cover a significant portion of the cost of the procedure and associated hospitalization. He simply could not afford it.

I was irate and vowed to Gilbert I would do everything I could to find a way for him to have this procedure without the financial stress. Years before, I was fortunately successful in fighting his insurance company when they denied him an insulin pump device that his doctors thought would best control his diabetes. I wasn't going to sit by after all those years of work to keep his heart healthy, only to let a treatable situation like diabetes get in our way. Gilbert tried on his own, but his temper got the best of him as he wrestled with the insurance company.

"They don't want to talk to me anymore because I get pissed off," he told me.

After two weeks of letters and making calls up the ladder to the medical director of Gilbert's health insurance company, we finally got a call from a representative of the insulin pump company. "I don't know what you said to whom, but all of sudden, we received approval for Mr. Tremain's insulin pump." Gilbert's health and mood improved tremendously after this, and I was determined to do battle once again for his defibrillator.

Gilbert often bragged to my students and staff, "I have had three cardiac catheterizations in total, and I never went to sleep for any of them." Despite his bravado, when a vascular surgeon wanted to insert a catheter with a small camera to see if malfunctioning valves in his leg vessels were the cause of the now-constant swelling of his 70-year-old legs, the ever-skeptical Gilbert hesitated. When the surgeon kept insisting that he pursue the catheterization, Gilbert first had a few questions for the surgeon. He wasn't quite satisfied about the purpose of the procedure. Applying the common sense that had kept him alive and well against all odds, he wanted to know if the surgeon actually had new valves to replace any bad ones he might find with the catheterization. If not, Gilbert simply saw no point in playing around just to look.

He made an appointment to meet the surgeon in person to review his questions. When he arrived, he was told that the surgeon was stuck in the operating room. After some time went by, the doctor's nurse offered to call into the operating room to relay Gilbert's questions. Gilbert recounted the experience to one of my medical students.

"You see, dear, I first wanted to know where he would place the catheter. I was told that it is typically put in the left groin. When I asked him over the phone call into the OR what he was going to do about the scar tissue from previous operations, he was unsure and told me he would get back to me later. That was unacceptable. Even worse, I didn't get his call until two weeks later. You see, in my file, I made it a point to specifically state not to call me between 1:30 and 4:30 p.m. because every day I help my wife with her regular doctor's appointments. Wouldn't you know it, he called me at 3:30 p.m., and I of course missed the call. When I called back right after my wife's appointment, the nurse said the surgeon was now unavailable. She said that it was just a simple procedure and didn't know what all the fuss was about."

When the nurse went on to give Gilbert a list of steps to prepare the day before, he abruptly stopped her. He admitted, by that point, he had become a bit too uptight. He calmly but sternly told the nurse to relay to the doctor that the procedure was not happening.

"You guys just don't seem to be able to get your act together. I have been patient and asked reasonable questions that have not yet been answered by the doctor. The surgeon himself has not even taken the time to read my file to see when I was available to talk on the phone. Anyone that is so incapable of listening, responding, and following a simple request certainly will not be going anywhere near my groin with a scalpel." As he hung up, he was well aware that his bluntness was probably one of his downfalls. But he had no tolerance for anyone's poor performance and never hesitated to tell them so.

FOSTER SOCIETAL PROGRESS THROUGH UNITED PHYSICIAN LEADERSHIP

Despite all of the existing and potential problems in American society's approach to healthcare, I remain hopeful that we still have a tremendous capacity to move forward in a positive direction. Unlike in other countries, where physicians are relegated to functioning purely as civil servants, the tenuous authority wielded by American physicians renders them uniquely poised to play a major part in the evolution of our health system. To secure this authority and privilege, we ultimately have to lay down our psychological shields and economic weapons, drop our defensive posture, and swallow a little humble pie. We can only hope to lead others if we honestly focus on the roles doctors play when things go wrong, instead of reflexively blaming the "system" for our situation. This scapegoat approach only tends to further convince healthcare workers and the public at large that a physician-led healthcare system is a self-serving, fragmented, and powerless institution. Looking to the stars instead of our hearts to find blame creates mistrust and places our profession at a disadvantage when it comes to serving as effective advocates for meaningful healthcare reform.

In the November 1, 2019, Medical Society of the State of New York Newsletter, the presiding president of the society, Dr. Arthur Fougner, openly and rawly expressed this sentiment. "Do you recall the days when physicians dictated every manner in which medicine was practiced? I do. Today, those days seem just a lovely dream," he writes. "Patient care was once the physician's *raison d'être*. Now it's an inconvenient truth. Physicians are always the good guys, the nice guys, the ones who, when reimbursements are cut, are reduced to plaintively requesting, as Oliver Twist once did, 'Please, sir, I want some more.' Remember that moment in every Popeye cartoon when our sailor, finally at his limit, reached for his spinach, exclaiming, 'That's all I can stand 'cause I can't stand no more.' Would you rather just settle into Kübler-Ross's Acceptance and simply shuffle off to watch the sunset?"

If we physicians begin to stop seeing ourselves as the proverbial victims, we can then start to take a much-needed proactive approach. As a case in point, only when we face the reality that our field may create as many, if not more, medical problems than we solve, such as medication errors, infections, and addictions, can we truly begin to best address these unfortunate and frustrating products of our present practice patterns. Likewise, we cannot hope to tackle the frustration of poorly designed EMR systems—which break down inter-professional communications and tear us away from our patients and families due to the inordinate amount of time we now spend behind our computer screens and tablets—if we do not fully participate in and guide the design of future alternative solutions such as artificial intelligence systems.

As a physician, I also believe that we must also not shirk our historically unique role as power brokers in US society. We are entitled by society to maintain this leadership position, not through any selfish economic benefits we may procure but by promoting the welfare of our patients. American medicine uniquely evolved under a system intrinsically tied politically, socially, culturally, and economically to the pursuit of no less than our ideals of life, liberty, and happiness itself. Without health, how can any one of our patients ever truly and fully hope to achieve these ideals?

We physicians must stay the course, even when moving forward is tough and we feel alone. I sense that American society portrays a significant degree of indecisiveness in regards to our government's strategic goals for our healthcare system. Simply stated, we are a fickle people. This opens the door for distractions that erode our highest principles and hinder progress in improving how we care for each other. When faced with seemingly insurmountable challenges, we tend to hand off our responsibilities too quickly to those who reap the benefits at the cost of depriving others of their rights to equitably access quality health services.

When threatened individually, we tend to become selfish to protect ourselves and our loved ones. These actions contradict our most basic democratic principle that attests to the belief that when we lift up someone else in need, we all do better. With every sick patient under my care, I never give up trying to make and keep them well. I remain stubbornly optimistic. Similarly, because our healthcare system itself is in dire need of treatment, the medical profession must not conclude that, at its very core, the whole American healthcare system is irreparably broken and thus abandon any hopes it can be healed.

I am convinced that though the fundamental values of our healthcare system may be buried out of sight under deep piles of bureaucracy and waste, they remain vital and intact. Americans united must reclaim these values and bring them up to the surface and into the light for all to witness. We will then all see that the engine of our health system is still fundamentally good. We simply have a few flat tires and need a tune-up.

More to the point, we may realize that we have been driving this vehicle through too many side roads or, at times, even led completely off course. Because we now find ourselves hitting potholes and debris, resulting in even more flat tires and wear and tear, we can now admit to ourselves that we should not have steered off the main road in the first place. The engine in this analogy is clearly the prioritization of a patient-centered healthcare system supported by strong patient-physician relationships. This focus is what moves the system forward, and we must all ensure that it remains the driving force. Any entity with ulterior motives that threatens to veer us off course in our collective journey should not be welcome to come along with the rest of us.

Physicians and society in collaboration should publicly hold strong to the fact that these values are paramount to a successful healthcare system and accordingly guide our government in a direction that supports this particular road as the route of preference. If through our silence, we let anyone, especially our own government or corporations, create systems that steer us from our intended path, I suggest that every American should intellectually and philosophically consider themselves ultimately responsible for any accidents that will undoubtedly occur as we deviate off the main road. Physicians should still see themselves as the GPS system for healthcare and not relegate this responsibility to others unfamiliar with the best roads. When we give up this role, those we are supposed to guide will inevitably become lost and us along with them. When the medical profession allows those less capable to drive and guide without our experience, there will be more accidents and chaos than ever existed in the old system we are proposing to "fix."

As we finish our medical school education, all students pledge a solemn oath to uphold certain ethical standards, to include maintaining patient confidentiality and doing no harm to those we professionally care for in the future. This promise is based upon the principles exemplified by the Greek physician Hippocrates almost 2,500 years ago. As practicing physicians, we are ethically and legally bound to this oath by our society.

The reality is that, all too often, as soon as we leave our protected academic towers, physicians readily leave the standards of care we were taught in training. We become a ragtag army with little leadership and consistency. Even the most cursory postmortem analysis of our response to COVID-19 highlights the pitfalls of such a chaotic approach to a universally dangerous health problem. The lay public expected that the medical profession would deliver the same standard of care throughout our borders. They soon learned the hard way, through the tragic loss of life and economic stability, that health standards differed significantly between communities and states. Even higher institutions such as the Centers for Disease Control and Prevention, the Food and Drug Administration, and the National Institute of Health appeared to openly disagree on the best course of action against the pandemic. Fear and anxiety understandably reigned in this atmosphere, and the people needed their physicians to calm the waters. This inconsistency of healthcare standards needs to be addressed if physicians are to maintain any credibility and effectively treat the public. We must also not forget that healthcare belongs to everyone, and outside forces will have no choice but to take control back from the medical profession if they do not step up to address this critical issue.

The large corporations and government are keenly aware of the important role the health profession plays in this American experiment and often attempt to limit the scope of our influence over the general populace. In other words, we threaten these power brokers because they perceive that, through our profession's concerted efforts to serve the welfare of others, doctors "control" the highly valued and vital commodity of health. Doctors thus possess the political clout to dominate a large portion of our economic resources.

The Obama administration openly justified the need for the ACA[75] on the basis that our economy could never hope to recover and remain resilient if we did not address the impact of runaway healthcare-related expenditures. Physicians as individuals and collectively our profession must take both some of the blame and the credit for our role in this financial double-edged sword. On the other hand, we need to publicly counter the disinformation campaign of the other power brokers that portray physicians as responsible for the greatest proportion of healthcare-related costs and, as so blatantly demonstrated during the

75 Furman, Jason, "Six Economic Benefits of the Affordable Care Act," The White House, Feb. 6, 2014 (online), https://obamawhitehouse.archives.gov/blog/2014/02/06/six-economic-benefits-affordable-care-act.

COVID-19 pandemic, an institution that wants to take away people's freedoms.

To claim legitimate authority in the present, tangled healthcare reform debate fueled by selfish agendas, physicians must counter the perception that we are helpless puppets of an oppressive system. A unified, physician-guided health profession must step forward as advocates and leaders of an empowered patient community to transparently address the health system problems we face now and in the future. We need to create a strong positive narrative if we are to regain any justified control of society's health standards and expectations. As Gilbert so poignantly demonstrated by his experience with the vascular surgeon, we first need to tidy our own house before we can be invited to clean entire communities and the nation. If doctors cannot give patients the time to discuss why and how we plan to invade people's bodies with procedures and medications, why should they ever be granted society's trust to handle and guide the policies and direction of the healthcare system at large? Physicians professionally may also feel safer to remain within their own walls and reluctant to enter into the overwhelming outside political fray. If the larger house we call America is to remain intact, doctors have no other choice. Current reality dictates that the US medical profession needs to enter into base polemics to stand as a political force for good in the advancement of health for all.

As engaged physician leaders helping to create the map of our healthcare system, in conjunction with policymakers, we must apply the Hippocratic standards we swore to as we designate the best locations to place these roads. The only role of our local and federal governments should be to build and then keep these roads open and clear for everyone to access equitably. Government should never be granted the power to alter the course of this health system independent of society's wishes. The road we Americans choose to travel should be designated according to the best interests of all our people. The collaboration between the medical profession and laypeople, which is essential to mutual success, can only exist when doctors and patients freely engage together on the road. Through this process, this journey, we can best demonstrate that the moral and ethical compass of American healthcare is a good one, aiming upward to the True North. It is not forever broken. It just needs to be reinforced and brought back to the front lines in this war against disease that physicians and their allied healthcare professionals are especially well trained to fight.

Though there may be inherent problems and conflicts of interest with the advent of large medical entities, such as corporate-based hospitals or large, private practice mega-groups, they provide several advantages. Their sheer size provides significant clout in negotiations with several of the other major players in the healthcare business that a single physician or small group of doctors simply does not wield. In the early part of this millennium, as soon as these larger entities came into being in my geographic area of New York's Hudson Valley, the medical insurance companies I worked productively with for several years stopped sending representatives to my office.

"We simply do not have the resources to negotiate with groups of less than five physicians," my contact at Oxford Healthcare explained over the phone. "We appreciate and have enjoyed our relationship with you these past several years, but it has become much more efficient for us to work with the larger groups. They can best leverage good reimbursement rates with us due to their large volume of patients. You should probably consider joining one of them."

This leverage also applied to other aspects of running my office, to include working with office and medical supply vendors. When I eventually joined a larger entity of almost 400 physicians in 2016, I was amazed to see the costs of items as basic as paper or telephone fees cut by 50 to 75 percent overnight. I literally could tell some of my original vendors to take a hike if they did not relieve me of some of the outstanding debt incurred by the proportionately higher fees they charged my original four-physician practice. If they wished to continue doing business with me and expand to my now much-larger customer base, they had to demonstrate why I should still support their services with my new entity. Those that met me at least halfway on my old debts all continued to operate and grow significantly with me. Those that refused I quickly paid off and jettisoned from my business life. It is no surprise that many of these less cooperative entities are themselves now struggling or no longer exist. My membership in a larger entity clearly allowed me to survive the rougher economic times.

My relationship with the larger entity, sponsored by one of the most prestigious medical centers in the country—Boston Children's Hospital of Harvard University—also allowed me to return to my original larger academic world with better clinical recognition and support than when I was a standalone, small, private, community-based entity. After starting my education and career at Columbia University, followed by a clinical professorship at the Albert Einstein College of Medicine, I found myself detached from a prestigious teaching-institution for three years. In 2016, 18 years since coming to this New York suburban community, I returned to academia through this association with Harvard.

Whether I participated in a local community hospital project, referred patients to a world-class tertiary hospital, or called the New York State Department of Health, my affiliation with Boston Children's carried more weight. I would like to believe that it was purely my age, experience, and track record that spoke for me, but I recognize that many similarly experienced and qualified colleagues of mine did not have the same degree of influence as me simply because they remained with smaller and less worldly recognized entities.

Under Boston Children's, I could continue forward with many of the projects I envisioned years ago but was unable to achieve as a small medical practice bogged down by excessive costs and administrative duties. Over the past six years, I have expanded my clinical services in several more sites, collaborated on the development of new local children's hospital-based services, and solidified the scope of my role as a medical educator for a growing medical student community. I now work daily with the regional medical schools, residency programs, and nurse practitioner and physician assistant schools. I taught and increased my pool of community-based medical technicians for unique diagnostic tests, now branching into pediatric specialties other than cardiology.

Together with my original small cohort, the larger Boston Children's team is creating a regional consortium of specialists dealing with prenatal and perinatal high-risk pregnancies. We are officially part of the New York State registry for cardiac birth defects—a status which formerly was only attained by tertiary medical centers. Spewed on by the pandemic, we developed a robust pediatric telehealth service that reaches out more consistently to families less able to take time off to attend in-person doctor appointments and to patients in more remote regions. On the horizon are several potential exciting projects, including a local pediatric clinical and community health research center, as well as a series of diagnosis-based multispecialty clinics.

I cannot overstate my general sense of improved professional and intellectual well-being afforded by my partnership with a larger prestigious entity. I am so appreciative of the opportunity to discuss patient management with colleagues in the hallways of my office on a daily basis. Even my desire to return to writing medical essays has been reawoken. Most importantly, the range of medical services that I can provide my own patients and other children in their own community has been enhanced. This fact alone reassures me that I made the right choice to join the larger group.

As our society inevitably ventures into the realm of population health management discussed in the previous chapter, the reimbursement model of FFS is transitioning into a VBC approach. If physicians are to preserve any degree of clout in the American healthcare system, they must both fully understand and help guide the policies behind this transition.

The concept of population health encompasses the global healthcare services provided to all the patients of a medical practice, not just those who show up in the doctor's office, clinics, or emergency rooms. In an FFS system, the doctor is paid for the medical services of only the patients they actually see and touch in the office or hospital. The actual outcome resulting from the care rendered is never a consideration in this system. If the patient does well, they simply do not return or require fewer visits for this problem. If they do not get better, they simply return to receive and get billed for additional medical attention and testing.

In a VBC reimbursement scheme, the actual well-being of the patient is considered in the payment model. This requires that all the patients under a physician's care—whether they show up or not to the office—are evaluated and considered when calculating the final payments to the doctor or the medical institution for which they work. This VBC can increase these reimbursements by achieving improved population-wide outcomes. They can also be penalized financially for bad outcomes. These outcomes are all tracked using the EMRs. An alternative tactic available to the VBC system is the option to "share" the burden of health outcomes between the practitioners and the payors. Thus the practitioners and their employers are essentially provided one standard payment for a patient's diagnosis. The more complex the problem, the higher the reimbursement amount. If the medical practitioners improve the patient's care successfully, and at a lower cost than the standard reimbursement, they pocket the excess as an incentive.

If the medical providers are to survive economically and, I would argue, psychologically, through the transition to a VBC population health model, they must change their practice policies and patterns from an individual provider to a collaborative care team (CCT) approach. A large medical entity is more capable to provide such team services than a solo physician or small group practice. The concept behind a CCT is much more prevention-based than that of an FFS system. If a diabetic patient, for example, can be provided with regular home nurse visits, home blood sugar level checks, and nutritionist services, the likelihood they will crash into the office or hospital with a severe diabetic crisis is significantly reduced. A large multidisciplinary practice or clinic can also theoretically offer general and specialty medical care in a much more coordinated and streamlined fashion than separate independent small silo practices. Over a lifetime, the cost of providing healthcare to such a diabetic patient is minimized significantly by this more proactive CCT approach. If the reimbursements are set at an appropriate level, the potential exists for both the payors and the practitioners to benefit.

Stephen was a 14-year-old, strikingly handsome, five-foot-nine-inch boy who reportedly fainted in school two weeks prior. Until he was fully evaluated and cleared medically, he was restricted from returning to school and was home-tutored in the meantime. Upon arrival at my office, my team and I immediately noted that he was extremely thin. The mother commented that he lost about 20 pounds over the past month and now weighed in at 94 pounds. He had been restricting his diet to one meal per day and increased his aerobic exercise to two daily sessions of one hour each.

Most curiously, his mother obtained a video recording of his fainting episode through a hallway camera at the school. She played it for me on her smartphone. As I watched, I saw him rush out of his classroom door and walk briskly to the bathroom entrance just 10 yards up the corridor. She then fast-forwarded the video about 15 minutes later, just as he peeked his head out of the bathroom door. He suddenly leaped to the other side of the hall, landing against a row of built-in lockers. As he literally forced himself down the hall, back toward the classroom, he constantly clung onto the wall of lockers. Almost as if he were rock climbing, he gradually grabbed lower and lower onto each successive locker until, after eight yards, now virtually across the door from the classroom he initially exited, he finally lay completely face down on the floor. He was motionless for almost another 10 minutes as the school bell rang, indicating the end of the current class time. He was quickly discovered by some of his fellow students, and the teachers and school nurse were called. The video recording ended as he was roused and taken away in a wheelchair to the nurse's office out of range of the camera.

His mother was called by the nurse, and she met the ambulance as it arrived at the local hospital. There, he underwent observation and extensive testing for almost 12 hours. In the end, everything came up normal, and he was discharged home in baseline condition, weighing 114 pounds. They were advised to see his pediatrician and consider cardiology and neurologic evaluations. The mother's intuition also led her to subsequently request the video recording.

When Stephen arrived in my office, and after I reviewed the video, I knew that my successful evaluation could not be rushed. He was shy and obviously very hesitant to tell me what happened. I needed to earn his trust if I was going to help him. Because he was not verbally forthcoming, I knew I could take the condensed, efficient, and passive approach that many other specialists do and simply order a bunch of tests after a brief physical exam. The visit would take 10 to 15 minutes, and I could charge for these tests.

I decided to focus on getting him to talk, even though this entailed no extra fees for testing and would take up to 45 minutes. As I joked with him about other topics and occasionally patted his shoulder encouragingly, he began to warm up. Within 20 minutes, I consciously guided him back to the topic of school and his aspirations for a future career. He was obviously very bright and actually quite mature. I learned that his father had left him and his mother when he was only five years old. The mother then had to return to a full-time job, and Stephen often came home from school before she did. Recently, as he started the ninth grade, the mother noted that he began skipping school. This was very unusual for him, and she sternly forced him to return. She in fact made a concerted effort to drive him to school herself, even though this meant he arrived almost 20 minutes before school started. He also developed the habit of exercising every day in their downstairs home gym. A few weeks later, he began skipping dinner, saying he ate a late lunch.

I asked him about school and if he liked the ninth grade. He confided that he liked most of his classes but did not like the first-period class. This happened to be the very same class that he was attending during the video recording. I then ended my inquiries regarding school and moved onto my exam and reviewed his electrocardiogram. I reassured him that everything appeared to be normal so far and invited them to return in one week for a follow-up visit. As I did so, I pulled out a piece of paper to sign in front of him, indicating that he was cleared to return to school.

"Do I have to?" Stephen blurted out. "I am doing so much better with the home tutor. Can I just wait one more week?"

Applying my suspicions, I countered, "Would you like to return but skip first period?"

Stephen paused. "You can let me do that? Sure, that would be great." He finally smiled.

Over the next two days, I called the school nurse, principal, and the family social worker. As the discussions proceeded, it became clear from the school and other students that the first-period teacher had been publicly picking on Stephen from day one. Many of his verbal attacks were directed toward Stephen's body build and how he was out of shape. The other students admitted that they were very uncomfortable with these exchanges as well.

The principal confided that the teacher had a history of similar interactions with colleagues and other students. At the next visit, Stephen confessed that he was very frightened by this man and was trying to get into better shape and lose weight to make him stop criticizing him. The school psychologist thought that this young man without a father figure may have been particularly sensitive to such attacks by a male authority figure. She also surmised that this disturbed man probably instinctively sensed this vulnerability. The teacher was fired the next week and brought up on legal charges as well. He would hopefully never teach again or work with children.

Two months later, Stephen was back to his baseline weight and loving school.

Over the years, my clinical style in caring for patients has been recognized by patients and colleagues as both compassionate and effective. Recently, I again came across medical literature describing the term and importance of "emotional intelligence." This concept embodies the philosophy of patient care that I practice daily and which I wholeheartedly applied in Stephen's case. I learned objectively that I may indeed have a significantly high level of this emotional IQ (EQ), which did not develop in a vacuum. I likely modeled my EQ through a combination of the nurturing interactions with my parents as well as the examples set by some of my most esteemed medical education mentors. I practice in this way both because I truly care and because it works. I also strive to teach this approach to my own students as a conscientious clinical maneuver. I explain, when it comes to interactions with patients, "Care enough to be curious. Be curious enough to show you care."

Recently, this EQ has piqued the interest of healthcare policymakers[76] as a potentially effective skill for patient-centered care models. They recognize that the physicians who take the time to apply this approach have an objectively higher level of patient well-being outcomes and spend far less money in the process. In Stephen's case, I ordered no tests and literally submitted FFS invoices to the family's health insurance company at a fraction of the level that a testing-based, 10-minute visit would cost. I in turn was able to spend the necessary time with Stephen because I was relieved of many of my former operational burdens of practice management by my new large-scale employer's organizational infrastructure.

Whenever I took the same time-intensive EQ-based approach with a patient in the past, I was obliged to either swallow the resulting loss of patient volume and revenue or work twice as hard to make up for this deficit. Under Boston Children's, my new business model freed up many hours per week formerly dedicated to my management duties. They also negotiated higher FFS reimbursements with the insurance companies while lowering my overhead costs. The resulting liberated time allowed me to see a greater volume of patients and, when the circumstances dictated, appropriately spend more time with them. The former excessive economic pressure was off of me, and I could apply my clinical style more freely.

The large entity also has the potential to provide population-based health resources, such as social services and home nurse visits, that

76 Birks, Yvonne F. and Watt, Ian S., "Emotional Intelligence and Patient-Centered Care," *J R Social Med.*, 100 (8): 368-374, Aug. 2007, https://www.ncbi.nlm.nih.gov/pmc/articles/PMC1939962/.

complement my clinical care. This type of operational approach better shields individual practitioners from extraneous bureaucratic, operational, and financial stressors and promotes skills such as emotional intelligence. Thus, the large entity and the individual clinician have the potential to function in a symbiotic relationship that benefits everyone—patient, provider, and business. The individual clinician can and should avail themselves of the operational infrastructure and population health resources provided by the larger entity. The larger entity should likewise support and strengthen the individual providers' most valuable assets so they can do what they do best—provide emotionally intuitive, health-promoting, patient-physician relationships.

Unlike the approach taken by many large corporate entities, the validation of clinical factors and skills such as EQ reveals that there is actually no advantage to altering the fundamentals of patient-centered care in favor of perceived time efficiencies and high volumes of patient visits and procedures. This productive collaboration between the individual doctor encouraged to apply their best EQ and the well-run large entity has the potential to thrive within the paradigm of a population health-oriented healthcare system.

I attend medical conferences several times each year. Though the stimulus to break from the daily routine and seek out some forum for further education stems in large part from credentialing requirements imposed by health insurance companies, many of my colleagues and I look forward to the academic stimulation these events provide. As with other professions, a component of these conferences is indeed social and allows for political networking with old and new colleagues. I always come away from a pediatric cardiology or even one of my wife's adult gastroenterology conferences with new information regarding advancements or novel discoveries. Here I find a renewed appreciation for the academic side of medicine, especially the pure high-caliber research that provides the empirical evidence to move us all forward.

For weeks after these conferences, my mind hums with new ideas for clinical research that will further some of the work of others most relevant to my patient care. Over the past two decades, I have been regularly invited to several conferences as an expert and educator to speak about some of my own clinical work and experiences. This adds a whole new dimension to these conferences for me because, as a speaker, I can engage in formal question-and-answer discussions or debates with my co-speakers and the audience. In this intellectual and collegial environment, my colleagues and I push ourselves to expand our minds and hearts so that we can continue to become better physicians, not for ourselves, but to better serve our patients and communities. If physicians are to be perceived as authorities to guide the health of individuals or the public, regular attendance to such forums of continuing education must be sustained.

Through the vehicle of these continued medical education conferences, I am relieved to notice that, for the most part, physicians still place a high value and emphasis on research that improves patient and community health outcomes. In the 2010s, aspiring physicians and other clinicians have more technology-driven tools potentially at their disposal than ever before to achieve these lofty goals. However, such resources are not free. Regretfully, in the United States, as with other disciplines in our society, such as the arts and environmental protection, the priority level granted to medical research[77] is too often dependent on the whims of a particular state or federal government's administration. The level of government-derived financial

77 Achenbach, Joel; McGinley, Laurie, Goldstein, Amy; Guarino, Ben, "Trump Budget Cuts Funding for Health, Science, Environment Agencies," *The Washington Post*, Feb. 10, 2020 (online), https://www.washingtonpost.com/science/trump-budget-cuts-funding-for-health-science-environment-agencies/2020/02/10/9c8dd784-4c2d-11ea-b721-9f4cdc90bc1c_story.html.

support such as research grants is directly dependent on the politics and macroeconomics of the day.

Private entities such as the AMA have to play a much bigger role to subsidize important research when government priorities are dragged elsewhere or during times of financial strain. I find it hypocritical and ignorant when politicians promote healthcare reform as a major component of their campaigns, only to later question the need for research funding. In doing so, they make it all too clear that they do not understand that research is fundamental to healthcare reform and the evolution of the medical sciences. It is time for all healthcare providers to step up as leaders of healing to reinforce the importance of supporting the creation and implementation of technologies through sound, evidence-based research. As physician scientists, we must reclaim control of advancements in healthcare from the realm of shallow politics. This effort requires physician advocacy at all levels of government so the pilots of healthcare can advocate for the best design and operation of the planes that carry our health services to all in need.

Healthcare and medical care, though interdependent conceptually, are not identical in practice. At risk of oversimplifying their distinctions, healthcare encompasses the policies and mechanisms by which medical care, such as drug treatments or surgeries, are actually made accessible to patients and communities. Medical care practiced in isolation without an effective healthcare delivery system is a purely intellectual and practically useless venture. Likewise, the pursuit of pure medical research without any mechanism to facilitate the application of the end products or discoveries to ultimately help treat or cure someone is basically biological research in a vacuum.

This is not to discredit the value of pursuing pure research without the Damocles sword of productivity or economic profit constantly hanging over a scientist's head. Discoveries brought to life in this unadulterated manner often have applications that would not have been foreseen if a blinded focus aimed in only one direction—such as one disease—was the only envisioned scientific motive. Thankfully, many wise people today and their institutions have realized that research and development (aka R&D) can be mutually compatible. Together, R&D can promote the advancement of medical science by facilitating the rapid transitions of scientific theories to discoveries and ultimately to practical applications.

I have worked at several institutions of higher learning, as well as with private enterprises, where leaders created environments to facilitate pure research while simultaneously providing the necessary resources to bring the scientific discoveries born in these protected spaces to the real world. With the application of the Internet and very powerful computer-based technologies over the past two to three decades, the speed with which hypotheses lead to new scientific knowledge that positively impacts all areas of science and medicine has increased exponentially.

While training to be a pediatric cardiologist in the late 1990s, I spent several months working in the animal research laboratories at Columbia. While there, I witnessed many remarkable physicians of repute make scientific discoveries that quickly became part of the standard of care for clinical medicine. One of these physicians was the young heart surgeon, Dr. Mehmet Oz, who was one of the principal investigators at the Columbia Institute of Comparative Medicine. He had been a mentor of mine in medical school, and we occasionally worked together in the care of mutual patients.

"What are you studying with all those pigs?" I asked him one late fall day when he and I were the only two people still hanging around the lab.

"Interesting you ask. Since you are a pediatric cardiologist, you probably will be quite interested in this work. We are trying to figure out why some kids who have been hit hard in the chest by projectiles like baseballs suddenly collapse and die. We think the heart basically gets stunned and has a concussion, but we are not sure how this leads to death. We are using the animals to recreate a model of this real-world situation so that we can better understand, prevent, and treat children faced with this event."

Dr. Oz described the phenomena known as *commotio cordis.*[78] Because of similar research in Columbia and other institutions such as Boston's Tufts University, it was discovered that a projectile, such as a small hard ball, hitting a child's chest at over 30 miles per hour could cause the bottom of the heart to suddenly begin to quiver erratically. This abnormal electrical heart rhythm pattern, known as ventricular fibrillation, prevents the bottom chambers of the heart—the ventricles—from squeezing in the normal coordinated fashion in response to regular signals from the top of the heart. If not corrected immediately, the child will not receive sufficient blood supply to the body, collapse, and die within seconds. The clarification of the mechanism by which *commotio cordis* killed led to the sports industry modification of baseballs, bats, lacrosse equipment, and chest protectors, as well as the awareness of the need to immediately implement CPR to an unconscious victim of such an impact.

Years later, I joined a New York state and nationwide parent advocacy group as a medical director to screen and educate children and their families to prevent and recognize sudden cardiac arrest and death. Two of the nonphysician leaders of these remarkable programs, known as Heart Screen New York[79] and Parent Heart Watch,[80] an energetic and beloved Long Island couple, Karen and John Acompora, repeatedly expressed their regret that such scientifically based research was not

78 Link, Mark S., "Commotio Cordis: Ventricular Fibrillation Triggered by Chest Impact-Induced Abnormalities in Repolarization," *Circulation: Arrhythmia and Electrophysiology*, 5: 425-432, Apr. 2012, https://www.ahajournals.org/doi/full/10.1161/circep.111.962712.

79 "Home: Heart Screen New York," Heart Screen New York, https://heartscreennewyork.com/.

80 "Parent Heart Watch: Sudden Cardiac Arrest in Youth Prevention: SCA," Parent Heart Watch, https://parentheartwatch.org/.

in place to prevent the death of their own son from *commotio cordis*. Together, physicians, investigators, clinicians, researchers, and non-medical community members formed incredibly effective advocacy institutions, such as The Marfan Foundation and The Muscular Dystrophy Association. Because of physician leadership in research and advocacy groups, countless lives have been and will continue to be saved.

I would argue that, today, clinicians—not purely profit-motivated people—hold both the legitimate right and the means, if they so wish, to harness and control the applications of their discoveries to advance medical care. They can only do so if they also actively help guide the policies by which these discoveries may become part of healthcare. We must be wary and appropriately cynical of the intentions of the proverbial venture capitalists who lurk in the hallways outside the medical research laboratories, hoping to make a quick buck off of any new discoveries.

In the next generation, we need to focus much more attention on the dynamic between medical treatments and cures and how they are actually delivered to our people. In doing so, we should not become preoccupied with catering to transient political agendas and corporate shareholders who live for moments of power and wealth without a vision for the long term. This is not to neglect or underestimate the potentially favorable impact that political entities and capitalism can have on the speed and direction that medical and healthcare will take. With the right physician leadership and proactive use of these amazing technological tools now available, a free society with good government and industry representation can overcome many of the misguided political and greed-motivated obstacles.

I reiterate that where healthcare goes, a society will go. If this were not so, then our current-day politicians would not be so focused on healthcare reform as of late. Sadly, their constant focus upon economics in isolation from the goal of achieving the best healthcare outcomes deters the well-meaning efforts of many medical professions and policymakers. To address this disconnect, I have made a concerted effort to attend meetings where physicians better align with their political representatives and thus achieve mutual goals that address both quality and cost. Such forums attest to the recognition that politicians cannot be successful in healthcare policy and delivery without healthcare professionals leading the way.

Fortunately, though publicly and repeatedly threatened, the emphasis on physician leadership has not been completely abandoned in this era of healthcare reform. An engineer cannot build the best airplane without consulting the best pilots. The best pilots cannot be called the "best" just because they fly high and fast, but also because of a sound and enduring safety record and principles that they promote while on the ground. Society has to ultimately choose what kind of pilots they want to transport and guide them to their desired destination. Along the way, we must also never forget that in a true democracy, the good pilots strive to allow anyone to choose to be a passenger, not just those who can afford a high-priced first-class ticket.

Like many Americans in 2019, I found myself earnestly trying to tease out the policy differences amongst the 2020 presidential candidates regarding their comprehension of the problems that erode the American healthcare system and how they plan to address them. As I read and listened to their words on the campaign trail, it became all too clear to me that the forest had been lost in the trees by both the current and potential leaders. There was far too much intellectual capital focused on bureaucratic minutia, such as statistics, data procurement, and endless protocols—the individual trees. Such endless details tend to render the audience numb and distract their attention away from the big-picture reality that the well-being of the whole community remains far from ideal—the forest.

I believe that we should avoid becoming lost in the tangled woods as we navigate through the solutions to our healthcare deficits. I agree wholeheartedly that improving individual and population healthcare outcomes while reducing costs are rational and worthwhile objectives. However, doing so by increasing and overemphasizing the relative importance of the bureaucracy buries physicians under piles of menial tasks that drag them away from direct patient care. This approach is not logically sound.

For any forest to be healthy, the soil must be nutrient-rich. The forest of high-quality healthcare is best ensured when the soil that feeds and nurtures it is nutrient-rich. My career taught me that the standards that allowed the American healthcare system to be so exceptionally fruitful have always been rooted in the rich soil of our high-quality medical education. To produce high yields of the best-quality medical professionals, student physicians and allied health professionals need to start their careers with sound training according to a strong and consistent curriculum. I remain satisfied that, despite constant assaults by profiteers, the fundamental role and standards of medical education remain virtually intact.

A quality education best promotes doctors inclined to consistently obtain a thorough medical history and examination as the launching pad for each of their patient encounters. When a physician is well-trained in the first place, this history and physical exam-guided approach to clinical care assures the most appropriate use of testing and medications by a doctor. There is no easy access to diagnoses and treatments hidden somewhere deep in the magic woods of computer algorithms or smartphone applications. It is the hard work of tilling the soil through training and dedicated practice that ultimately achieves the best healthcare outcomes. Technologies such as advanced diagnostics and EMRs, standards of care provided through best practices or guidelines, clinical protocols and policies, and continuing education during one's career all work best when supported by a strong foundation of education.

Medical education within a supportive healthcare environment that does not lead the physician away from the bedrock principles of patient care is a critical component of physicians' abilities to maintain legitimate authority at the helm of our healthcare system. If sound education is well-reinforced by a united community of medical educators and practitioners, then there remains less need for any outside entities to come into our professional sphere to recreate the wheel or keep doctors "in line."

I remain optimistic about American physicians' abilities to be leading advocates for meaningful improvements in healthcare. I see many medical education institutions and my students implementing the core education principles upon which the advances that originally elevated America's medical reputation were made. They seek a return to the original soil that produced revolutionary therapies such as those which allowed a young Gilbert Tremain to grow old with a high quality of life.

As one of my graduating fourth-year medical students so eloquently wrote in a thank you letter to me after being accepted to the residency program of her choice, "I was originally so hesitant to stick it out and finish medical school. I was disheartened because it appeared that the medical field recently wandered so far off course from my vision of being a doctor that I would never be happy professionally. I saw so many of my mentor physicians swallowed up by computer reports and bureaucratic documentation that they were unable to spend quality hands-on time with their patients. Thank you for sharing your patient-focused approach and for pushing me not to give up hope that I could still be the kind of doctor who really gets to know their patients."

I am so proud of this young physician and so many of my students who believe and understand that a strong patient-physician interaction is the source of the rich soil that promotes the best medical education.

All the myriad of manifestations that healthcare reform pursues, such as ACOs and legislation such as the ACA described in previous chapters, operate best when they support meaningful interactions between doctors and their patients. These policy efforts deplete this life-sustaining soil of nutrients when they carelessly try to replace it.

I am well aware that the roller coaster of ever-changing political biases, and the myriad of systems spawned from them, are at times very frustrating for young and seasoned physicians alike. I earnestly wish that there was a strict separation of healthcare and politics similar to America's professed goal of separation of church and state. Despite these challenges, I remain confident that American physicians still have the upper hand intellectually and technologically as long as they strive to refocus their efforts on achieving the highest-quality patient-based healthcare system. I am also convinced that regardless of the economics, no sane political entity in any free society such as the United States would feel obliged to undermine or interfere in a top-10 level healthcare system, especially in a country as complex as ours.

The truth is that, in today's complex world, the government would rather focus on other things such as national security, infrastructure, the environment, and employment. They would be thrilled to leave the bulk of the management of healthcare to medical professionals. However, even if we had a relatively low-cost healthcare model, if America continues along our current path of a healthcare system ranking internationally in the 30s, our government and policymakers are forced to intervene. Reason dictates that in such a low-level healthcare system, the individuals themselves who receive this suboptimal healthcare will be disgruntled and demand better from their political leaders.

To return to the plane analogy once again, even an airline with cheap seats will go out of business if the passengers are sufficiently unhappy during the flight. If patients cannot look to the medical profession for guidance in improving healthcare, they cannot be blamed for turning to the less-equipped political entities for assistance. They need the government to step in and address the inadequacies of healthcare that foster a destructive divide in mutual respect and loyalty between politicians and medical institutions at multiple levels in our society. This led to the public display of a very dysfunctional and ultimately devastatingly poor American response to the COVID-19 pandemic.

The challenge for healthcare professionals in this free society is to be seen as servants who step up to the plate to improve the standards of our healthcare. Physician leaders in America are challenged by their communities to remain focused on delivering the highest-quality healthcare products to patients. People do not want their doctors to accept or follow the politicians' tactic of streamlining the healthcare delivery system to the point that it becomes impersonal, empty, and meaningless for patients. Americans want their doctors to remain autonomous professionals dedicated to humane and emotionally rich patient care, not mindless public servants.

A miserable airplane flight by an impersonal robot remains unsatisfactory even if the destination is wonderful. The truth is and always has been that together physicians and their patients are the only ones who hold the key to success in the arena of healthcare reform. The challenge is to build this high-quality healthcare system using all the tools available in this rich land while never letting go of the core of the system—a close patient-physician relationship. We physicians, regardless of our place of practice and the challenges that face us, each in our own little or big way, must decisively and continuously move forward as advocates for a constantly improving healthcare system. Together, with the experience and guidance of those more senior physicians, along with the vitality, enthusiasm, and intellect of those younger disciples of medicine, there is no effective impediment that can deter us from enabling our healthcare system to reach its full potential to serve our people.

DISTILL LESSONS FROM LEADERS

How could I have almost forgotten my much-anticipated meeting with Patrick Dollard? Thankfully, I set up this appointment months in advance and put it in my electronic reminder calendar. I just returned from a much-needed family break to Europe. My flight landed late the night before. As my alarm reminder sounded, I looked down at my phone to see the scheduled appointment later that afternoon with the president and CEO of the institution where my monthly morning clinic was taking place that day. It would be a long first day back to work.

Jet lag kicked in on that dreary, overcast December morning in 2019 as I drove the hour-long journey northward through the winding hills. Each month for over a decade, I had come to the Center for Discovery—a remarkable institution focused on novel approaches to caring for children and adults with severe neurologic impairments. Ever since my first visit to the Center, I was instantly captivated by the dedication and forward thinking literally embedded in the walls of the myriad of environmentally compatible buildings strategically and ever-so-thoughtfully placed throughout the hillsides of the campus. The staff at all levels exuded a contagious focus and warmth, and I readily agreed to offer my clinical services to the patients and residents there.

It occurred to me several months earlier that the general philosophy of the Center for Discovery was not only unique amongst its peers, but also very much aligned with the values I struggled for years to elucidate. The Center came to represent a striking microcosm of some of the best approaches and solutions to our nation's healthcare needs as a whole. Here the elements of good nutrition, collaborative care amongst caretakers and clinicians from multiple disciplines, evidence-based therapies, and a consistently warm residential environment seamlessly combined for the benefit of the Center's many residents.

I met Patrick Dollard for brief moments over the years at fundraisers and administrative meetings. I heard him speak to audiences about his general ambitions for the Center, but I now welcomed the opportunity to talk with him specifically about his visions for healthcare after all his years of remarkable leadership.

When I reached Mr. Dollard's office, I was struck that it was basically a large attic space turned into a workshop. Sitting across a large round table with room for 12 was Patrick Dollard. He graciously invited me to serve myself from some of the buffet-style lunch offerings, which had been grown onsite and prepared at the Center that day. This well-groomed, middle-aged gentleman with an immaculate mustache and gentle but firm manner was as comfortable in a suit with Fortune 500 entrepreneurs and ground-shakers as he now was in jeans and a casual shirt with papers spread all about on the table in front of him. This ship's captain sat at King Arthur's round table with two assistants he introduced as part of his visionary team—their presence requested in anticipation of our interview.

"When I first arrived here in the early 1980s, the focus in healthcare of people with severe handicaps was on treating the sickness, not the well-being or health of the whole person," Patrick began. People were not initially seen as people at all. They were considered "vegetables," a word used often to describe them, which was later replaced with "retarded," and, more recently, "demented." Patrick realized that physicians and others were *trained* to think in this way. Nurses, however, were trained differently and understood the concept of wellness much better.

He eventually expanded the original 30 employees to over 1,600 full-time staff with a focus on nursing and residential caretakers with an overarching holistic approach. He emphasized that, as the Center focuses on addressing the whole person, factors such as where these people live and the food they eat are priorities. As the Center grew, Patrick recognized that the economic realities of healthcare were undergoing significant changes. Basic operational costs were becoming exorbitant.

"In the past, surgical colleagues of mine could cover their annual malpractice insurance premiums with the reimbursements they received for about every four operations that they performed. Today, it takes over 90 operations for the same surgeon to earn enough to cover just this malpractice expense. This does not include the ever-rising costs of other increasingly numerous operational requirements."

As the staff grew, so too did the overhead. He therefore needed to be creative to stay ahead of the curve and keep the Center alive, growing, and productive. During our conversation, we realized that we both had taken a similarly aggressive approach to our practices by consciously choosing to provide as many of the clinical, educational, and diagnostic services as possible within the confines of our respective facilities. Patrick took these methods to soaring heights by creating therapeutic environments for his patients to live, learn, and work, to include establishing a farm on the campus to source the food for all residents and staff, as well as the local community.

To this day, it is common to see a child in a wheelchair at the farm with the animals or plants that are raised in their sustainable, organic, and biodynamically certified Thanksgiving Farm. Their Center Ridge Campus is New York's first residential and therapeutic campus specifically designed for autistic adolescents. They also established the nation's first environmentally sound clinic registered with the US Green Building Council—The Discovery Health Center—and have their sights set on expanding their research center and building a pediatric specialty hospital for their residents.

By working with local and state government agencies, Patrick has improved the local economy through employment and collaborative projects while simultaneously reducing the costs of providing healthcare to a highly complex patient community. Between 2011 and 2016, the Center reportedly created an over $1 billion economic impact for

New York State. All this activity readily explained the mass of papers and drawings stretched out on the round table between us.

Though outpatient pediatric care has improved for a majority of the population and thus reduced the need for hospital-based inpatient services, the children attended to at the Center are in need of continual care and dependent on others for all their daily living needs. Patrick understood very early on that the burden of caring for many of these individuals could be too great for any individual or family to bear.

As the local pediatric hospital wards shrank in the name of healthcare reform—while operating under the pressure of very restrictive, cost-containment-oriented reimbursement systems known as diagnosis-related groups (DRGs)—Patrick read the proverbial tea leaves and was already employing a population-health approach at the Center. His entire *raison d'être* focused on keeping his wards healthy within the Center's environment and out of hospitals where they would be treated as a DRG—not a person. My own sense is that the nation only recently caught on to the value of the model that the Center has been implementing for decades.

When I asked him where he thought the U.S. healthcare system was—and should be—heading as we ended the decade, he responded, "I watch hospital systems." Almost all single hospitals, he said, even those that had been local, regional, or national institutions, now became part of a larger multi-hospital system or network. These large corporations have amalgamated hospitals, clinics, and practices under one large umbrella. "I sincerely hope these important institutions don't end up just being ripped apart," he stated with an air of frustration.

He went on to explain that he anticipated that the new big players in town would include the large multi-chain pharmacies and urgent care centers. These entities have demonstrated that they can keep their parking lots around the state and nation full. They have a captive audience. He emphasized, "To stay competitive, the large hospital networks and multidisciplinary practices are naturally going to have to merge in some fashion with these corporate pharmacies and urgent care centers."

Patrick went on to explain that he had come to recognize that there was a silver lining to the impact that these large mergers created. They now supported his promotion of this trend toward large venture capital participation in US healthcare. "If we could harness this momentum, we could make some real impact in much-needed areas of social reform such as juvenile detention," he expressed with excitement. "We could reverse more recent historical trends that institutionalized young people and made a profit for some in the process. With properly directed venture capitalism, we could tackle issues such as prison reform and focus on keeping kids out of jail."

"How do you foresee the Center playing a role in such reshuffling and merging of healthcare institutions within this capitalist model?" I pressed him.

In a manner typical of big thinkers, he responded with another question. "What happened to the lifespan of those with one of our most commonly affected neurodevelopmental abnormalities, Down syndrome or Trisomy 21 syndrome? In the 1980s, their average lifespan was 28 years old. Today they live well into their 60s with a good quality of life. What changed over this time? The evolution of institutions like our Center for Discovery, which worked to deinstitutionalize them as patients and instead chose to create a home environment that could treat them as people while meeting their many needs. We thus relieved the burden of the single families that were trying to keep their loved ones home and out of the standard facilities despite not having all the necessary resources."

"You have given them a new home while keeping the family together," I added.

"Yes, and thus the Center has now found itself in a unique position of being in our own lane, especially with the coming of our new hospital and research center. We created a climate and a culture that is healthy for our residents and employees alike. We learned to address the whole team if we are to be successful. We can be a role model and a leader for care for all types of problems that affect neurodevelopment or interrupt our emotional and neurologic well-being, including the all-too-common stress and anxiety disorders."

Patrick introduced me to the concept of "radical kindness." One of the most important lessons to learn from working with the disabled, he said, is that these people need to be seen as a valued part of our society. When we, as caretakers, approach them in this way, we, ourselves, experience such a strong positive emotion that it "radicalizes" us.

I felt this from the moment I first visited the Center years before but never heard it explained so poignantly. Patrick was giving rationality to the intense feeling that all of us who worked at the Center shared nonverbally. In our constant efforts to care for people with such complex medical and social issues, we ourselves were changed for the better. This radical kindness became a part of who we were as people and professional caregivers. This realization was indeed powerful and remains so.

Patrick stressed that, though this work was at times hard and the rewards not always obvious, we should never give up our efforts because this could quickly reverse our progress and take us many steps backward. Whether working at the Center or in a nursing home, medical professionals all face this tendency to back off or give up.

These lessons could extend to other healthcare-related issues of our society, such as the weight of longevity with our aging population. Systems such as assisted living centers can collapse under the pressures associated with providing appropriate care for this increasing portion of our population. Patrick's solution is, again, to focus on the whole person, the whole caregiving team, and the whole of society. This collaborative spirit can best support our efforts to do the right thing by our elders.

"We also need to flip the conversation to social justice in healthcare," he added. "If we fix poverty, we as a society fix healthcare."

I could not have agreed with him more and told him that I said as much in the section of this book about American society's role in healthcare. Patrick is committed to addressing poverty within the rural community surrounding the Center. Sullivan County, New York, has a higher-than-average percentage of citizens living below the poverty line. If this cycle of poverty could be broken in some way by the efforts of the Center, then the health of the whole regional population could improve. Thus, Patrick remains dedicated to employing and training local residents at the Center.

In the process he also invested almost $15 million dollars per year into employee-related healthcare. Through this investment, he gained insight into their most important health issues, including mental healthcare and opioid addiction. From this vantage point, Patrick intends the growing Center to be a resource for the community at large and not just for their disabled residents. The Center has clearly become a vital part of the region's efforts to attain improved population health.

Patrick sees some hope in the fact that Big Pharma's hold on communities such as Sullivan County is now being challenged through public lawsuits. Public opinion in this power struggle is shifting toward those less fortunate, and Patrick intends to ride this wave of sentiment on behalf of his community.

"We also have to get out of our political silos if we are to make any meaningful progress as a society," Patrick warned. "One of the enlightening aspects of working at the Center has been to bring together at the table an advisory board, a group of people with disparate political views all focused on the same thing. Some are from the extreme left and others from the extreme right politically, but when they meet together here, they are all centered by the shared fact that they each have a kid at the Center. Here we work best and need left, right, and center to be aligned by such common goals."

"Perhaps it is this very idea that is embodied in your name—The Center," I suggested. Patrick chuckled. We both agreed that it would be nice if society as a whole could be "centered" on such a common mission when it comes to our healthcare.

Though we agreed that technology can "fix" someone, only a true clinician can "heal" them. Patrick believes that our society developed deep-rooted and high expectations for medical technology. "Ever since the first heart transplant, Americans accepted technology as a given when it comes to providing and advancing healthcare. They are very comfortable with it," he explained. He cited the example of Senator Bernie Sanders who "just had a heart attack, undergoes a procedure, and bounces right back onto the campaign trail for president. Years ago, this would have meant the end of the campaign, but today, people do not think of this as implausible. We are in a new, accepted reality when it comes to combining healthcare and technology."

Patrick boasted respectfully, "The Center was an early pioneer in extending occupational and physical therapy to a broader patient audience." Initially, such rehabilitation therapies had a narrower target audience and were just meant for work-related matters or athletes trying to get back on the field. Early on, the Center foresaw the benefits of occupational and physical therapy for their disabled population and made them an integral part of their program. As the Center expanded, they always incorporated new biomedical technologies grounded in neurodevelopmental sciences.

"As we look forward to our new hospital and research center, the Center will be working hand in hand with our colleagues in the technology industry. Through such partnerships, the Center will continue to align with all disciplines who are in some way dealing with brain dysregulation so that everyone can benefit from the work we have done and intend to do in the future with autism and anxiety. We will continue aligning with national groups such as the military, who deals with our veterans' post-traumatic stress disorders, researchers in brain development, and those addressing dementia and Alzheimer's in our aging population. We have much to contribute and learn about how stress and anxiety impact many areas of our health.

"The Center is also working with plant-based pharmaceuticals through collaborations with the SUNY Department of Agriculture," Patrick continued. He intends the Center's research facility to be instrumental in investigating the scientific basis for the therapeutic impact of THC and CBD. He will thus counter the current fad-based approach, vulnerable to being curtailed by government authorities and those in the pharmaceutical industry more interested in cashing in than truly helping people. "We at the Center need to lead with sound scientific evidence and get out ahead of this trend," he argued, "if we are to appropriately and responsibly influence our culture to understand and embrace the potential of the many new plant-based therapies."

IN SERVING, WE DISTINGUISH OUR PURPOSE

People who choose to become doctors have always displayed a strong inclination to take science into the real world. This "internal scientist" is one of the last hallmarks that distinguishes physicians from other clinical colleagues, such as nurses and physician assistants, who tend to be more purely hands-on and practical in the application of their skills. This emphasis on the scientific basis of physician training is the rationale and foundation for premedical course requirements at all undergraduate colleges. In medical school and beyond, many physicians are encouraged to maintain one foot in the science laboratory, the other in the clinical world—sharpening their clinical craft while nurturing their own intellectual needs.

These "servant scientists" use science and research to improve the health outcomes of their own patients. They remain dedicated to their scientist roots even as they leave the lab to work with patients. In maintaining this mindset, they are in a unique position to seamlessly apply the ever-evolving evidence-based knowledge from the laboratory bench to actual patients.

If a physician chooses to remain purely technical, a scientist in the lab, they no longer function as a physician. If, on the other hand, they abandon their scientific foundations, they can continue as clinicians but must depend on others' knowledge with regard to the medications and devices they use in their daily practice. They become the James Bonds of their profession, using cool gadgets designed by others for the benefit of their patients.

The "Batman model," which I unabashedly promote, on the other hand, allows doctors to design their own tools, often in collaboration with others, which they then put to use combatting the "criminals" they face in the form of disease. This servant scientist model has typified the careers of some of my most esteemed teachers and colleagues. In the NICUs of my training program, my professor physicians divided their time equally between teaching, research, and caring for patients. They melded these components of their professional lives into one seamless and comprehensive whole. It was eye-opening to watch these creative physicians interact with the medical device industry representatives who came to the medical center to work with them.

In one circumstance that stands out in my memory to this day, a company designed a machine to provide breathing support for the sickest newborn babies based upon the work of one of my teachers, Dr. Jen-Tien Wung. A soft-spoken and entirely patient-focused physician, Jen—as he was known to all of us—was unique in many ways, not the least of which was that he combined an education in anesthesia, obstetrics, and pediatrics to tackle the medical conditions of these littlest humans. When the company brought this respirator to the hospital for him to see, they told him it was designed to provide breathing support based on his research. Specifically, they designed it to administer very fast breathing rates at a very low pressure so as not to over-inflate, and thus burst, their fragile lungs.

They were now ready to test this respirator in the real world. For physicians at other institutions around the country, they provided very strict guidelines on the machine's usage and for which particular babies it could be used. They granted Dr. Wung free rein to use the device as he saw fit, however, allowing him to demonstrate its full potential and provide valued feedback for future modifications.

Over 25 years later, I still remember him staying up for many nights in a row as he employed this high-tech respirator like a virtuoso musician to save the lives of several very sick infants. In his hands, human intellect and machine merged into one single and powerful entity dedicated to the highest calling—serving others in need.

More recently, I had the opportunity to work with a heart surgeon named Dr. Khanh Nguyen, who exemplifies the servant scientist's drive to push forward against current standards defined by rigid protocols and algorithms. During many open-heart surgeries, a special machine is required to allow the part of the heart being fixed to remain still and empty of blood. These heart-bypass machines revolutionized the field of adult and pediatric heart surgery several decades ago. For the littlest of our patients, however, there remained an inherent problem—the tubing that runs between the machine's pump and the patient needs to be full to keep it bubble-free. This requires so much blood that there may not be enough left for the baby. This long tubing also increases the risk of introducing irritating substances or inflammation into this plumbing circuit, which can cause life-threatening blood-clotting problems. As you can imagine, this can significantly impact a baby's chances of survival and recovery, even when the operation goes smoothly.

Despite this frustrating situation, many medical centers doggedly continued using the standard bypass system with several feet's worth of tubing. My colleague, Dr. Nguyen, on the other hand, decided that this situation was not acceptable and went to his home workshop to tackle the problem. Over the years, he designed and then built a series of bypass machines with ever-decreasing tube lengths between the patient and the pump unit. When he arrived at a version where the machine was only inches behind him during the operation, he decided to take the bold step of bringing the whole pump unit off the floor and onto the operating table itself.

He did not stop there. He returned to the drawing board and designed a way to attach the pump to the side of the table, just above and out of the way of the space that he needed to perform the operation. He thus eliminated the tubing altogether, and this in turn eliminated the problems inherent in the standard bypass design. The medical device industry then stepped in to make this bypass design commercially available. Da Vinci himself would be proud.

Over the last several decades, the field of computer science has become a very popular college major, spawning an explosion in technical innovation in a myriad of industries. The medical profession has been somewhat behind the curve when it comes to incorporating computer technology into routine clinical functions. Many patients with computer science degrees told me that even the software used by current EMR platforms is outdated and clunky at best. They remark that even the most basic applications for online shopping are much more sophisticated and user-friendly. This archaic software leads to daily hassles, which in turn lead to our own blood pressures rising several times each day.

On the other hand, computer science is at the threshold of altering the landscape of medical care at multiple levels. Technologies such as three-dimensional reconstructions of the body's organs, including the brain and heart, allow for planning and rehearsing complex surgeries and other interventions in a much more noninvasive fashion. This virtual surgery rehearsal paradigm will speed up these procedures while reducing trauma to surrounding organs and tissues. As an education tool for such procedures, the possibilities are limitless. Physician servant scientists should lead the way in exploring the myriad of possibilities that computer science can bring to clinical medicine.

As gene-based technologies advance, physician servant scientists are responsible for many recent breakthroughs in therapies and cures for some of our most historically stubborn medical conditions. Doctors have returned to the lab to develop gene-based therapies to attack cancers, potentially revolutionizing the way cancers are treated. For the first time, the possibility of eradicating certain cancers now appears to be less science fiction and more reality.

Most recently, doctors have applied the full resources of genetic technologies against one of the oldest blood-borne diseases in the world—sickle cell anemia. This disease is so intrinsic to the medical world that all medical students learn the basic concepts of genetic disorders using sickle cell anemia as the model. They learn that, over centuries, a genetic variation initially protected some individuals from infection with the parasite that causes malaria. The variant gene changes the shape of the protein hemoglobin that carries oxygen in our red blood cells. This ultimately changes the entire shape of the red blood cell from a soft sphere to a thin, elongated sickle that can clearly be seen through a microscope. The malaria-causing parasite cannot live easily in the sickle cell, and thus the patient becomes resistant to it.

This genetically advantageous adaptation was passed on from generation to generation over many hundreds of years in areas of the world infested with malaria. Now people were not dying prematurely from malaria, but there was a frightening price to pay for achieving this immunity to malaria. These sickle cells have a high tendency to become stuck in the small blood vessels of the body and cause significant and often crippling painful episodes known as "crises." Despite the genetic basis for the disease being known for decades, the medical therapies for these crises are rooted in hydration, medication-based pain management, blood transfusions, bone marrow transplants, and treatment of superimposed infections. For those suffering from this disease, treatment has been something of a horror show. The primary problem of sickling was not being addressed.

It was not until 2019 that scientist physicians returned to the research bench to address the genetic roots of this problem. In the process, they recruited the most unlikely accomplice, the human immunodeficiency virus that causes AIDS. They removed the harmful genetic codes from the virus and replaced them with normal codes for the hemoglobin of healthy spherical red blood cells to replace the code that causes sickling. Miraculously, the first few test patients with some of the most severe manifestations of this disease became symptom-free as microscope slides with their blood indicate that the sickled cells were virtually eliminated. As a physician, I find this very moving, and I believe it was only made possible through physicians returning to the servant scientist model.

Gene testing for inherited diseases, as in many of my own heart patients, and in situations such as breast cancer, also has proven more of a model for empowering patients than the initially feared vision in which genetic information invariably commits an individual to a "death sentence" that they cannot change. If physicians return to being better advocates for evidence-based scientific discoveries, they can use this genetic information to essentially act as a "crystal ball" and see what may lurk around the corner regarding their own health. This should then allow their patients to take preemptive steps that can alter the ultimate course of their lives.

If someone knows that they carry a strong family-based gene for breast cancer, for example, they can avoid carcinogens such as cigarettes that easily convert their gene into the cancer-producing mode. Many women, following the impassioned and brave example of celebrities such as Angelina Jolie, may decide to undergo prophylactic surgeries at a certain stage in their lives to prevent these cancers from even starting.

Physicians are obligated to become familiar with such gene-based technologies and their applications on behalf of their patients. The more that physicians approach these resources with the philosophy of a servant scientist, the more available these therapies become. This paradigm intrinsically provides the intellectual basis for allowing scientifically based medical care to become fully integrated into our healthcare system itself. Physicians stand in a unique position amongst their clinical colleagues to maintain and promote this approach and thus reaffirm their true integrity and authority within the American healthcare system, if they so choose.

The servant scientist model also supports the inherently American concept that the promotion of individuals' well-being is an integral component of ensuring the well-being of many. I have always been moved by the value system that leads Americans to literally send out the Coast Guard and spend exorbitant sums of money to search for a single missing or trapped individual. Recently, I attended a presentation of a clinician scientist that exemplified this ideal of focusing upon a single individual, even when it is initially not apparent how others may benefit.

This enthusiastic young physician-scientist recounted how he identified the cause and developed the ultimate treatment for a child with a degenerative and lethal genetic defect in their metabolism that had never been described before. As a clinician, he began by taking an exhaustive account of this patient's personal and family history and symptoms. He concluded that he had no more than one year to find a cure before the child would be permanently damaged and eventually die.

Standard computer-based systems to identify abnormalities in genetic patterns were not helpful. He, therefore, returned to his laboratory with blood samples from this patient and spent weeks combing through her genetic code in excruciating detail. Once he identified the potential genetic coding problem, he understood that the patient was unable to make certain proteins used to protect and maintain the health of her nerves. He then created in the laboratory a scenario in which the correct gene pattern could generate a sufficient amount of the normal protein to replace the flawed one.

To use his discovery, he had to apply to the Food and Drug Administration for the right to create a medication that could benefit only one patient in the whole world. This process actually consumed the majority of the child's remaining year of health. Unwilling to take no for an answer, he persevered and was finally able to give the unique medication to his patient before the year ended. In undertaking this Herculean task, he punched a figurative hole in the scientific and medical universe by establishing a model for finding causes and treatments of orphan diseases that may affect only one person.

We in the audience were not only blown away by his achievement but also proud to be citizens of a country where this idea was conceived, let alone achieved. When we saw the final slides with pictures of his healthy young patient, there wasn't a dry eye in the crowd.

THINK OUTSIDE THE BOX

In our meeting, Patrick Dollard laid out a very coherent vision for healthcare. As I hoped, he extolled a set of principles that could be scaled to a broader audience and encapsulated many of the ideas I incorporated in this book. The following 10 points summarize these principles:

1. **Physicians need to be leaders** if we are to maintain any influence over the future of our society's healthcare. Patrick clearly believes that the Center's results earned him the right to lead the expansion of their methods into treatment of areas such as anxiety and stress-related illness. He understands that this requires collaboration as well as continual dedication to maintain any leadership capacity.

2. To lead effectively, **physicians need to fight our own prejudices and be constructively critical of ourselves as individuals and a profession**. We need to deemphasize our current bias toward treating diseases in favor of treating people. Only after doing so can we begin to honestly assess where we are now and where we should go in terms of healthcare reform. Patrick says that moving forward will require a different way of thinking than we have used over the past couple of decades. Doctors must overcome the outside pressure to emphasize volume over quality. Only when we do can we be creative enough to find real solutions to difficult problems, like how best to support the health of our aging population and encourage death with dignity by employing strategies such as end-of-life palliative centers.

3. **Duality of thinking must stop** so that we can find our collective common center. Doctors cannot allow ourselves to disconnect from each other's disciplines and the communities we serve because of stubbornly held prejudices. Such silos only weaken our collective potential to address the many issues we face and thus place us at the mercy of others less equipped to tackle these problems. Divided, we invite less capable forces into our midst who will focus on the financial bottom line. This can be best achieved by emphasizing teamwork, including consideration of others' roles and opinions regarding the administration of healthcare. Patrick emphasizes that it is important for this team to bridge various disciplines, including generalists, specialists, technicians, therapists, and technologists.

4. **We must address caretaker burnout at all levels**. Anyone—whether a family member or a health-related professional—can be overwhelmed by the responsibility of caring for someone disabled with neurological difficulties or experiencing end-of-life consequences. Doctors and nurses attending to life-threatening acute or chronic illnesses are vulnerable to depression and anxiety. Physicians need to be more cognizant and proactive in this regard if we are to survive as a profession. Patrick thus believes the protection of his staff is critical to the Center's ongoing ability to care for their medically complex residents. Through employee support groups and continuing education forums, as well as a network of mental health professionals, he ensures that his employees feel valued and taken care of, which in turn ensures the integrity and effectiveness of their work.

5. **Medical institutions should play a major role in addressing social inequities in their communities**. The Center proactively addresses poverty at the entry-level positions of their staff with endowments specifically dedicated to their salaries and benefits. They view the Center as a vital asset to the economic well-being of the region. The US medical system, through hospitals and other healthcare-related facilities, clearly influences local economies, but unlike other countries such as Canada, this influence is left to the private sector and not a national-level commitment. The United States has yet to consistently agree that healthcare reform should be a force for social justice and focuses, instead, on cost containment and profits.

6. Patrick warns that **we must not let ourselves be hijacked** by entities such as Big Pharma, the National Rifle Association, and politicians. These entities function in a different—and selfish—reality that they try constantly to impose on the public. Like an oil company in the midst of an obvious massive oil spill, they are quick to claim that "there is no issue here." Like the Wizard of Oz, they make pronouncements while standing behind a curtain, hoping we won't notice. This book is designed to stimulate thought and to nudge people

to think for themselves and not blindly accept what we are told by corporate-sponsored media. Only then can the curtain be pulled back to see the power brokers as they are—their true motives revealed—so that we can limit their influence over this critical healthcare dialogue.

7. **Observational and emotional IQ skills are necessary** to achieve quality healthcare outcomes. They translate well when working with all patients but perhaps are best learned and strengthened by caring for people with disabilities such as autism. These people have much to teach us about being the best physicians possible. Through our interactions with those with communication difficulties, we learn to better communicate ourselves, which will only improve our ability to holistically diagnose, treat, cure, and heal. Working with people who need a lot of care puts us more in touch with our own need to be in the service of others.

8. **We must learn from other medical disciplines and models around us**. Patrick is concerned that the field of pediatric psychiatry, for example, focuses on pharmacotherapy and has diverted away from other modalities and interventions such as occupational and physical therapy, nutrition, and counseling, while pediatric cardiology and hematology has expanded from the purely technical to incorporating more holistic approaches, such as exercise and meditation. Our patients do better—and at a lower cost—when we communicate across our disciplines with the goal of collaboration on their behalf.

9. Within the next decade, **our healthcare efforts should prioritize institutions focused on brain–body health**. This is our next public health frontier and the only way that we will tackle the larger issues such as racism, prejudice, gun violence, drug addiction, and domestic terrorism. Isolating mental illness from other medical disciplines, in particular, is artificial at best and dangerous at its worst. Society requires and deserves a more holistic approach.

10. Ultimately, **we all need to focus on healing—not treating or curing—as the foundation of this craft we call medicine**. Our

founding mentors understood this best—they were not yet overwhelmed by the pressures of technology, market forces, and politics. If we are to achieve true "reform," we first need to step back, reassess, and regroup as a collective to reclaim our role as healers.

I admit I have always been somewhat idealistic in my view of what Americans can do with creative thinking. We are the people who first proposed that a leader could step down and hand over control peacefully to their successor. We launched the era of the automobile and the airplane. We take national pride in being the first nation to place a man on the moon. We even claim the birth of the Internet as our own. So why are we so stumped when it comes to solving the problems of our healthcare system?

In large part, our impediments are part and parcel of our complex democracy. In other words, the fact that this has been so difficult is not the problem—it is the point. The formulation of something as important as healthcare in a society as vast and diverse as ours—with all of its accompanying idiosyncrasies, flaws, conflicts of opinion, and beliefs—is not supposed to be simple if it is to be effective for all of us. It is also not supposed to be etched in stone but rather planted in rich soil and tended to dearly as it grows with us.

As a practicing physician who has been on the ground and in academia for almost a quarter of a century, I have several general solutions of my own. I propose two of them here, not as completed works ready for prime time but in the hopes that they might possibly engender further collaborative discussions that may ultimately bear some fruit.

A NATIONAL HEALTH ADVISORY COMMITTEE

Our current healthcare system in many respects appears to be a patchwork quilt instead of a uniform blanket. This may be *apropos* as it may simply reflect the diversity of our nation. However, this complex quilt does not currently appear to display the integrity of a well-sewn blanket. My sense is that this is because many of the constituent components are not necessarily working together on the same blanket. At times, they even appear at odds with each other. Component pieces include the American Medical Association, the National Institutes of Health, the Centers for Disease Control and Prevention, the Food and Drug Association, private industries, hospital corporations, academic medical centers, Planned Parenthood, state medical societies, state departments of health, the surgeon general, and the US Department of Health and Human Services, just to name a few. Even for a seasoned doctor, the list is staggering, and the actual roles of each are not always clear.

Each of these organizations operates somewhat independently and is clearly beholden to different entities. Many of these agencies are appointed by and/or report to the federal government. Others answer to shareholders. Many have lost their credibility, trustworthiness, or relevance over the years. The AMA, for example, mainly functions as an advocate for its physician members. It is well recognized worldwide for its major role in research, journal publications, and public health. However, as succinctly explained by Alex DelVecchio of the TechTarget Network, "The AMA sometimes joins forces with other organizations such as the Centers for Disease Control and Prevention to ask for changes or updates to existing health policies that affect the day-to-day work of American medical workers and patients."[81] In essence, even the AMA, with all of its physician members and research, can at best only request for others to listen as they make their recommendations. It therefore is inclined to seek more clout by bringing others to the table for important matters. This is like the pilots' union bringing in

81 DelVecchio, Alex, "American Medical Association – Definition," *TechTarget*, March 2015, https://www.techtarget.com/searchhealthit/definition/American-Medical-Association-AMA?Offer=abt_pubpro_AI-Insider.

the engineers to convince the Federal Aviation Administration that alterations to a plane are potentially needed for safety purposes. We see how well that has gone recently with Boeing.

To complicate matters further, the current standards of care for many of our medical conditions are available through guidelines disseminated by the different medical fields. The expert panels that provide these guidelines are recruited for this advisory purpose as old standards come into question. Typically, these guidelines are not revised for more than a decade. This includes basic issues such as the diagnosis and treatment of hypertension. The newest guidelines were published in 2017 and had not been updated in 14 years. Once created, these guidelines are published in medical journals for dissemination. For many physicians, it is virtually impossible to keep up with, let alone implement, these guidelines in their daily practice. Ten years after publication of the Sudden Death Screening Guidelines, reports indicated barely 30 percent of doctors caring for children and young people were even aware they existed.

Some, but not all, EMR software systems may include the relevant guidelines as a reminder in a patient's chart. Large mega-group physician practices such as Northwell can better equalize and enforce the access to the current guidelines than smaller groups. The new term "best practices" was even coined to represent this process within the larger groups and hospitals. This best-practices approach made some clear improvements in raising the bar of care, but the level of implementation remains variable and in large part organization-dependent.

Tragically, I have come to realize through my work as a medical expert in legal matters that doctors and hospitals often first learn of these guidelines only when they are sued for not following them, resulting in the injury or death of a patient. Physicians actually despise these guidelines because they feel it makes them more vulnerable to litigation. They contend that the guidelines are not always applicable in every situation, but this does not stop the lawyers from using them against the physician by waving them in the jury's face.

Given so many different entities with different agendas, combined with difficulties in disseminating medical standards of care, it makes sense to me to create one independent health advisory committee for the entire nation, free of conflicts of interest. Its members would come from diverse backgrounds, including some of the already existing organizations, but be beholden only to the health and welfare of the people. Like an international court, it would strive to remain free of boundaries and operate on behalf of humankind. Like the separate branches of our government, it would be autonomous in its advisory powers and should possess administrative and enforcement powers if it is to be effective. In this way, our healthcare will be as separate from the state and the politics of the day as our founding fathers intended for religion.

The composition of this National Health Advisory Group would remain consistent and include physicians, public health officials, researchers, journalists, computer scientists, ethicists, the disabled, clergy, laypeople, and businesspeople. Each member would be nominated by a standardized recruitment process and have a term limit of about five years. This group would identify and regularly update the best current evidence-based national standards of care in detection, prevention, and treatment for our most common and important health problems. They would derive these standards in conjunction with medical experts who would report regularly to this body. These standards would be continuously disseminated throughout the nation to create a more consistent and uniform approach within our healthcare system, including clinician education.

If new problems arise that need urgent attention—such as the COVID-19 pandemic—this advisory body would recruit the necessary agencies to assist with formulating targeted recommendations. With a click to the committee's website, anyone could familiarize themselves with these standards using this one national source. They could also be readily incorporated into existing databases of all EMRs and pop up when applicable.

Most importantly, this National Health Advisory Committee would reestablish the public's trust in the healthcare system. In this body, they would see a nonpartisan collaborative group—not beholden to industry, profits, or government—communicating effectively and working entirely on behalf of all our people as equals. The patchwork quilt would be made stronger and more reliable.

INCORPORATION OF THE MENTORSHIP MODEL OUTSIDE ACADEMIA

Certain fundamental principles cannot be ignored. One of them is that it takes a strong foundation to build a strong house. In medicine, this foundation has always been the education of our students through a mentorship model. Every medical student is implicitly aware of the concept and the value of "see one, do one, teach one." This tradition dates back to the time when, like other craftsmen, an aspiring physician lived with a reputable doctor and his family as an apprentice, working up through the menial tasks in hopes of someday striking out independently.

As the profession became more organized and advanced, the education requirements and expectations became more onerous. Thus was born the university model of medical education, which culminated in the receipt of a diploma certifying the student's capabilities. Soon even this was not sufficient, and further years of formal academic training in hospital settings were added—the internship, residency, and fellowship years. In an era of increasing complexity in the medical sciences and technologies, this education process is still rooted in the mentorship model. Like a well-organized newspaper company with its hierarchy of young reporters all the way up to the editor-in-chief, or like the organization of the military from corporals to brigadier generals, medicine relies on senior physicians teaching the next generation.

Somewhere along the way, as more physicians left the academic centers and started their professional careers in more remote sites, we veered away from the mentorship model and became increasingly oriented toward a self-reliance model. It was impractical to stop and make a telephone call to a professor in the city when a patient case became more complex. Standards of care did not disseminate to these doctors as readily as in the urban areas where the teaching centers resided. Regular conferences and meetings provided a means of refreshing and updating one's knowledge base, but not everyone was able or inclined to avail themselves of these opportunities. You were on your own, and this required establishing an independent standard based upon trial and error, innate talent, and experience. A not-too-subtle divide between academic and nonacademic physicians was clearly evident when I left the city in the late 1990s to start my practice in the suburbs of New York.

As communication technology arrived in the 1980s, physicians were granted ready access to current medical knowledge and standards. Some physicians were hungry for this knowledge and others less so. Younger physicians took it for granted that technology would be a part of their daily practice as part of their arsenal. This hodgepodge of learning soon highlighted the different standards of care among physicians.

Recently, insurers and hospitals forced continuing education requirements upon all physicians. Large practices, too, jumped on this bandwagon. However, much of this education is more bureaucratic than actually informative. Physicians can sign on to a website and take a computer module-based course that provides an electronic stamp of completion. These course requirements have become ubiquitous and take hours away from patient care. Physicians are now required to complete at least 10 such courses, either hands-on or computer-generated, annually. This is in addition to ever-increasing American Medical Boards' requirements and reexaminations.

Much of this is viewed by physicians as more reflective of medico-legal and bureaucratic requirements than a source of genuine education—a waste of their time and energy. It is not, therefore, surprising that physicians have become so resentful of this process that they are fighting back through their organizations.

In thinking back upon the origins of our profession, I found myself yearning for simpler days. I return often to the sense that reform in healthcare does not always have to be completely new but can build upon well-tested and effective foundations. In this sense, *reform* becomes *return to form*. The mentorship model in medicine not only works well but remains at the core of our psychology and philosophy. When we lose touch with it, the system unravels like a hundred strands of loose string we are trying to reshape into a cohesive ball by adding extraneous education requirements. Why not simplify things and bring the mentorship model with us into our daily professional lives?

Using technology, such as social media platforms, we could hardwire a mentorship hierarchy throughout the nation. The leading experts in a field would sit at the top of this pyramid of knowledge and experience, advising those with progressively less experience. This living knowledge pyramid would extend from academic centers all the way down to the remotest communities. This network could extend internationally for more rare circumstances. Like a well-run organization, every physician would connect to someone as a designated mentor for any given clinical circumstance simply by entering all of the relevant clinical information into the network's database.

Today, it is up to the individual physician to determine whom they call to discuss any particular case. I have the good fortune to have maintained relationships with several leading experts in my field who are also very approachable. As I advanced my own career, I increasingly find myself serving as a mentor to others. Not everyone is as fortunate.

This national mentorship resource is not only technically feasible today, it has several innate advantages. It opposes the current tendency to force out older physicians with a great deal of experience because they cannot physically keep up with the high patient-volume demands. Instead, these senior physicians would see fewer but more complex patients, leaving more junior physicians to handle less complex cases more quickly. Any doctor knows that it just takes one difficult patient case to throw off the whole day's schedule. This system would be more efficient in the end without sacrificing total volume.

Keeping more experienced physicians around longer into their careers also creates the first step of the mentorship pyramid as a living local resource. These mentors could be further reinforced by attendance at forums designed to disseminate their wisdom. Eventually, this national mentorship resource would pull all the loose ends of the ball of string back into the core, eliminating the need for excessive testing and education requirements. Finally, this approach is also innately more constructive, cohesive, and proactive than the current mechanisms, which tend to be defensive and divisive in nature.

CONCLUSION

BE CURIOUS ENOUGH TO SHOW YOU CARE

One of my medical students, Christine Tholany, became genuinely interested in Gilbert Tremain's life story. There soon developed a mutual admiration between Gilbert and Christine. Though I have to admit that I was just a bit jealous of the time that Gilbert was spending with my student, inside, I was laughing with joy. Gilbert was now imparting his wisdom to the next generation of physicians. To see them together was pure magic—a taste of which I now share with you, the reader, in the excerpt from Christine's notes below:

> *Dr. Fethke held a seminar at the hospital a few years back, and he invited me to attend in the afternoon. It was about the longevity of the younger patients that he and his colleagues were now treating and the fact that these patients were often not following up with cardiologists regularly because back then it had not been possible to put in valves right away during their first operations. However, since new procedures were allowing valves to be put in sooner, they were now seeing an upsurge of patients in their 20s and 30s that had been lost to follow-up, but were now good candidates for the latest procedures. They were also talking about how, as congenital heart doctors, with the success of the field, they were fortunately getting to follow*

patients with cardiac defects throughout their lives. I had just turned 70 at the time of the conference. Before the day of the conference, Dr. Fethke asked my permission to introduce me to the room of attendees, and when he stated that I was 70 years old and had Tetralogy of Fallot, everyone in the room turned to look at me in disbelief. They had never seen someone living at my age who had this condition.

It has been a wonderful life. I have two children, three grandchildren, and five great-grandchildren. I spent a lot of my time raising my family, working, and volunteering. I was always taking care of somebody else. I never worried about myself. I was a volunteer firefighter for 50 years. It is impossible to be a firefighter and not run into some dangerous situations. Luckily, I have never been hurt very badly. I just did what had to be done. I was also on the Cliff & K rescue team for about five years. I jumped off the sides of some pretty high ledges to get down to caves that were dark, cold, and wet. But if someone is stuck down there, then you have to go rescue them. That is the way I have always been. If it has to be done, then I get it done no matter what. I did a lot of crazy, interesting things in my life because I just did not let anything get in my way.

Today, Tetralogy of Fallot is not even considered one of the toughest congenital heart conditions to treat. When I was born, they had figured out what it was about, but no one had figured out what to do about it. And then they started playing with it. Over the course of two operations, I got to have my heart chopped, carved, and sewn. There are not too many people alive today who can say they had both operations since it was not long after I had my first surgery that there were talks about doing both surgeries in one shot. Before Dr.

Malm performed my second operation, he remarked, "There are a lot of things that have happened. Now, this is more like having your appendix taken out." It has come so far. And it comes farther every day.

If the telling of my story has been helpful in any way to someone—patient, family, doctors, or nurses—dealing with congenital heart disease, then it was worth the time and the effort of this old man. I wish you all well.

America's diversity is both its strength and its vulnerable Achilles' heel. As we strive toward our highest ideals of open and equitable access to our nation's resources, our rich tapestry makes it all the more difficult for our policymakers to navigate through the complex web of priorities championed by each unique community. Yes, many of us identify ourselves as belonging to more than one such community, and this creates the hope and possibility that we will increasingly respect and appreciate each other regardless of our differences. There are, however, two vital resources we all share in common.

Each and every one of us, regardless of our race, gender, religion, and culture, needs access to nutrition and healthcare. Because we are all stakeholders in our healthcare system, I believe that any reform of this system by definition must address the needs of each community in a manner that adheres to and promotes our highest democratic principles. It is for this very reason and at this particular moment in history, with so many hard divisions drawn between our diverse communities, that I have done my best in my daily work, public advocacy, teaching, and with tireless effort through this book to demonstrate that healthcare belongs to everyone. For the health system to serve us all equitably, all members of society, not just the medical professionals, must gain a sufficient understanding of the elements and dynamics of this complex system to participate in its evolution. Doctors must teach their patients, students, and laypeople. Politicians must include their medical professionals and constituents in the formation of health policies. Each resident and citizen of our land must step up to demand knowledge and guidance from their healers. I sincerely intend that this book serves as a catalyst for such noble activity.

As I sit facing south in our New York apartment, overlooking the expanse of civilization embodied in downtown Manhattan, Queens, and Brooklyn, I cannot help but chuckle with awesome fear and respect regarding the irony of the catchphrase, "Hindsight is 20/20." Here in this original epicenter of the COVID-19 pandemic, almost three years since the first large-scale impact of this assault of nature assaulted our eastern shores in early 2020, the streets are still less crowded with tourists, and the peoples' resiliency still dares to reveal itself through the intense eyes above their variety of face masks. Like a cold shower waking us up to the reality of the day, the year 2020 will forever live as a harsh reminder that our healthcare system was far too vulnerable. If we vow to never forget the 2,977 souls that died on September 11, 2001 within the exact same landscape that I view at this moment, then surely the over one million Americans that died since early 2020 as a consequence of our poor response to the COVID-19 pandemic should urge us to reflection and action so that this tragedy may never happen again.

I often suggest to my students and young patients, when making important health and career decisions, they play a mental game with themselves. I ask them to imagine themselves 20 to 30 years in the future, looking back over their shoulders at the current, younger version of themselves.

"What do you see?" I ask. "Is the older you proud and happy with the choices the younger you made?" They don't have to give me a response. The answer is personal, like a secret wish that belongs to no one else.

It is my hope that, after reading this book, my readers are in a somewhat better position to pose this hindsight question to themselves. Whether you are a physician, medical student, or a patient, it is time to decide what you want the future of our healthcare system to be. Together, these collective choices will shape our nation's physical and economic well-being. What will the future-you tell your younger self about the choices we make here and now?

YES, I STILL WANT TO BE A DOCTOR

"The doctor will see you now," uttered the quiet Japanese hostess in direct translation from the nurse. My sister-in-law, Pom, looked nervously at the back of her hand, now swollen, red, and very itchy. She and her husband, Kai, went for a long hike in the Japanese countryside the day before. Upon return to their inn, they noted a discrete, elevated red spot surrounded by some mild redness the size of a dime on Pom's right hand. It was mildly itchy, but not painful, so they decided to just watch it.

The next morning, the redness was still there, and the hand was a little bit more swollen. Pom, a dentist, and Kai, an obstetrician, were both seasoned attendings and instructors from large New York City academic centers. Though born in Thailand, they had been American citizens for years and culturally were definitely more American than Thai. As they prepared to leave for their next destination—the small city of Kanazawa on Honshu, the large main island of Japan—they began to feel somewhat concerned that Pom's hand was not getting better. They admittedly also kicked themselves for not packing any basic medications. They decided to see how things looked when they returned to their inn in Kanazawa because it was more likely to have a modern clinic.

By the time they ate and settled into their room in Kanazawa, Kai noted that Pom's hand was actually much worse. She tried not to draw attention to the matter, but later in the evening, the concern level led them to ask their hostess at the inn—a middle-aged, energetic woman named Yuki—if there was indeed a medical clinic nearby. It now already approached midnight, and Kai considered delaying the next leg of their trip until someone attended to Pom's hand. Because they planned to leave early the next day to stay at a remote monastery, they all agreed that she should have her hand evaluated as soon as possible before they left. Yuki stepped in and graciously insisted that she walk with them to the 24-hour local hospital clinic. The couple humbly accepted.

Upon arrival at the pristine clinic, Yuki further offered to stay and help them fill out several pages of paperwork written in Japanese. Kai and Pom chuckled between themselves that, so far, the process seemed very similar to the American system. Then the situation took a different course. Yuki informed them that the clinic wanted to know if they would pay in cash for the visit before they left. Because they were well aware that their American medical insurance would not cover international non-emergency care, they confirmed that they were in fact obliged to pay in cash.

A nurse dressed in unremarkable standard scrubs then came into the waiting room to escort them to the exam area. She spoke not a word of English as she ushered them with her hand signals into the 10-by-10-foot room decorated in the minimalistic style of a comfortable Japanese home. They sat down on the two chairs across from a non-descript desk positioned on the far end of the room. After the nurse exited, closing the door behind her, the three of them remained in this very clean, well-lit space for another 10 minutes before the nurse returned to speak with Yuki at the door.

"The doctor will see you now," Yuki translated. An elderly gentle-man in a white, cleanly pressed smock-top uniform with buttons on the side and a stethoscope over his shoulder walked in, quietly trailed by the same nurse. As he walked toward the desk, Yuki bowed to the doctor and nonverbally indicated that Pom and Kai should do the same. The doctor then sat at his chair across from them. Through the assistance of Yuki's translation, he asked a few limited questions about where this happened and when. He then asked Pom to lay out both hands on the desk and proceeded to gently, but thoroughly, examine them both. After no more than five minutes, he stood, bowed again to Pom and Kai who now knowingly reciprocated, and exited the room.

"It's done? Is he coming back?" Kai frowned with his Western defenses in full physician mode.

"Will we be able to ask him what he thinks is going on with my hand and how to treat it before we leave?" followed Pom.

Yuki translated matter-of-factly that the doctor's portion of the visit was finished, and he prescribed some medicine they could retrieve as they left. "The doctor does not explain such matters, but the pharmacist will," Yuki explained. The nurse then directed them to the pharmacist office down the hall.

As instructed, the pharmacist, who spoke some broken English, was indeed very informative and helpful. The doctor surmised that this was likely some form of insect bite, and Pom was having an allergic reaction. Even the English names of the two different pills he had prescribed were not recognizable at all, so the pharmacist reached up on a shelf and produced an old version of the American *Physicians' Desk Reference*. After dusting it off, they all stood around the book together and eventually identified the medications as a relatively esoteric but safe non-brand-name steroid and antihistamine. The pills worked like a charm, and as they headed out to the monastery the next day, exhausted but relieved, Pom's hand was already almost completely back to normal. En route, they discussed their remarkable experience with Japanese urgent care.

"Wow. That was wild. The doctor was treated with immense respect by everyone. We didn't get to talk to him after the exam, even though we are American medical professionals ourselves," reflected Pom.

"Yeah, I wonder what would happen if we tried this same approach with our patients back in New York. Would we ever get the same level of respect?" laughed Kai.

"Sure, like that will ever happen," chimed in Pom as she stretched her fully healed hand to greet their host at the monastery.

Yes, I want to be a doctor. These are words that some might repeat to convince themselves that they made the right career choice. For others, these might be a way of convincing oneself that they should continue on the same career path that they had so happily chosen many years before despite the ever-increasing pressures and stresses that continue to arise in the field. Yet again, for others, this may be a quick brush-off response to those more junior people asking a more senior student whether or not they themselves should also consider becoming physicians.

For me, in the end, there has never been any question in regards to whether or not I either wanted to become a doctor or desire to continue being a physician, teacher, and mentor to others. Seeing young people and my students, while volunteering at the local ambulance corps or emergency room, smitten by the intoxicating sensation of helping someone survive a severe accident that may have ended their life—filled with the sense of an incredible ability to possibly change the ultimate outcome of life or death—I remember anew similar feelings in my own past as I began to enter a career to hopefully help others on both a small and large scale.

As of the writing of this book, our nation is in the midst of a decades-long struggle with the question of healthcare policy and delivery to our citizens. During the approximately seven years that I have been writing this book, the issues regarding healthcare have become even more mainstream topics within the consciousness of American society. There appears to be a strong tug-of-war across the political, economic, and ethical spectrum, with nothing more precious than our nation's healthcare riding on the line. There does not seem to be a more pertinent time in my recollection to personally address and responsibly reflect upon the choices we make as physicians moving forward within this present arena of tumultuous uncertainty. Perhaps this is the very reason I persevered with this project of reflection—writing down my ideas and thoughts that occurred upon many a discussion and quiet moments traveling between hospitals and my medical offices.

Who am I? Just a doctor who cares deeply about and loves what he does. Simply because I care, I remain curious about the many things that influence my patients and how I can best serve them. My curiosity leads me to explore, learn, and challenge myself and others to always constructively question the *status quo* and ask how we can help to make things better. I am also a teacher who earnestly wants to reach others and perhaps help them to achieve the joy of being a physician or other allied healthcare professional.

Most importantly, I am an American citizen who, like others, remains concerned about the current and often frustrating dialogue about the future of US healthcare. I am not a world authority on the subject but someone who has tried to practice medicine for several years in an ever-changing environment. After over 20 years of a clear labor of love in this field, I realize that recently, many people now ask me to comment on several very complex questions.

My students ask, "What is it that makes someone like you want to become a doctor, and what is it that can be done to assure that healthcare in our country will continue to be of high quality and stimulating and rewarding for those presently practicing as well as for those future physicians to come?"

My patients and non-physician friends seek insight regarding how to navigate the present, very confusing US healthcare landscape and are uneasy about where this system is heading. A common theme amongst everyone involved—physicians and the general public—is that they feel powerless and left behind in this overwhelming struggle to shape the American health system.

Over the past almost 30 years, I trained and worked in some of the higher institutions of learning in our country. I also had the opportunity to provide basic healthcare, as well as more complex subspecialty care, in developing countries such as Guatemala and South Africa. I worked with colleagues from all over the globe and of all backgrounds, including medicine, nursing, the technical field, public health, law, journalism, administration, and government. There has always been the common theme amongst these colleagues of a desire to change and positively impact an individual's life so that they may return to their loved ones better than we found them. Some of these colleagues are leading experts in the world and within their own fields. Others are less in the limelight and more focused upon the delivery of care at the ground level.

My own views, and those of these caretakers and public servants, are clearly the sum of our interactions with each other and those we care for. It has always been my goal to absorb and represent well the best aspects of the skills that I learned from these valued colleagues. What do we learn about ourselves and our values when we encounter other ways of practicing medicine, like my in-laws, Pom and Kay, did in Japan? In the end, medicine is a continual apprenticeship that evolves and develops every moment from such exchanges.

There is no debate that the stakes are high for all parties when it comes to the ultimate manifestation and direction that healthcare reform will take. It is thus in dedication to my patients and students that I took the very first steps in organizing my responses to their questions through writing. My goal with this book and during my years of practice has been consistent and simple.

Within this unique democratic environment we call the American experiment, the answers to such important questions as healthcare reform are best found when we enter into a public discourse empowered by knowledge. With this book, I invite you the reader to join me in seeking to identify that which makes our American healthcare system unique to us as a people. My aim has been to lead you toward your own determination that this system is ultimately worth nurturing, rather than discarding it without due consideration. I remind my students and patients daily that, to find an answer to any important question, we first must feel curious and emboldened enough to step up and ask the question clearly and thoughtfully. If through my writings and daily work with all those I encounter, I am in some way able to stimulate a passionate discourse and shed some light on possible solutions to many of these questions, I will consider myself fortunate. As a physician educator, I thus intend to persist until sufficient evidence arises to confirm that my endeavors have been worthwhile.

As with anyone who spends the majority of their time focusing on a particular area of expertise, one begins to realize that when we begin to look both in retrospect and with the proverbial "third eye," our life has indeed been an accumulation of experiences that hold possible meanings for others and the future. I make no claim that this book and its contents are based upon specific intensive research in the field of healthcare policy or other administrative areas of medicine. On the contrary, I endeavored to present the sentiments of many of my own colleagues who continue working in the forefront of healthcare delivery.

As with any battle—in this case, that against disease—there are always soldiers on the front lines. These front-guard warriors often wonder whether those at the higher echelons truly understand what is going on at the ground floor. It is for this reason that I attempted to describe this battlefront for those making policy, those on the receiving end of healthcare, family members and friends of physicians, and those seeking to possibly enter this profession. From this frontline vantage point, this first of several planned books addresses the very influential roles in healthcare played by our uniquely American institutions and our society at large. If this book proves to be motivational, or it clarifies any questions or concerns on the part of those involved, then this project will have been a small success. In the end, all that those involved in the delivery of healthcare should strive to achieve is that we deliver this care effectively, compassionately, and honestly.

At the center of our endeavors to address our healthcare issues, our focus should always be on the best interests of those we care for. Throughout the book, I have woven the stories of the most influential individuals I encountered in my career—my patients. I chose to spread out the biography of my oldest patient—Gilbert Tremain—throughout this book. His story is the essence of my field of pediatric cardiology, and I owe much of my philosophy regarding the art of medicine to my relationship with him.

In balance and because of my wonderful patients that I have been fortunate to meet during my career, I consider the more positive experiences to have far outweighed the negative ones. These wonderful interactions have been the motivation for my continued push forward professionally on a day-by-day basis, as well as my impetus for completing this book. Too often, the downsides of any experience are more often publicized than the positive elements. It has always been my conclusion that success and happiness in one's career do not come from the big leaps but through the smaller steps that consistently and reliably lead us forward.

The exercise I despise more than any other is running. The exercise I love the most and cannot get enough of is running. It's this paradox that keeps me motivated and fascinated enough to keep running. I'm not fast by any means, but I can keep going as long as I have the time. I found that if I look down as I go, instead of ahead, I don't get discouraged about how far I have yet to run. I focus on the pavement or path directly beneath my feet or just one or two steps ahead, not the horizon. I become absorbed in the moment, and before I know it, I am at the end. That is not to say that I don't look up now and then to see what lies ahead, but I do not become so preoccupied with it that I forget to appreciate where I am and how far I have come.

In many ways, I applied this same philosophical and practical approach to being a physician. The psychological discipline that I developed through exercise enabled me to continue through the multitude of changes, barriers, and frustrations of our ever-changing American healthcare system. I always tried to focus on the current moment as my driving force. These moments were plentiful and personally enriching as I worked with my patients, colleagues, community, and students. It was these very same precious moments that became the impetus to every once in a while look ahead to where I was heading.

This process and the fact that I still truly love the profession I chose is ultimately also a main source for my desire to write this book. In so doing, I hope to inspire and inform those who still want to remain involved in the destiny of our nation's healthcare system. For those with a passion for helping others, I encourage you to choose the health profession as a field. If you are a student with a calling, I hope you found a spark of motivation somewhere in these pages to persevere in your own goal of becoming a clinician, even if you have been admonished by others that this would be too difficult or impossible.

If you are a disillusioned practitioner in the early or middle part of your career, I sincerely wish that this work somehow reached you and gave you some kernel of strength to continue onward. If you are a seasoned caretaker toward the end of your working years, I hope that you know that we are all sorely in need of your wisdom and knowledge to be passed on to those behind you so that we can maintain the integrity of our profession. If you are a layperson, policymaker, or in an allied healthcare field, my invitation into the lives of frontline physicians like myself remains open so that we can all come together with mutual insight and compassion.

As a practitioner, I earnestly tried to explore, navigate, and explain the forces in our unique American healthcare environment so that we can all be more cognizant of our present situation and thus proactively shape our future. It does not make sense to enter a profession without some understanding of the realities of the environment in which you will work. Yet somehow physicians are expected to leave their clinical education and enter the workforce naïve to the very real elements that could either help or hinder them in their day-to-day battle to heal their patients. All the elements and experiences of my life, both positive and negative, merged to make me the physician that I am still working tirelessly to improve upon. In taking the risk of so honestly portraying myself in this book, I clearly intend to express to the reader that a physician is, at their core, a human being in the service of other human beings. Doctors are no more important to our society than those we serve. We therefore would do well to listen to and include the wisdom and energies of our patients if we are to be successful.

If, after reading this book, a reader can now or still answer a resounding "Yes" to the question of whether or not they want to be a doctor, then my efforts have been worthwhile. If others are encouraged to join other aspects of the medical field, such as nurse practitioners, physician assistants, nurses, technicians, administrators, educators, or computer programmers, then please know that we are truly in need of your contributions. As discussed in this work, we still have a long way to go in fighting the battle against both biological and psychosocial disease in our country and the world. I argued that physicians and their clinical colleagues must regain and maintain their prominent role in this endeavor by collaborating more effectively than ever with our patients. It is this same patient–physician relationship that is being challenged and undermined by the most recent manifestations of healthcare reform.

As Paul Starr eloquently demonstrated in his fundamental review of American healthcare, we physicians are at risk of losing the cultural and moral authority of our profession if we abdicate our original duty and responsibility to maintain and disseminate the standards of medicine to other people. This role is not an outdated and empty historical artifact. It is the core of what has made our American health system so unique in the first place. With this model, we helped expand the paradigm of equality and liberty itself. We must not allow politics or pure economics to erode the foundation of our system. We owe it to ourselves and our patients.

"I hope that he is OK. What could make someone want to do such a thing?" reflected our harried, red-faced young waitress as she wiped the sweat off her brow and paused for a moment from disinfecting the table next to ours.

"He reportedly is just crazy. Good thing that he didn't actually hurt anyone. It's upsetting, but in the end it's just a nuisance, and we'll all be OK," claimed a pleasant, middle-aged woman seated at another nearby table.

It was barely eight in the morning, and this packed little hotel dining room buzzed with conversation about the events of the night. It was the late spring of 2021, Memorial Day weekend. Like many of the other hotel guests, my wife and I came to Portland, Maine, as a testament to our ability to leave the confines of our homes just as the travel restrictions related to the COVID-19 pandemic lifted. It didn't matter that a literal monsoon poured nonstop with unseasonably cold rain down the northeast coast for the entire weekend. People were just happy to get out and feel more normal again. Holding back the windswept rain with our umbrellas, Viyada and I walked back the three blocks, giddy from a delicious farm-to-table dinner experience.

As we approached the hotel, we noticed a couple of policemen waving flashlights over the small, open-air hotel lot where our car was parked.

"Thanks for keeping an eye on the cars here," I politely remarked to one of the officers.

"No problem. I wish we were just here for a routine check on everything, but the truth is that we are looking at the cars in this area for signs of damage. Is one of these cars yours?" He gestured with his flashlight.

"Why yes," I replied, now stopping to join him in the middle of the lot and point to our car. "That little SUV over there."

As the beam of his light swept our tires, I felt a sudden punch to my gut. The front driver's side tire was completely flat. "Looks like he got you too," sighed the rain-soaked young officer. "We had received reports about a man vandalizing cars in this area for the past couple of hours. Looks like he went around slashing dozens of car tires. We caught him with a knife in hand just five minutes ago after a brief chase. He is known in this area as someone with psychiatric problems. No one was injured, but this is some mess he created tonight."

After we left our contact information with the policeman, I paused to inform the hotel receptionist about the situation. Momentarily stunned as she processed the implications of this news, she thanked us for letting her know as she picked up the phone to notify her manager.

With the telephone receiver perched on one shoulder, she gestured to me. "I'm so sorry this ruined your night. The hotel will take care of everything for you. Thanks for letting us know. This would have been horrible to discover in the morning just as our guests are checking out."

Restless with thoughts about early-morning car repairs, we were most thankful for the sedative effects of the bottle of wine we shared at dinner. As I stepped into the small hotel lobby the following day, the same receptionist greeted me warmly.

"Thanks to your heads-up, we have been up all night making a list of our guests' cars with flat tires. The manager and our crew were up since 4 a.m. out there in the rain trying to order replacement tires and removing the damaged ones."

As I walked around the side of the building, this small lot and the entire block looked like a disaster zone. There were three AAA tow trucks with long lengths of red air hoses crisscrossing the street and running between at least 15 jacked-up cars with one or two missing tires. The crowd of people was a mixture of policeman, hotel bellmen, guests in sweatpants, and gawking onlookers all centered around the hotel's general manager and his building supervisor.

"Which one is your car?" the obviously fatigued and unshaven general manager asked as he warmly greeted me. "We want to help get you on your way as soon as possible. "

Over the next two hours, we learned that at least 70 tires were slashed by the now-jailed and infamous perpetrator. Within 10 hours of his escapades, at least 200 other lives were briefly turned upside down. Dozens of guests stood helpless in the lobby. Others were ushered into the small little hotel restaurant for a free breakfast served by an unsuspecting and understaffed crew. The hotel employees found themselves all cross-covering different positions as the night crew stayed on to help.

Our understandably stressed-out waitress was actually the hotel greeter. Her two assistants were from the housekeeping staff. They ran back and forth to help the cooking crew make toast and flip eggs, as the guests intermittently peeked out the window to the street below to check on the status of their cars. Rental car companies and taxis were called to urgently take guests to the airport so they would not miss their flights. Two bellmen, still in their maroon uniforms, drove pickup trucks full of tires, damaged and new, ushered back and forth between a local Ford dealer to help with repairs. Families were contacted by increasingly anxious guests spilling over into the meeting rooms. Many would not be home as planned. Could someone pick up the kids from Grandma's? The dogs would have to stay one more night in the kennel. Additional personal days would have to be taken at work.

Later that day, the storm finally broke, and the bright, warm sunshine bathed the land and sea. As we cautiously drove Route 1 northward along the scenic Maine coastline for over 150 miles to our Bar Harbor destination, the spare temporary donut tire humming against the pavement, I reflected upon the events of the prior 12 hours. In the midst of all of this unforeseen busy human activity, what struck me most was a calmness that pervaded the entire affair. Unlike my recent sense of the pandemic over the past several months at work and through the media, there was no public vitriol, anger, or outrage. There was no self-centered and entitled yelling at the hotel staff. What a welcome relief.

The people I saw were supportive of each other and clearly relieved that this "crazy, troubled man" had not hurt or killed anyone. Even more amazing was that almost everyone was truly concerned about the mindset and well-being of the man himself. They referred to him simply as a person with problems. They didn't assume anything about who he was or try to pigeonhole him into a particular category based on race, age, or socioeconomic status so that they could somehow distance him from their own lives. To the contrary, his plight somehow emotionally brought everyone closer to their own realities. It was as if, after over a year of pervasive societal stress in the midst of the scourge caused by COVID-19, enough people reached a collective empathy to say to themselves, "You know, I have been there too. I can see myself getting to the point where I just need to lash out to relieve all this pent-up stress." Was it possible that we had truly come through this pandemic with a new sense of and sensibility for other people? As our acting waitress expressed so well, she had hope.

In response to this forced pause in our lives due to the COVID-19 pandemic, I too hold out hope. I hope that Americans hit the reset button on our priorities, including healthcare. I hope that, perhaps more than before the pandemic, we all now understand that the mental, physical, and spiritual wellness of each person is vital to the well-being and success of the American pursuit of life and liberty.

If, as a local Portland, Maine, artist so succinctly encapsulated in a retrospective creation commenting on our interconnectedness during the pandemic, "Healthcare Is at the Heart of Democracy," then we as a people need to ensure that our individual and collective hearts remain strong and unbroken. Perhaps I remain fundamentally idealistic when I grasp for even a glimmer of light and hope in the compassion expressed by the people who cared less about their personal property, the slashed tires, than they did about the mental wellness of a man whose quality of life had been beaten down low enough to commit such a blatant call for help. In caring to consider this man's plight, these people gave me hope that, though admittedly on shaky ground, our American values are not a light that has yet been fully extinguished. To the contrary, if we understand anew that the solutions to our deepest problems are attainable only when we truly care enough to recognize someone else's health needs, then in our endeavors to help them, we once again light the torch for all to see.

As the spring of his 75th year approached, Gilbert Tremain passed away, not specifically from his heart but from the combination of diabetes and vascular disease. The last six months of his life were not his best, but through it all, his rebellious streak continued to shine. He complained that very few of the doctors he was forced to visit knew anything about him as a person, let alone all the health issues he tackled.

"Except for you, Doc, the others are not like my old-time docs—Dr. Humphreys and Dr. Malm. They don't really hear what I'm saying and instead just push medications on me and send me out the door in 15 minutes. If they have their way, they'll certainly end up killing me."

As he grew shorter of breath with each step and started to retain fluid over his whole body, the twinkle in his eye remained his most endearing feature. He had in fact played the role of Santa for several of our patients' holiday parties. When he once asked me why I cared so much about him, that I was always trying to find ways to make his life better and longer, I told him I had a vested interest in keeping my best Santa around as long as possible.

His heart was actually fairly stable over the past 10 years. His irregular heartbeats did not become more prevalent, making the need for implanting a defibrillator device less of a concern. The leak in the valve that Dr. Humphreys and Dr. Malm operated on in 1964 remained unchanged. He constantly admonished me to not feel like I had to take action just because I found something on a test. Because he was one of the oldest people alive with his cardiac condition, there was very little data by which to make decisions. For over 15 years, every time I thought maybe I should do something, he urged restraint and patience.

"I feel fine, Doc. If my heart has taken me this far, messing around with it may only make things worse. I will tell you if I start to feel bad and something should be done."

I remember this advice, and I learned more from him than I did from any textbook or teacher I ever encountered. None of the things I was concerned about ever became prominent enough that I regretted our shared decisions to not intervene.

Gilbert Tremain was ever the explorer, the maverick, blazing a path of common sense, while never losing his passion for life. He had little tolerance for those who would not stop to listen and *care*—he spared no words or decibel of his voice in telling them so. He was described as a most difficult patient by many, but I—and the nurses in our practice who cared for him—knew he was simply afraid to find himself dependent on clinicians that his instincts told him not to trust. His instincts were his most powerful weapon against illness and served him well, taking him further beyond the 10 years that his parents were told he would live.

As he walked into my office with his now-blind wife, for whom he became the main caretaker for over 10 years, he looked more tired than I had ever known him to be. At the prior visit, he was attended by one of his daughters for the first time. She was obviously concerned about his declining health. He had always been so strong and stubbornly self-reliant that she was at a loss as to what to do for him.

Now on this, his last visit with me, he explained that she had not come this time because he did not wish to burden his children. He knew that he had been difficult at times with them and many of the clinicians who tried to help him along the way. He was too proud to rely upon anyone, and it was too late to change now. If it was his time, then he had made a good run of life and would go out on his own terms. I gave him my usual big hug, though his return hug was not as strong as usual. I never saw him again, and we received the news about two weeks later that he passed away surrounded by his large family.

With Gilbert's passing, the gates to a wonderful era of American healthcare closed as well. His life remains a perpetual testament to what is possible. He warned me to never forget that these accomplishments were possible because doctors and patients worked together, side by side, as equals. He stressed that he was kept alive by wonderful technology and skills, but he was able to live a full life because of the strong partnerships with his physicians. He was wary of any doctor who did not listen well or even try to know their patients. He explained that only through caring enough to better know someone could real trust be achieved and healing occur. This fundamental truth could not be replaced by prescribing medications, ordering tests, or performing interventional procedures. He made sure I understood the crucial facet to success within this collaboration between patient and doctor. I promised him I heard everything he said to me over the years, and I would not forget.

As this book ends, I now realize that I have been writing it for him all along.

ACKNOWLEDGMENTS

As with any project of intended value and meaning, there are countless people who shape the motivation and support the perseverance to see it through to completion. Thus, in this, my first foray into serious writing, I must humbly and proudly admit that I have many people to thank for their contributions to this book. I here mention just a few and apologize if I have unintentionally left anyone out. If so, please know that this in no way implies that I am not sincerely grateful.

My students have been my muse regarding the topics and much of the material content. Their constant and appreciated inquisitiveness have prompted me to explore the many concerns—both intellectual and emotional—that they are experiencing as they head towards a career as health professionals in this current and often-confusing environment.

My patients, especially those whose stories I have included in some form in this project or my other teaching work, continue to motivate me every day to push forward alongside them as they bravely face the challenges of serious heart conditions. It has been an honor to be involved in their lives for almost three decades. I owe a particular debt of gratitude to Gilbert Tremain and his family, as well as Emaan Ali and her mother, who continue to reach out so the lessons of their lives can be a benefit to so many others.

I am fortunate that the voices in my head that continue to guide my clinical thought processes and standards originated with wonderful mentors including physicians, nurses, and ancillary medical professionals. Amongst the most potent memories have come from Dr. Welton Gersony, Dr. Thomas Stark, Dr. Alan Hordof, Dr. Daphne Hsu, Dr.Howard Zucker, the late Dr. John Driscoll, and Margaret Challenger.

My most esteemed colleagues have supported my efforts to maintain the legacy of the founders of my field of pediatric cardiology. In this light, I continue to appreciate the support and collaboration of Dr. Michael Gewitz, Dr. Robert Pass, Dr. Sameh Said, and the late Dr. Khanh Nguyen. The clinical and clerical team at Boston Children's Health Physicians has blown the wind in my sails that urged me to launch this labor of love. Thank you for having my back.

I started out with a lot of passion to share my experiences in healthcare through writing. Without the patience and guidance of my original editor, Jennifer Margulis, I would never have become a true storyteller and author. The publishing team members at Paper Raven books—especially Morgan Gist MacDonald, Rachel Martorano, Heather Preis, M.A. Hinkle, and Charlotte Zang—have turned all my work into a reality so that the power of my pen (actually a keyboard) may help educate interested readers, stimulate thought and dialogue, and ultimately call people to participate in the constructive reform of our healthcare system.

Without a strong foundation of family and friends, no truly meaningful effort is ever possible. To my wife, Viyada, and my sons, Daniel and Christopher, I owe their tolerance of my constant inquiries and their breath of enthusiasm as I grew to become a better writer. I am so fortunate to have my family and many close friends and neighbors, at home and abroad, as my cheering squad for this now very public expression of my thoughts and dreams for a better tomorrow.

www.ingramcontent.com/pod-product-compliance
Lightning Source LLC
Chambersburg PA
CBHW062109020426
42335CB00013B/899